The Human Use of Animals

THE HUMAN USE OF ANIMALS

Case Studies in Ethical Choice

SECOND EDITION

TOM L. BEAUCHAMP, PhD
Professor, Department of Philosophy
Senior Research Scholar, Kennedy Institute of Ethics
Georgetown University

F. BARBARA ORLANS, PhD
Senior Research Fellow, Kennedy Institute of Ethics
Georgetown University

REBECCA DRESSER, JD
Daniel Noyes Kirby Professor of Law
Professor of Ethics in Medicine
Washington University

DAVID B. MORTON, PhD, MRCVS
Professor Emeritus, Department of Biomedical Science and Ethics
The Medical School, University of Birmingham, England

JOHN P. GLUCK, PhD
Professor Emeritus, Department of Psychology
University of New Mexico

OXFORD
UNIVERSITY PRESS
2008

OXFORD
UNIVERSITY PRESS

Oxford University Press, Inc., publishes works that further
Oxford University's objective of excellence
in research, scholarship, and education.

Oxford   New York
Auckland   Cape Town   Dar es Salaam   Hong Kong   Karachi
Kuala Lumpur   Madrid   Melbourne   Mexico City   Nairobi
New Delhi   Shanghai   Taipei   Toronto

With offices in
Argentina   Austria   Brazil   Chile   Czech Republic   France   Greece
Guatemala   Hungary   Italy   Japan   Poland   Portugal   Singapore
South Korea   Switzerland   Thailand   Turkey   Ukraine   Vietnam

Copyright © 2008 by Oxford University Press, Inc.

Published by Oxford University Press, Inc.
198 Madison Avenue, New York, New York 10016

www.oup.com

Oxford is a registered trademark of Oxford University Press

Library of Congress Cataloging-in-Publication Data
The human use of animals : case studies in ethical choice / Tom L. Beauchamp [et al.].—2nd ed.
    p. ; cm.
Includes bibliographical references and index.
ISBN 978-0-19-534019-8
1. Animal experimentation—Moral and ethical aspects—Case studies. 2. Animal welfare—Moral and
ethical aspects—Case studies.
[DNLM: 1. Animal Welfare—ethics—Case Reports. 2. Animal Use Alternatives—ethics—Case Reports.
3. Animals, Laboratory—Case Reports.] I. Beauchamp, Tom L.
HV4915.H85 2008
179'.4—dc22   2007020916

Printed in the United States of America
on acid-free paper

Preface to the Second Edition

This second edition of *The Human Use of Animals* carries forward our long-standing commitment to the view that human interactions with animals need to be guided by continuing ethical reflection, analysis, and discussion. In the previous volume we presented and analyzed cases that covered topics of research, education, food and farming, companion animals, and religious ritual. There was a particularly strong emphasis on research issues in that volume, and we came to think that it was a slight overemphasis. Research issues continue to have a major presence in the current volume, but we have added sections devoted to conservation concerns and the use of animals in entertainment. In particular, we now include cases on endangered species, zoos, circuses, and "sport" fighting. Given the ever-increasing importance of factory farms, we have added a case in this area on hog farming. While the introductory chapter discusses many of the same moral notions discussed in the first edition (moral status, ethical theory, animal minds, evolutionary theory, and the moral ground of research oversight), this introduction has been considerably expanded, updated, and made relevant for discussion of the cases.

We have attempted to present the case studies in an objective, balanced, and considered manner. Our goal has not been to reach a particular moral conclusion but to spark reasoned debate about moral questions. There is no question however, that it is difficult to write narrative-based cases, while raising moral questions, without the intrusion of some form of value judgment. Even selecting certain facts, while not pursuing others, involves an evaluative appraisal of their relative importance.

All five of the authors from the first edition have remained involved in the current volume. As a consequence, the nature of the chapter revisions and chapter additions reflect the evolution in our own thinking about the ethics of human uses of animals. The updating and rewriting involve very significant change. Not a single page in this book remains as it was in the first edition.

Tom Beauchamp's move to the first authorship position in this edition arises from Barbara Orlans's generosity of spirit. She realized that Tom had to take over the day-to-day management of drafts and to lend a final hand to all parts of the redrafting efforts of others. There was simply no other way to organize the work. All of us recognize, nonetheless, that Barbara remains the motivational center and ethical heart of this project, as she has been since we started working together, now 15 years ago.

We were hugely assisted in this edition by Sven Peterson and Paul Naquin, two research assistants who were assigned the work of doing first drafting of the four new cases in this volume: "Humane Housing for Hogs," "Winky and Wanda at the Detroit Zoo," "Ringling Brothers' Big Cats," and "Bonobos: Humans' Closest Relatives Face Extinction." Peterson wrote the first and last, as here listed, Naquin the other two. We recognize with great appreciation and admiration their work in both researching and first-drafting these four cases. Without their work, this volume would have been delayed by several months.

The present volume has been improved by the extensive reviews of the first edition and the critiques of our colleagues. Special thanks go to Bernard Rollin and Charlene McIver, and to Raymond Frey for discussions since the first edition.

Preparation of this manuscript was benefited by the generous support of the Panaphil Foundation. Work on these cases over the years has also been supported through a grant (SBE 91-21191) from The National Science Foundation (Ethics and Values Studies Program) and by financial support from The Kinnoull Trusts. Once again, Moheba Hanif has contributed able and important editorial assistance in the preparation of this manuscript, as did Stacylyn Dewey and Patrick Connolly, our student assistants throughout the project.

About the Cover

The monkeys depicted on the front cover are Stumptail Macaques (*Macaca arctoides*) who were part of a larger social group that had been formed for the purpose of studying their unique social behavior. The mother, "Rose," was purchased from an animal importer who had trapped her in Cambodia or Vietnam and shipped her to the United States. The baby, "Virginia," was the first infant born in the newly formed colony, and the companion, "Granny," was acquired as a "surplus" animal from the Los Alamos National Labs in Los Alamos, New Mexico. Her research history was not provided at the time of transfer, ostensibly for security reasons. The picture was taken in 1981 by one of John Gluck's student lab assistants, and John wishes to thank Trish for the gift of the photograph. We all wish to thank her for capturing this scene.

The confined pigs depicted on the back cover are in a typical 2007 factory farm in the United States. The techniques of farming are as described in the case study of pig farming, chapter 2. The sows weigh 500 to 600 pounds. The image was provided to the authors, with permission for use in this volume, by Diane Halverson and Marlene Halverson, with credit for the photograph to Marlene Halverson/Animal Welfare Institute. The farm is a pig factory in the midwestern United States. No company mentioned in the case study in chapter 2 should be associated with this photograph.

Contents

Interested Parties and the Political Landscape, 139
Ethical Issues, 141

PART V. RELIGIOUS USES OF ANIMALS

9. Animal Sacrifice as Religious Ritual: The Santeria Case, 149

    The Ritual Sacrifice in Santeria, 150
    Responses in the Hialeah Community, 151
    The Supreme Court Decision, 152
    Animal Use and the First Amendment, 154
    Ethical Issues, 155

PART VI. ENDANGERED SPECIES

10. Bonobos: Humans' Closest Relatives Face Extinction, 163

    Who Are the Bonobos? 164
    Human Threats to Bonobos, 166
    Strategies for Preserving the Bonobos, 167
    Ethical Issues, 170

PART VII. BIOMEDICAL RESEARCH AND COSMETIC TESTING

11. Head Injury Experiments on Primates at the University of Pennsylvania, 177

    The Use of Baboons in Research, 177
    The Laboratory Raid, 178
    Protests by Animal Protection Sympathizers and NIH Policy Decisions, 180
    Ethical Issues, 181

12. What Does the Public Have a Right to Know? 188

    Issues about Access to Meetings, 189
    The Legacy of PAWS' Legal Challenges, 191
    Legal Battles and Legal Reasoning in Precedent Cases, 193
    Ethical Issues, 195

PART I

INTRODUCTION

1

Moral Issues about Animals

Humans use animals in a dazzling variety of ways. The fish and meat on the table for dinner come from farms, fish markets, and butchers. Many items of clothing are from the leather industry, the animal dye industry, and the fur trade. Circuses, zoos, and trained-animal fights (such as cockfights) are parts of the entertainment industry. Many cosmetics have been safety-tested on animals, and the pharmaceutical and chemical industries each year expend millions of research dollars on millions of animals in toxicological studies. Hunting and fishing are considered by many to be relaxing and pleasurable. Companion animals can reach to the level of "man's best friend." These examples touch little more than the surface of the human use of animals.

All reflective persons find it difficult to determine precisely which of these uses of animals are morally justified and which are unjustified. Most of us are more than a little confused about how to make our moral views consistent. For example, we tend to be upset when we learn about abuses of and neglect of companion animals, but when we read fundamentally identical reports about the conditions of farm animals such as pigs and cattle, many simply regard these creatures as "animals." It seems that companion animals have more moral significance to us than the source of our bacon, but why, and can such views be made coherent?

Some think that questions about the moral place of animals and their rights are of very recent origin, but in fact they are ancient—dating at least from the time of the Pythagoreans.[1] The most extensive and imposing ancient account was that of

3

the Neoplatonist philosopher Porphyry (3rd–4th c. A.D.) in his influential treatise *On Abstinence from Animal Food*.[2] The most revolutionary ancient source was probably Plutarch's "Whether Land or Sea Animals are Cleverer" and "Beasts are Rational."[3] Also very influential was Aristotle's thesis that humans alone have intellect or reason— though many animals are intelligent[4]—and the denial by the Stoics that significant language, reason, virtue, and even real emotion can be attributed to animals.[5]

This impressive body of ancient thought was carried into modern discussions. For example, the landmark *Historical and Critical Dictionary* authored by French philosopher Pierre Bayle (first published in 1697) engages the history of the discussion, citing a large number of authors—ancient, medieval, and modern—who discuss whether animals have souls, whether they deserve some form of moral consideration, and whether animals reason.[6] Contemporary struggles with justifying the use of animals are often not fundamentally different from those of ancient times. The issues today, as in the past, address whether something about animals makes them morally considerable, and, if so, what humanity and justice permit us to do with them. However, even this way of framing the questions is subject to spirited controversy. Many people think that questions of humanity and justice have nothing to do with our treatment of animals.

The cases in this book are intended to serve as a source of reflection on these and many other questions about human-nonhuman interactions. The goal of this introduction is to provide a framework for moral thinking about human-nonhuman relations. In the next section, problems about the nature of morality, professional morality, and the moral community are discussed. In the second and third sections, psychological and biological questions about animal minds and Darwinian theory receive attention. In the fourth section, issues about the moral status of animals are examined. In the fifth section, some relevant types of systematic moral philosophy are considered, followed by the sixth and seventh sections, which treat issues in the justification of our treatment of animals and our approach in law and institutional committees to the evaluation of research involving animals.

MORALITY, PROFESSIONAL MORALITY, AND THE LAW

The term "morality" refers to a body of learnable standards of right and wrong conduct that are so widely shared that they form a stable, although incomplete, set of social conventions. As a social institution, morality encompasses many standards of conduct, including moral principles, rules, and rights. Moral directives are transmitted across generations. All persons living a moral life grasp the core dimensions of morality. They know not to lie, not to steal others' property, to keep promises, to respect the rights and liberties of others, not to kill or cause harm to innocent persons, and the like. All persons committed to morality are comfortable with these rules and do not doubt their relevance and importance. They know that to violate these norms is unethical and will likely generate feelings of remorse as well as subject violators to moral blame by others.

Like natural languages and political constitutions, core parts of morality exist before we become instructed in the relevant rules and regulations. As we develop and mature, we learn moral responsibilities together with other social obligations, such as legal obligations. Eventually we learn to distinguish general social rules of law and morals from rules binding only on members of special groups, such as those rules that bind only members of the veterinary profession. That is, we learn to distinguish general *social morality* from more specific moralities such as a *professional morality*.

Social Morality

The set of norms shared by all persons committed to morality constitutes what is often called "the common morality." The common morality is not merely *a* morality in contrast to *other* moralities. The common morality applies to everyone, and all persons are rightly judged by its standards. The following are examples of standards of action (rules of obligation) found in the common morality: 1. Don't kill; 2. Don't cause pain or suffering to others; 3. Prevent evil or harm from occurring; 4. Rescue persons in danger; 5. Tell the truth; 6. Nurture the young and dependent; 7. Keep your promises; 8. Don't steal; 9. Don't punish the innocent; 10. Obey the law.

In recent years, the favored language to express this morality has been "human rights," but standards of obligation and virtue are no less important.[7] It would, of course, be absurd to suppose that all persons do, in fact, accept the norms of the common morality. Many amoral, immoral, or selectively moral persons do not care about or identify with moral demands. Nonetheless, all persons in all cultures who are committed to *moral conduct* do accept the demands of the common morality.

The problem is that there are many distinct moralities comprising moral norms and positions that spring from particular cultural, philosophical, and religious sources. One reason that ethical norms governing human uses of animals vary so significantly from society to society, and even from person to person, is that rules about the permissible treatment of animals are not a part of universal morality. That is, no part of common morality has a specific focus on animals and on what veterinarians should and should not do. Universal common morality only supplies the core moral concepts and principles on the basis of which we can and should reflect on the appropriate treatment of animals.

It is obvious that many moral norms, whether pertaining to animals or to groups of humans such as health professionals, are not shared by all cultures, groups, or individuals. Whereas the common morality contains general moral norms that are abstract, universal, and content-thin, particular moralities present concrete, nonuniversal, and content-rich norms. These moralities include the many responsibilities, aspirations, ideals, sympathies, attitudes, and sensitivities found in diverse cultural traditions, religious traditions, professional traditions, and institutional settings. Views about the moral treatment of animals have always been forged in these contexts, and likely they always will be. At the same time, the common morality serves as the basic source for reflection on the place and treatment of animals.

Professional Moralities

Many professions have specific moral codes and traditions. These codes often vary legitimately from other particular moralities in how they handle many subjects. Persons who accept a particular morality often suppose that they speak with an authoritative moral voice for all persons. They operate under the false belief that they have the force of the common morality (that is, universal morality) behind them. The particular moral viewpoints that these persons hold may be morally acceptable and even praiseworthy, but they do not bind all other persons or communities. For example, persons who believe intensely that the California condor must be allowed to survive or that eating meat is immoral may have very good moral reasons for their views, but they cannot claim the force of the common morality for those views.

Professional obligations, such as those of veterinarians, are specific to the work of the professionals within the scope of the rules. Just as there is a general common morality across society, with shared principles and rules, so most professions contain, at least implicitly, a professional morality with widely shared standards of acceptable behavior. In professional contexts some measure of morality is transmitted informally, but formal instruction and attempts at the codification of professional morality have increased in recent years. These efforts have addressed many problems of ethics in professions engaged in research involving animal subjects—most prominently in codes of professional ethics, codes of research ethics, and government-sponsored reports and rules. (These codes are discussed in the section "Alternatives, Government Regulations, and Committee Review" below.)

Particular codes written for groups such as veterinarians, biologists, physicians, and psychologists usually spring from attempts to discover and develop an already inchoate morality that is accepted in the profession itself; it is an attempt to specify, explain, and expand the inchoate morality. A professional code usually emphasizes role obligations, which may be obligations either to animals or to other humans. (For examples, see the cases in chapters 3, 6, and 8.)

The following types of responsibility are often cited in codes and federal regulations pertaining to the use of animals:

RESPONSIBILITIES TO ANIMALS

Avoidance and reduction of unnecessary pain, deprivation, and suffering

Welfare protection by improving the animals' environment

Searching for alternatives to the use of animals through replacement models

Setting institutional policies and performing professional review

RESPONSIBILITIES TO SOCIETY

Avoidance of unnecessary harm-causing activities

Disclosure of risks to human health and to the environment

Public disclosure of procedures involving animals

Maintaining public trust

RESPONSIBILITIES TO EMPLOYERS AND FUNDING SOURCES

Codifying responsibilities in formal codes of ethics

Protecting privileged information

Reassessing policies, goals, and commitments

Adhering to contracts, laws, and professional standards

RESPONSIBILITIES TO PROFESSIONAL COLLEAGUES

Reporting data, methods, studies, and results in publications

Reporting unacceptable behavior and conditions to authorities

Mentoring by teaching ethical responsibilities to new colleagues

Promoting professional standards through written codes of practice

This outline of topics is only a representative list, not an exhaustive one.

Law and Morality

The "morality" of many actions and policies is commonly thought to be determined by whether the law prohibits the relevant form of conduct. Many violations of law are often called "ethics" violations. The reason is that the law is often the public's agent for translating its morality into explicit social guidelines and practices and for determining punishments for offenses. Case law (judge-made law expressed in court decisions), statutory law (federal and state statutes and their accompanying administrative regulations), and international law (law from treaties and agreements among nations) set standards for science, business, medicine, health care, and many facilities. These sources have deeply influenced moral discussions.

Moral evaluation is, nonetheless, very different from *legal* evaluation. Issues of legal liability, costs to the system, practicability within the litigation process, and questions of compensation demand that legal requirements be different from moral requirements. The law is not the repository of our moral standards and values, even when the law is directly concerned with moral problems. A law-abiding person is not necessarily morally sensitive or virtuous, and from the fact that an act is legally acceptable it does not follow that the act is morally acceptable. For example, when women and slaves were denied many basic human rights, these acts were morally unjust despite the fact that the law upheld them. It is commonly argued that much the same is true at the present time in many human uses of animals.

In sum, many actions are not illegal that turn out to be morally unsustainable.

ANIMAL MINDS

At the root of many of the issues addressed in this introduction and throughout this book is a rich body of empirical and theoretical issues about animal minds. Some of these issues are psychological. Among the best known philosopher-psychologists is the American pragmatist William James. He once wrote: "Other minds, other worlds. . . . My world is but one in a million alike embedded, alike real. . . . How different must be the worlds in the consciousness of ant, cuttle-fish, or crab!"[8] This is the problem of animal minds.

Most observers of animal behavior today agree that many animals have capacities to understand and have developed complicated, sometimes elaborate forms of social interaction and communication. Little agreement exists, however, about the levels and types of mental activity in these animals or about the ethical significance of their mental lives. The more we are in doubt about an animal's cognitive and affective life, the more we may find ourselves with doubts about the animal's moral significance; conversely, the more we attribute to an animal in the way of cognition and affective states, the more we are likely to upgrade the animal's status.

Historical Background in Philosophy

These questions have a long history, again reaching back to the ancients. For several classic philosophers, including Aristotle and Immanuel Kant, animals have *intelligent minds* but lack *reason* or *speech*. Other philosophers, including Pierre Bayle and David Hume, held that animals have both minds and capacities of reason but still may lack capacities such as moral judgment. Finally, some philosophers—René Descartes being the prime example—have viewed animals as lacking all mental capacity, all feeling, and even consciousness. This view suggests that animals, being devoid of minds, are no more than matter in motion, lacking not only moral sensitivity but mental sensitivity as well. Descartes and Hume will receive consideration now. Kant will be considered later (in the subsection "Kantian (Deontological) Theories and Obligations to Animals" below).

Descartes

Descartes (1596–1650) was the major figure whose views Charles Darwin later had to confront—and presumably to refute. Unlike Darwin, Descartes found profound dissimilarities between human and nonhuman creatures. He argued that nonhuman creatures lack the capacity to feel pain and do not have minds in the normal sense of the word. Animals are automata who:[9]

> act naturally and mechanically, like a clock which tells the time better than our judgment does. Doubtless when the swallows come in spring, they operate like clocks. The actions of honeybees are of the same nature, and the discipline of cranes in flight, and of apes in fighting. . . . All [animal motions] originate from the corporeal and mechanical principle.

Descartes's mechanistic theories of the physical world derive from his conviction that the natural sciences can provide explanations of complex physical phenomena. Nonhuman animals, Descartes thought, are simply parts of the physical world, thus their actions can be exhaustively explained without reference to mind. Descartes thought that the lack of language and abstract reasoning in animals provides sufficient grounds for a lack of mind. While Descartes agreed that animals and certain machines sometimes look as if they are acting and emitting sounds that resemble human speech, he thought that only a nonphysical mind could creatively use language to respond to novel circumstances through sophisticated abstract thought. Animals, by contrast, fail to move beyond the particularities of sensual experience and reactions based on instinct and conditioning—the mechanical principles of their nature.

Descartes offered several clarifications of and qualifications on his views, the following among the most important:

> Please note that I am speaking of thought, and not of life or sensation. I do not deny life to animals, since I regard it as consisting simply in the heat of the heart; and I do not even deny sensation, in so far as it depends upon a bodily organ. Thus my opinion is not so much cruel to animals as indulgent to human beings—at least to those who are not given to the superstitions of Pythagoras—since it absolves them from the suspicion of crime when they eat or kill animals.[10]

On the basis of this theory, Descartes argues that humans are absolved of any crime or guilt in killing, eating, and experimenting on animals. This account was accepted by many scientists and philosophers of the seventeenth and eighteenth centuries, but many also dissented from it. They argued that animals are conscious and do feel pain, though not all viewed such pain as a matter of moral concern or as a form of cruelty. After all, if humans rightly have dominion over animals, how could any respectable use of animals, such as medical experimentation, violate standards of good stewardship?

Descartes influenced theologians in need of a theodicy (a theory to vindicate the goodness of God in the face of evil). They needed to account for animal suffering. In light of Descartes's theories, they could maintain either that there is no animal suffering or that the suffering involved is a proper exercise of human dominion—possibly even a human moral obligation. These views were as powerful in England as in France—the two major countries at the time for new discoveries in both science and philosophy.[11]

Hume

A powerful alternative to Descartes was offered a century later by the Scottish philosopher and historian David Hume (1711–76). Hume regarded Descartes's views as an example of the excesses of adherence to a dogmatic and speculative philosophical theory. Though Hume lacked access to the theory of evolution, he anticipated some features of later Darwinian thinking about animal minds. He acknowledged that humans are far superior to other animals in advanced capacities of reasoning, but he set out to show fundamental similarities in experience, memory, inference, understanding, and reason:

> Animals, as well as men, learn many things from experience, and infer, that the same events will always follow from the same causes. By this principle they become acquainted with the more obvious properties of external objects, and gradually, from their birth, treasure up a knowledge of the nature of fire, water, earth, stones, heights, depths, &c. and of the effects, which result from their operation. The ignorance and inexperience of the young are here plainly distinguishable from the cunning and sagacity of the old, who have learned, by long observation, to avoid what hurt them, and to pursue what gave ease or pleasure. . . .
>
> In all these cases . . . the animal infers some fact beyond what immediately strikes his senses; and this inference [of reason] is altogether founded on past experience.[12]

Hume attributed rationality, or at least the capacity to reason, to some animals, on the grounds that these animals are significantly like humans in the principles of their nature, their patterns of learning, and their powers of inference. Hume cited, as evidence of thought, the capabilities of many animals to adapt in order to obtain food, to develop and implement ingenious strategies, and to use tools. Hume claims that differences in species are generally of *degree* rather than *kind*. Nonetheless, humans do seem unique in their capacities of morality, criticism, politics, law, and religion, and Hume regards nonhuman animals as lacking the capacities to participate in the rich array of cultural activities and in forms of reasoning such as demonstrative reasoning. Accordingly, Hume confines his attention to the limited thesis that many animals love, hate, enjoy, suffer, and the like, and that they reason by making causal inferences. He also maintains that the passions of animals are directed at many of the same objects at which human passions are directed. For example, animals learn, as do we, that certain objects are to be feared, and their fear is then directed at those objects.

Hume attributed more than rationality to animals. In *A Treatise of Human Nature*, he included whole sections on topics of *love* and *pride* in animals.[13] He discussed sympathy and cooperative schemes in the animal world. In each case, he found the capacities of nonhuman animals analogous to human capacities. He argued that a philosophy with a proper breadth to grasp mental powers would have to explain animal cognitive skills along with parallel human skills. Likewise, we would have to explain the "evident" continuities between the human and the animal, as well as the discontinuities, such as the nonhuman animals' apparent lack of a sense of virtue and vice.

Prior to Hume, the prevailing view in philosophy and theology had been that human beings are fashioned in the image of God and occupy a status above nonhuman animals in the hierarchy of nature. Hume suggested that humans are more closely aligned with the animal kingdom than the kingdom of God and that humans are as much a part of the natural realm as are the other animals. His legacy, in the end, was to move as far as anyone before him to a naturalistic explanation of both human and nonhuman minds, an explanation that used similar categories for the human and the nonhuman.

Contemporary Issues

Close observers of animal behavior today agree with Hume that many animals have capacities to understand and have elaborate forms of social interaction and communication (whether these qualify as having a language or not). Intelligence and adaptation in animal behavior, as explored by ethologists and psychologists, are often inexplicable without acknowledging that animals exhibit understanding, intention, thought, imaginativeness, and various forms of communication. Certain facts of *mental* life in many animals do not seem any more in doubt than facts about *physical* processes in these creatures. That a dog feels sick or that a bear is angry is often not more doubtful than that a child is sick or a spouse angry. We may not know the nuanced character of mental states in others, but we are confident that we have correctly attributed at least some mental states such as pain to animals.

Donald Griffin (American professor of zoology, 1915–2003) argued in his influential books *Animal Thinking* and *Animal Minds*[14] that the complex actions of animals, which are often novel in the circumstances, suggest adaptive and creative forms of judgment. Typical examples are innovative forms of defense, use of tools, adaptation to sudden and threatening changes in an environment, intentional movements and sounds to communicate or convey feelings, creative forms of play, construction of shelters and prey-catching devices, and the like. Griffin attributes consciousness, self-awareness, and emotion to animals, based on the many forms of animal behavior that Griffin argues cannot be explained unless we attribute mental states to the animals.

If capacities such as intention, understanding, emotion, choice, belief, and thought are attributed to animals, they are thereby credited with properties relevantly similar to human capacities. Therefore, some argue, they merit whatever moral protections humans enjoy by virtue of having the same properties.[15] However, we understand very little about the inner lives of animals, or even about how to connect many forms of observable behavior with other forms of behavior. For example, we have difficulty understanding the concepts of intention and choice in animals because animal behavior is so different from human behavior; there are therefore gaps in our understanding when we attribute intention or choice to animals. Forms of communication are similarly difficult to grasp. We understand little about how animal noises (for example, those of killer whales) relate to animal behavior, or why these noises occur under one set of conditions but not others. It is difficult to peer into the mental life of another species, even one as close to us in the evolutionary scheme as other primates.[16]

Neither evolutionary descent nor the physical and functional organization of an animal system (the conditions responsible for its having a mental life) gives us the depth of insight we would like to have in understanding the animal's mental states. Even the most careful scientific observation of behavior often does not yield adequate understanding. When we have as full an explanation as can be obtained under current scientific standards, we still have to decide about an animal, as with a brain-damaged human, whether the individual really has mental states such as understanding and intention or is merely acting *as if* he or she had such states.

The behavioral and life sciences together with the philosophy of mind shed only limited light on animal mental states—such as alleged depression or happiness—and on questions of whether animals act intentionally by planning to trap their prey, build nests, and protect their young. (Several chapters in this book deal with this issue; see especially chapters 4, 6, 10, and 14.) There remain many questions about what we are entitled to infer based on our limited knowledge about physiology and behavior, as well as how this knowledge would affect our thinking about ethics.[17]

DARWIN AND EVOLUTIONARY THEORY

In the face of radical disagreement among great philosophers such as Descartes and Hume, Charles Darwin stepped forth with a theory that was as philosophical as it was scientific and as revolutionary as any in the history of science. In *The Descent of Man*, he catalogued many similarities in mental ability between humans and apes.[18] He observed that "it is a significant fact, that the more the habits of any particular animal are studied by a naturalist, the more he ascribes to *reason* and the less to *unlearnt instincts*."[19]

We have seen that prior to Darwin many biologists and philosophers argued that, despite clear anatomical similarities between humans and apes, humans are distinguished by the possession of *reason, speech,* and *moral sensibility*. Darwin thought, by contrast, that there is ample empirical evidence that animals have powers of deliberation and decision making, excellent memories, fertile imaginations, and even moral emotions. Darwin therefore criticized the hypothesis that major cognitive differences separate apes and humans in the respects proposed by thinkers such as Descartes.[20]

In Darwin's theory, complex biological structures and psychological functions are shared in the evolutionary struggle. From basic biology to memory and inference, remarkable continuities are present across the species. Any animal able to use mental abilities to choose between alternative forms of behavior is likely to be advantaged in the evolutionary process. It would be odd, Darwin suggests, if only humans had achieved any measure of the massive evolutionary advantage given by advanced mental structures. Darwin rejected all accounts that hypothesize large gaps between the species. He adopted instead a continuity model of connections between species.

Degrees of Mental Power

Darwin argues that despite "enormous differences" in *degree* of "mental power" between humans and apes, no fundamental difference exists in *kind* between humans and many forms of animal life. His hypothesis is that apes are highly intelligent and are similar to humans in emotional responses such as terror, rage, shame, and maternal affection. They are also similar in character traits such as courage and timidity and are even similar in the use of systems of communication that approximate human language and human conceptual abstraction. Moreover, Darwin argues, a greater gap exists in the intelligence level of apes and marine life than between apes and humans. In nature we find "numberless gradations" in mental power, with apes and humans on the high end. In a revealing sentence, Darwin maintains that "it is a pure assumption to assert that the mental act is not essentially of the same nature in the animal as in the man."

Darwin also challenged features in the abovementioned views about self-consciousness and higher-level cognitive abilities. He wrote in an 1872 work on emotions in animals that

> It may be freely admitted that no animal is self-conscious, if by this term it is implied, that he reflects on such points, as whence he comes or whither he will go, or what is life and death, and so forth. But how can we feel sure that an old dog with an excellent memory and some power of imagination . . . never reflects on his past pleasures or pains in the chase? And this would be *a form* of self-consciousness.[21]

Language

Darwin has interesting, though underdeveloped, views about language. He takes it as proven empirically that animals communicate through sounds and gestures. He says that "the habitual use of articulate language [verbal speech] is peculiar to man, but he uses, in common with the lower animals, inarticulate cries to express his meaning, aided by gestures and the movements of the muscles of the face." Darwin notes that "our cries of pain, fear, surprise, anger, together with their appropriate actions, and the murmur of a mother to her beloved child are more expressive than any words." These forms of expression Darwin regards as shared by humans and many species of animals. He judges that animals such as parrots and dogs can respond to and make associations with articulate sounds, much as humans do. (See the classic case of the African Grey parrot named Alex discussed in chapter 4.)

Darwin also thought that animals possess "mental concepts," including abstract or general concepts. When you say "squirrel" and your dog begins looking in trees and circling, according to Darwin the dog has an abstract idea of a squirrel ("a general idea or concept") and an idea that "some animal is to be discovered and hunted." Part of Darwin's motivation in this argument is to show that rational abilities in humans are the products of natural selection, as they are for other animals. Therefore, we do not need a special account (such as God's infusion of a rational soul) in order to explain the human species.

Darwin comes to the conclusion that human language is different from that of other creatures, but only by degree. The acceptability of his conclusions depends on how much is packed into the concept of a "language." On a minimalist view, a language is a system of conventions that allows communication to occur among members of a community. Clearly animals have this measure of "language." But if a more enriched notion of language is used, requiring syntactical rules, sentences, true and false statements, creative use of conventional symbols, and the like (as Descartes may have assumed and as many after him have assumed), then perhaps no animals other than the human animal will qualify.

Use of this enriched notion of language suggests that if nonhuman animals have nothing corresponding to syntax in a language, then there is a sharp break in the evolutionary scheme. Darwin offers no refutation of this hypothesis, but he does indicate that he is leery of all sharp-break theses. He tried to account for major differences in terms of the complexity and developed character of the brain, which he thought more advanced in humans than in animals. He accounted for differences in rationality similarly. Just as some psychologists today speak of several different forms of intelligence or IQ, Darwin thought several forms and degrees of rationality could be found in animals: means-to-end reasoning, spatial perception, capacity to improvise and cope successfully, manipulation of the environment, desires and beliefs joined together in action, sensing and avoiding harmful conditions, etc.

The Moral Sense (Conscience)

In chapter 3 of *The Descent of Man,* Darwin argues that the human moral sense, or conscience, is itself the product of evolution. "Social instincts," meaning dispositions to act in certain ways, have become fixed in human nature so that "the moral sense is fundamentally identical with the social instincts." These instincts allow us to set aside self-interest to act in the interests of others. The moral sense or conscience is an advanced sense of obligation and a form of sympathy that can be extended to a larger social group. Darwin finds it "the most noble of all the attributes" found in the human animal: "I fully subscribe to the judgment of those writers who maintain that of all the differences between man and the lower animals, the moral sense or conscience is by far the most important."

Darwin thought that this mental and moral capacity is not without analogues in the nonhuman animal world. Darwin argues that nonhuman animals have emotions such as love and sympathy, both for their kin and their larger social group. They have social instincts, enjoy companions, are sympathetic with the plight of those to whom they are close, help their fellows, knowingly risk their lives, grieve in the loss of life, and are gratified by others' approval of their behavior. Darwin thus thought of animals as having altruistic dispositions, even if lacking in the higher level of conscience.

Although Darwin did not develop a detailed theory of the motivational structure of animals, he did maintain that animals act beneficently—that is, for the benefit of others (of their family or species). He argued that just as we can correctly attribute beneficence to humans based on their behavior, so we can do the same for animals. His examples come from community organization, affection in companionship, play, mutual or reciprocal provision of services, mothers caring for offspring, the adoption of helpless orphans, caring for the wounded or invalids, attending to elderly parents, feeding the blind, and intentional exposure to danger in order to protect others—all found in various communities of nonhuman animals.

So convinced was Darwin of the validity of his inferences that he attributed extraordinary, selfless acts of bravery to animals and referred to these acts as involving moral *heroism.* He believed that some animals can act altruistically, even if they have no conception of altruistic behavior and no rules of obligation requiring such behavior. Although Darwin lacked sophisticated ethological and psychological studies on which to base his theories, it is evident that he would regard many of the studies conducted in the twentieth and twenty-first centuries as confirmations of his views.

In summary, Darwin looked less for differences across species than for similarities. Whatever moral, physical, and mental qualities humans possess evolved through a gradual series of processes that similarly occur elsewhere in nature. The faculties of reason and speech are no different in their evolutionary origin than the tooth of the snake, the fin of the fish, and the beak of the buzzard:

> The difference in mind between man and the higher animals, great as it is, certainly is one of degree and not of kind. . . . If it could be proved that certain high mental powers, such as the formation of general concepts, self-consciousness, etc. were absolutely peculiar to man, which seems extremely doubtful, it is not improbable that these qualities are merely the incidental results of other highly advanced intellectual faculties. . . . The half-art, half-instinct of language still bears the stamp of its gradual evolution.

Thus Darwin, who was conversant with eighteenth- and nineteenth-century moral philosophy, seemed to deny that animals make moral judgments, while affirming that they have moral dispositions. For example, he thought that animals do not truly make judgments of blame when they are punishing their peers for misbehavior, but that they do have passions and dispositions of love, affection, and generosity.

Moral Implications in the Aftermath of Darwin

Darwin's biology and psychology challenge the traditional idea that human beings have magical capacities that distance them from the rest of the animal kingdom—so-called human dignity. We are not, from Darwin's perspective, "the rational creature," as Aristotelians, Cartesians, Kantians, and other philosophers had suggested; we are but one among all the other rational creatures. This thesis about rationality across species is a consequential moral matter, because it throws into question the received view that human beings are fundamentally different and deserve unique or sole moral consideration.

Darwin's theories have stimulated discussions about whether morality in an analogous sense to human morals is found in some parts of the animal world. The term "morality" was defined previously in this chapter as a body of learnable standards of right and wrong so widely shared in society that the rules form a secure body of social conventions. Darwin and others note that many animals live in communities that require conformity to basic norms of communal life, much as human communities do. However, whether there is good evidence of real morality in nonhuman animals is controversial. Some observers believe that it is little more than human fantasy to suppose that animals act morally; other observers find close similarities between the behavior of humans and nonhuman animals.[22]

One difficult question is whether animals have a capacity to make moral *judgments* about members of their social group—for example, when those members are violating fixed expectations of conduct and deserve punishment or some form of rebuke. That animals intentionally reprimand and punish members of their group seems clear, but whether they use moral standards and make judgments is less certain.

If one understands morality in terms such as the various substantive rules mentioned early in this chapter (e.g., keep your promises), together with the adoption of an impartial attitude, then it seems unlikely that animals have such a morality. At least it is doubtful that they have a morality that involves applying rules and acting impartially. But perhaps they do act morally insofar as they act lovingly, protectively, and generously. Conceivably, animals "act morally" in some respects but lack critical capacities of acting morally in other respects.

These issues, first raised by Darwin, continue today in fresh forms, both in biology and in interdisciplinary discussions between philosophers and biologists. Evolutionary biologist Marc Hauser and primatologist Frans de Waal, among others, have presented empirical work suggesting that the great apes possess genetically shaped dispositions toward moral behavior, act in accordance with rudimentary moral rules in communities, and have moral capacities such as sympathy as well as moral emotions such as empathy.[23] De Waal has controversially suggested that human morality is likely descended from conditions of primate sociality. Though this discussion mirrors Darwin, it is today being developed in a notably different scientific context.

MORAL STATUS

Problems about whether animals act morally, whether they are part of the moral community, and whether they have higher-level mental capacities are connected to human attitudes and assumptions that have been at work for centuries.[24] Claims of human supremacy and rightful dominion have been particularly influential. For example, in the first chapter of the first book of the Bible, God is reported to have granted humans dominion over animals.[25] Based on such passages, animals have been treated as not having any moral (or legal) *standing* or *status*.

On another account, animals have little or no status, because we owe obligations only to the humans who *own* animals, not to the animals owned. On this account, if you poison your neighbor's barking dog or a ferocious tiger in a circus, you violate a moral obligation that you have not to destroy an owner's property, but you do not violate any obligation to the animal. The neighbor is injured; the dog and the tiger killed are not injured. Your neighbor's animal has no more moral value than your neighbor's plants. If you poison the animals or the plants, you have wronged the neighbor only, not the animals or the plants.

Many people find this conclusion counterintuitive, and many judge it offensive. Others think these questions are difficult to judge because they are at the outer boundaries of moral concern—that is, we here find ourselves on the borderlines of how far our moral concepts reach. As is the case with questions about moral obligations to future generations of humans and obligations to the environment, we find it difficult to confidently provide moral answers to such questions. To sort through these issues requires that we examine several underlying issues about moral status.

What Is Moral Status?

The basic moral question is, "Which individuals and groups are entitled to the protections afforded by morality?" Terms like "status" and "standing" have been transported into ethical discussions from law, where "standing" is "one's place in the community in the estimation of others; one's relative position in social, commercial, or moral relations; one's repute, grade, or rank" (*Black's Law Dictionary*). Animals have been given almost no legal standing or status in British and American systems of law.[26] However, recent discussions about fetuses, infants, the brain damaged, the mentally retarded, and animals have appropriated the terms "standing" and "status" while stripping away their distinctly legal meanings. In moral philosophy, to have moral status is to deserve the protections afforded by the basic norms of morality. In a *weak* sense, "status" and "standing" refer merely to any status, grade, or rank of moral importance. In a *strong* sense, "status" and "standing" are used to identify those who have rights or the functional equivalent of rights. (For examples of such an attribution of rights, see most cases in this book, but especially chapter 10.)

The mainstream approach to the question of what *kind of entity* merits moral protection has been to ask which *properties* of the entity qualify it for moral protection. Some say that there is one and only one property that confers moral status. For example, some say that this property is *human dignity*—a fuzzy notion that moral theory has done little to clarify.[27] Others say that another property or perhaps several other properties are required to acquire moral status—for example, sentience, rationality, or moral agency. Each such property has been developed by one or more writers as a general theory of moral status. Most theories have been framed in terms of either distinctively human properties or properties of sentience and other psychological properties such as emotions. Each type of theory of moral status has several subtypes and a considerable body of supporting literature.[28]

Human and Cognitive Criteria of Moral Status

The first type of theory, based on distinctively human properties, has long been attractive, because it supposedly distinguishes humans in the relevant ways from animals and justifies why we traditionally allow human interests to rank higher, have more value, and count for more whenever they are in conflict with the interests of animals. Much recent discussion about moral status has centered on the criteria for being a *person,* under the assumption that only persons have the relevant distinctive properties needed for moral status.

An example is found in *The Great Ape Project,* as originally conceived by Paola Cavalieri and Peter Singer.[29] They argue that the great apes are *persons,* just as humans are *apes.* It is no accident that a central theme of their project is the *personhood* of the apes. The more properties an animal possesses that approximate the properties of persons, the higher it appears the status of the animal would be. A widely shared view today is that if animals have capacities of understanding, intending, and suffering (or even of having desires, preferences, and other such psychological capacities), these properties confer *some* moral status.

Most theories of this sort do not restrict themselves to mere human biological and species criteria. The theories usually feature certain *cognitive* properties. ("Cognition" here refers to processes of awareness and knowledge, such as perception, memory, thinking, and linguistic ability.) Properties found in various theories of this first, or cognitive, type of theory include: (1) self-consciousness (consciousness of oneself as existing over time, with a past and future); (2) the freedom to act and the capacity to engage in purposive sequences of actions; (3) having reasons for action and the ability to appreciate reasons for acting; (4) the capacity to communicate with other persons using a language; and (5) rationality and higher-order volition. Any entity having such higher-level properties has moral status, and this status confers moral rights.[30] In general, the claim is that individuals have moral status because they are able to think about their lives through their cognitive capacities and are self-determined by their beliefs.

Suppose that dogs and ducks lack some critical property on this list of five properties. Which property do they lack? A property often cited is self-consciousness, or a conception of oneself as persisting through time. Animals, many believe, lack this capacity and so lack the ability to plan for the future and to understand the past. The hypothesis is that although animals exhibit goal-directed behaviors such as building a nest, they do so without any sense of self, which is thought to be essential to personhood or to any condition that confers moral status.[31]

Critics of this type of theory deny that there are *morally* significant cognitive differences between humans and animals and ask why cognitive criteria get special consideration over other criteria such as sentience. They also note that theories appealing to cognitive properties may in the end confer moral status on many nonhuman animals. Capacities such as intention, understanding, desire, preferences, free action, systems of communication, and beliefs need not be *distinctively human,* because many animals may exhibit significant levels of these capacities. As long as a theory requires sufficiently high-level cognitive criteria such as abstract, deductive thinking for moral status, then nonhuman animals likely will not be able to qualify for significant status. But if one appeals to other cognitive capacities, such as intention, understanding, desire, having preferences, and having beliefs, then perhaps animals will acquire some significant range of moral protections.

A major worry about theories of moral status that attempt to find a cognitive set of properties is that the set identified is simply tailored to one's preconceived and favored moral position that only humans deserve such status. From ancient Hellenic times to the present, people who were refused a certain social standing (slaves, women, and the like) were declared to lack some morally relevant property and therefore failed to qualify for full moral status. Over time, views about the moral rightness of these social norms changed, and the moral status of these groups changed even though none of their relevant properties had changed. That is, moral perception was widened even though the properties of the individuals did not change at all. In this way, women and many minority groups who had been denied significant moral status had moral status conferred on them by society. The worry today is that animals may be in much the same situation. They fail to satisfy reigning social criteria of status precisely because the criteria of moral status (including laws in many countries) are tailored specifically to deny them a substantive status. The literature on cognitive criteria of moral status is especially worrisome in this regard.[32]

Noncognitive Criteria of Moral Status

This opens the way to a second type of theory. Perhaps some creatures deserve moral status if they do not possess any form of cognitive capacity. Perhaps a *noncognitive* property confers some measure of status.[33] At least two kinds of properties deserve consideration: (1) properties of sensation (or perception) and (2) properties of emotion.

First, consider sensation. As Jeremy Bentham long ago pointed out, the capacity to feel pain might by itself be sufficient for conferring a significant moral status, and pain is not a cognitive criterion. Lack of personhood did not for Bentham imply a lack of moral status. (See the section on Bentham's utilitarianism below.) In a recent extension of such ideas, Donald Griffin argues that there is no good reason to place much weight on the distinction between perceptual awareness in animals and a reflective consciousness in humans, though traditionally we have made sharp distinctions between the two that affect animals' moral status. Griffin argues that there are multiple levels of mental activity that are shared across species, from basic pain receptors to intentionality.[34]

Second, consider emotion. The emotional lives of animals have long been avoided in scientific literature, where attributions of emotion, intention, and the like have been criticized as an unscientific abandonment of critical standards and precise measurements, as well as an importing of anthropomorphism. Yet many good reasons exist for attributing a range of emotions to animals. The basis is as good as we have for the attribution of pain and suffering to these animals. In Griffin's early work, *The Question of Animal Awareness,*[35] and in the popular bestseller *When Elephants Weep: The Emotional Lives of Animals,*[36] we find returns to Darwin's idea that animals experience love, joy, anger, fear, shame, compassion, loneliness, and many other emotions.

These noncognitive properties of sensation and emotion may be sufficient by themselves to confer some form of moral status. However, it remains unclear what *level* or *degree* of status is gained.

Speciesism

One widely discussed issue about moral status is speciesism, a notion first advanced by Richard Ryder and later popularized by Peter Singer.[37] A speciesist is generally thought of as one who believes that the interests of members of the species homo sapiens are to be favored over the interests of any other species.[38] However, *generalized* speciesism has nothing to do with the particular species homo sapiens. Any bias in favor of any species just because of species membership is an instance of speciesism. If one prefers dogs to ducks and deer merely because of species membership, one is a speciesist. A creature's moral status obviously could be determined entirely by speciesist considerations.

The term "speciesism" is typically used pejoratively by analogy to racism and sexism. In this usage, speciesism is understood as an improper failure to respect the lives and rights of other groups merely because they are other than human or other than a favored species. Just as gender, race, IQ, accent, national origin, and social status, for example, are not relevant properties in morals, neither is species. "To each according to species" seems as morally irrelevant and unfair as "to each according to one's skin color."

However, speciesism need not be understood in this negative manner. Some speciesists willingly and even enthusiastically accept the label if it is used to mean placing a moral priority on members of the human species. Some speciesists point out that humans have a natural feeling of kinship and closeness with members of their own species, just as some human family members have natural feelings of closeness to other family members.[39] In both cases, natural feelings create stronger obligations to members of the relevant group—the family on the one hand and the species on the other. This claim may be correct, but it is difficult to assess what it proves. Does the argument justify all forms of action based on close-knit relationships? For example, can military persons favor military persons, members of the upper class members of the upper class, members of one race the members of their race, members of one gender the members of their gender? If one can detect an unjustifiable bias in these schemes of personal closeness, is speciesism invalidated?

One possible defense of speciesism is that certain properties associated with the human species—in particular, the cognitive properties discussed previously—give humans a special moral status; it is not species membership alone that justifies special treatment for humans. From this perspective, it just so happens that those who possess these properties are of one species. This argument runs the risk, however, of permitting (or even demanding) the same treatment for members of the human species who lack these same properties—such as the mentally handicapped and the brain damaged—as for nonhuman animals.

MORAL PHILOSOPHIES

Many figures in the history of philosophy have attempted to develop a systematically organized set of moral principles together with a justification of the system—a moral philosophy that aims to organize and integrate the moral life in the form of a theory. Such a system would integrate virtually all the topics that we have thus far considered: the nature of morality, moral status, basic human obligations, and the like. The present section describes three general theories that have played and continue to play a significant role in the discussion of human uses of animals—namely, utilitarian theories, Kantian theories, and rights theories.

Some knowledge of these types of moral philosophy is indispensable for reflective study of the ethics of human uses of animals, because the field's literature frequently draws on the terminology, arguments, methods, and conclusions of these accounts. In almost every case in this volume, one or more of these theories is helpful in assessing the morality of what was done or should be done, what is permissible, and the like.

Utilitarianism and the Well-Being of Animals

Utilitarian theories have been the most widely discussed type of theory in the development of ethical issues about animals. Utilitarians invite us to consider the larger objective or function of morality as a social institution, where morality is understood to include rules of justice and other rules of the moral community. The point of the institution of morality, they insist, is to promote welfare by minimizing harms and maximizing benefits; there would be no reason to have moral codes unless they served this purpose. Utilitarians thus see moral rules as the means to the fulfillment of individual needs as well as to the achievement of broad social goals.

Utilitarians hold that an action or practice is right (when compared with any alternative action or practice) if it leads to the greatest possible balance of good consequences or to the least possible balance of bad consequences in the world as a whole for all affected parties. Utilitarians hold that there is one and only one basic principle of ethics: the *principle of utility*, which asserts that we ought always to produce the maximal balance of positive value over disvalue—or the least possible disvalue, if only undesirable results can be achieved.

Four conditions must be satisfied for a theory to qualify as utilitarian.

1. *The principle of utility*. First, the principle of utility requires actors to maximize the good. We ought in every circumstance to produce the greatest possible balance of value over disvalue (or the least possible balance of disvalue) for all affected parties—whatever that balance is and however it is distributed. For example, we ought to maximize the public benefits of scientific research, well-ordered zoos, veterinary medicine, public health measures, etc.

But what is the *good* or the *beneficial* or the *valuable* as the utilitarian conceives it?

2. *A standard of goodness.* Utilitarians say that the goodness of consequences should be measured by items that count as basic goods or utilities. Many utilitarians agree that we ought to look to the production of what is always and for everyone valuable for the condition of well-being—for example, health, security, freedom, and companionship and attachment. Such goods, or conditions of well-being, do not vary from one subject to the next. However, other utilitarians are a bit suspicious that there are such goods, and they interpret the good as that which is subjectively desired or preferred. In the ethics of animal treatment, this question about the *nature* of values might be thought of as less significant than issues about *whose values* will be considered, and whether they will be considered equally. The latter problem is one of moral status, and it should be kept distinct from the theory of *which values* are to be considered. In human life and in a wide range of animal life, it is vital to ask what conditions of well-being must be satisfied for them to have a decent life. For them, as for humans, conditions such as health, security, liberty, and companionship and attachment are essential to well-being, and therefore are basic goods.

3. *Consequentialism.* All utilitarian theories are consequentialist. That is, actions are morally right or wrong according to their good or bad consequences, rather than by virtue of any intrinsic moral features they may have, such as fidelity, friendship, or trust. In many cases in this book, we will see that certain consequences for human health and survival seem to matter more than anything else in determining how some people make moral decisions. However, many utilitarians consider consequences for animals to be also of basic moral importance. The growth of human populations often has severely negative consequences for animal life in the region, and in any broad utilitarian theory such consequences will be balanced along with consequences for humans.

4. *Impartiality.* Finally, utilitarians require that all parties affected by an action receive impartial consideration. In seeking a blinded impartiality, utilitarianism aligns good and mature moral judgment with moral distance from the choices to be made. A moral point of view is impartial in the sense that a moral judgment is formed without regard to personal preference and interest and also without regard to morally irrelevant properties such as how athletic or beautiful a person is. Unbiased evaluation without regard to race, sex, nationality, and the like is considered morally imperative.

But how about species? Can we morally prefer the members of our own species without running afoul of requirements of impartiality? A utilitarian holds that any partiality that is displayed toward particular individuals—such as members of one's own family—must itself have a strict utilitarian justification in terms of the public benefits of such arrangements of partiality. Similarly, partiality toward a species—any species—would need a utilitarian justification. (See the "Speciesism" subsection above.) Such a requirement of impartiality that embraced species impartiality would powerfully affect how animals are treated. If we must treat animals with the same impartial regard that we treat human persons, the effect would be to revolutionize many past practices.

Unfortunately, whether animals are to be counted and who is to be treated impartially are systematically ambiguous questions in many (though not all) utilitarian theories. Given this uncertainty about questions of moral status, we might obtain two very different recommendations from two committed utilitarians in a particular case: action *A* would be recommended if *only human* goods and interests were considered, whereas action *B* would be recommended if the goods and interests of *all affected animals* were to be considered. It is easy to imagine how different our environmental policies would be if we had to consider both the interests of animals and those of humans—especially if we had to give them equal consideration. There is therefore a general problem in utilitarianism about what constitutes "the general welfare" and "all those affected by an action."

The simplest alternative is to maintain that species properties and differences are irrelevant and therefore that the welfare of all sentient animals is to be considered. The morally relevant consideration, in this interpretation of utilitarianism, is who or what has the relevant experiences, feelings, pleasures, and the like—not what species it belongs to or what kind of being it is.

Bentham's Theory

Among the earliest and most significant utilitarian writings were those of British philosopher Jeremy Bentham (1748–1832). He offered historically influential thoughts that have been widely quoted in the animal ethics literature. Bentham argued that animals, like humans, have the capacity to feel pain and therefore deserve moral protections. He reasoned that despite important differences between humans and animals, there are also important and relevant similarities, the chief being the capacity of sentience—that is, the capacity to experience pleasure, pain, and suffering.

As we saw earlier, the capacity for experiencing pain was itself sufficient, for Bentham, to confer at least some significant moral status. This reasoning underlies a famous statement he made: "The question is not, Can they [nonhuman animals] *reason?* nor, Can they *talk?* but, Can they *suffer?*"[40] Bentham used his utilitarian moral theory as a way of grounding obligations directly to animals. We have duties to animals not to cause them pain and suffering, and these duties are independent of any duties we may have to the owners of the animals.

Bentham's thesis pushes the point that moral claims on behalf of animals do not in any obvious way have anything to do with the animals' intelligence, self-consciousness, personality, or any other such fact about them. It is pain, suffering, and overall welfare—not rationality or self-awareness—that provide the reason many critics of our uses of animals resist the way primates are used in biomedical experimentation, rabbits are used in cosmetics research, and chickens are raised for the market.[41] (Virtually every case in this book is concerned with issues of pain and suffering and with their moral importance.)

Contemporary Theories of Utilitarianism

Contemporary utilitarians such as Peter Singer maintain that many animals have desires and preferences about their futures and that they experience pain and suffering.[42] Singer argues that we need to justify our uses of animals on a basis that takes account of utility from the animal's perspective. This utilitarian perspective "makes it more difficult to claim that a genuinely utilitarian approach favors animal experimentation in general or as an institution," although "some individual experiments—those that do not involve any or very much suffering for the animal, and promise major benefits for humans or animals—may be defensible on utilitarian grounds."[43]

Another influential utilitarian thinker in debates about animal ethics in the last 30 years is Raymond G. Frey, whose view of the practical implications of utilitarianism are starkly different from Singer's. Frey argues that the value of any life, human or nonhuman, is contingent on its quality, and its quality is contingent on the goods in that life. Although animal life is typically not as rich and therefore not as well endowed with goods as human life, some animals have lives that are more valuable than other animals, including human animals. The lives of dogs, cats, and chimps, for example, are more valuable than the lives of mice, rats, and worms, and if the life of a human infant is less rich than the life of an adult chimpanzee, these infants have less moral status than do adult chimpanzees.[44]

This comparative-value and quality-of-life analysis allows Frey to maintain that (1) we should maximize utility for all affected parties, not merely the human species, and (2) for humans and animals alike, life is valuable only under certain conditions. Life progressively loses value as its riches or valued components are stripped away. As a life becomes less valuable, it has a reduced moral status that makes it increasingly more vulnerable to use in biomedical and behavioral research. Frey's utilitarian theory opens up the possibility that humans with a sufficiently impoverished or substandard existence may justifiably be treated exactly as we treat animals at the same level of existence. They can be used for research, mined for organs, etc.

On both utilitarian accounts—Singer's and Frey's—mere species membership should not be a factor in making moral judgments. It is not one's species, but the quality of one's life (its utility), and others' lives, that count. There is no consistent way to draw nonarbitrary *moral* lines based solely on species differences between human and animal life that will exclude one and include the other in the scope of justified activities.

However, these two utilitarians differ on numerous issues, largely because of their different assessments of the consequences of various practices. Utilitarians understandably will reach different conclusions about right and wrong depending on their views about the future consequences of a certain kind of act or rule. One very important difference is Frey's allowance of a more extensive use of both animals and humans than Singer's. Frey must, in consistency with his utilitarian commitments, countenance the use of not only animals but limited-capacity humans in biomedical research.[45] Frey is here acknowledging a breakdown of the lines that have traditionally distinguished human and nonhuman animals. If some nonhumans turn out to possess significantly more advanced capacities than customarily envisioned, their moral standing could and should be upgraded to a more human level. However, this possibility remains speculative and may be less important than Frey's thesis that because many human *lack* the properties that some animals possess, they are thereby rendered equal or inferior in moral standing to some nonhumans. If this conclusion is defensible, we will need to rethink our traditional view that these unlucky humans cannot be treated in the ways we treat relevantly similar nonhumans. For example, both animals and humans might be used without consent as human research subjects and as sources of organs.

Singer believes that an unattractive feature of accounts such as Frey's utilitarianism is that they allow some human persons to be drafted without consent as research subjects and then harmed or killed, just as we treat animals. Singer suggests that this line of argument leaves not a *narrow* but a *broad* range of human subjects unprotected:

> Certain categories of human beings—infants and mentally retarded humans—actually fall below some adult dogs, cats, pigs, or chimpanzees on any test of intelligence, awareness, self-consciousness, moral personality, capacity to communicate, or any other capacity that might be thought to mark humans as superior to other animals. Yet we do not think it legitimate to experiment on these less fortunate humans in the ways in which we experiment on animals.[46]

In the end, Singer favors an increase of protections for vulnerable animals and humans; by contrast, Frey favors increased access to both. In part their differences can be accounted for by the consequentialist character of utilitarianism. Singer and Frey have radically opposed conceptions of the consequences of adopting one set of principles and practices rather than another. If they could agree on the consequences of human experimentation, animal experimentation, vegetarianism, etc., they likely would agree in both theory and practice.

Many contemporary moral philosophers reject utilitarianism of all types. Two major reasons are that (1) utilitarianism requires too much unfounded speculation about consequences and lacks the backbone of any firm principle,[47] and (2) it requires a balancing of goods and harms that seems, on occasion, to violate rights or leave minorities vulnerable to abuse. Tom Regan uses a standard type of counterexample to utilitarian thinking:

> There is nothing wrong with a matador's painfully draining the life from a bull, for example, provided only that enough people find the spectacle sufficiently pleasant. . . . When it comes to how humans treat other animals, utilitarian theory seems better suited to defending rather than reforming the *status quo*.[48]

This type of problem with utilitarianism has driven many, including Regan, to look for a more satisfactory general moral theory. (Practical examples of this problem are found in almost every case in this book, but see especially chapters 5, 6, 7, and 8.)

Kantian (Deontological) Theories and Obligations to Animals

A second type of theory differs significantly from utilitarianism. Often called "deontological" (i.e., a theory that some features other than or in addition to consequences make actions obligatory), this type is now increasingly called "Kantian" because of its origins in the philosophy of Immanuel Kant (1734–1804).

Kant's Legacy

For Kantians, the rightness or wrongness of at least some actions can be determined *no matter what the consequences*. For example, if killing and disabling animals for "sport" is morally wrong, then activities such as hunting and cockfighting are *categorically wrong* and would be wrong even if many persons would be deprived of great pleasure or economic benefits by forbidding the killing. A bulwark is thereby erected against utilitarian balancing of consequences. Kant regards all considerations of utility and self-interest as secondary, because the moral worth of an agent's action depends exclusively on the moral acceptability of the rule on the basis of which the person is acting. An action has moral worth only when performed intentionally by an agent who possesses a good will, and a person has a good will only if moral obligation based on a valid moral rule is the sole motive for the action.

Kant's supreme principle, which he calls both "the moral law" and "the categorical imperative," is expressed in several ways in his writings. Most pertinent, for our purposes, is the requirement to never treat other individuals as means to one's own ends. Kant says, "Treat humanity . . . always as an end and never as a means only."[49] This imperative demands that we treat other persons as "ends in themselves," that is, as having their own autonomously established goals, and that we never treat others purely as the means to our own self-determined goals. Kant's principle does not mean that we cannot use human research subjects in nontherapeutic research, but it does mean that we cannot use them without appropriate consent and that the consent cannot be obtained manipulatively. He is silent on what his views might mean for how we conduct research with animals, but it is obvious that we cannot obtain consent from animals, and it is clear that they are not conceived as "ends in themselves" in Kant's account.

Kant does, however, address the status of animals and how, in general, they are to be regarded. He once stated his views on the illicit use of individuals as means to ends as follows: "*Unlike objects or animals,* humans are never to be used merely as a means to another's ends." "Animals," he says, "must be regarded as man's instruments, . . . as means to an end. That end is man."[50] From this perspective, animals have a reduced or instrumental value because of their status as subhuman, and this reduced value permits us to value them exclusively, or at least largely, in terms of their value to humans.[51]

Kant further argued that we have no direct obligations to animals, only indirect ones: "If a man shoots his dog because the animal is no longer capable of service, he does not fail in his duty to the dog, because the dog cannot judge; but his act is inhuman and damages in himself that humanity which it is his *duty to show towards mankind.*"[52] A person should not be cruel to animals, in Kant's theory, because such cruelty will make the person cruel in dealings with other persons, not because it violates an obligation to the animal. In short, Kant objects to ill treatment of animals because of the effect such behavior has on how humans will be treated.

Kant and many later Kantians have maintained that human dignity places humans in a privileged position in the order of nature. The idea is that humans have properties (rationality, souls, creation in the image of God, etc.) that place them in a fundamentally different category than animals. For example, only human beings intentionally perform actions that are motivated by *reason* and by *moral rules.* Animals are intelligent, but they do not act on moral reasons or exhibit a rational will. A person's dignity—indeed, "sublimity," Kant says—comes from being his or her own moral lawgiver, that is, from being morally autonomous.[53]

A major objection to Kantian theories (as well as other theories predicated on human dignity) is commonly referred to as the argument from marginal cases. Not all humans are rational and autonomous in Kant's sense, including young children and seriously brain-damaged humans. Such "marginal" humans are not ends in themselves and so seem not significantly different from animals. Therefore, it appears that they too can be treated as mere means to human ends, rather than as ends in themselves. This conclusion is obviously precarious for some humans who are weak, vulnerable, and morally incapacitated, just as it is for animals, because the protective qualities of dignity and moral autonomy are not present in these humans.[54] If there are obligations to these humans, what is the basis of the obligations, and why are there no obligations to similarly situated animals?

Kantians have had difficulty responding to this line of inquiry and remaining faithful to the full range of commitments of Kant's moral theory. However, we now turn to one theory with Kantian roots that attempts to overcome this problem while building exceedingly strong protections for animals.

Inherentism

This type of deontological theory is variously called "inherentism" and "the rights view" and has its primary exposition in the writings of Tom Regan. He views animals, like humans, as having significant value meriting moral protection because they are "subjects of a life." Each such individual has a life that matters to him or her, regardless of what others may think of his or her life. Regan adopts two features in Kant's philosophy. The first is the idea that basic to ethics is respectful treatment of the individual without regard to utilitarian consequences. The second is the idea that individuals are "ends in themselves" (despite Kant's own denial that animals are such ends). Regan thus defends what he calls "the postulate of inherent value" of animals.[55] Regan's conviction (sharply contrasting with Kant's) is that both humans and animals are experiencing subjects with their own *inherent value,* and therefore are owed respectful treatment. Regardless of any specific cognitive capacities, all experiencing subjects have a moral status that protects against their being treated in certain ways that reduce their lives to the status of mere resources for others. (For discussions, see the ethical-issues sections in the cases in chapters 2, 3, 4, 5, 7, and 11.)

Regan's postulate of inherent value rests on his view that it is arbitrary to exclude animals from the realm of creatures with inherent value once we recognize the power of the subject-of-a-life criterion. Like humans, animals perform actions and have beliefs, desires, perceptions, memories, a sense of the future, an emotional life, preferences, and welfare interests. This kind of life bestows rights on them (the right not to be harmed and a right of respectful treatment) and gives us obligations directly to them. Regan believes that moral beliefs that we all cherish (even if not originally fashioned for animals) support his contentions.[56] One need not stretch very far to see the sweeping and controversial character of these claims.

Regan rejects claims such as those of Frey that humans who have abundant intellectual, artistic, and moral skills have more value and can justly compel animals to serve human needs and interests.[57] Nonetheless, Regan's theory requires what he calls a fairly rich psychology for animals that includes beliefs, intentional acts, an identity over time, and the like. There is no inherent value for Regan without such properties, leaving his inherentism open to the problem that the lower the level of these traits, the less the inherent value would seem to be—a view somewhat similar to Frey's. However, Regan's theory strongly resists a utilitarian account in which values can be weighed, balanced, and traded off and in which the value of a life is related to the quality of life of the subject that possesses it.

Inherentism is, as Regan says, a "categorically abolitionist" philosophy.[58] It is thoroughly opposed to recreational hunting, sports that exploit animals, scientific research involving animals, use of animals for food, zoos that tightly confine animals, etc. That inherentism would radically reform contemporary human society is not questioned by anyone. The center of the dispute has been over whether this theory has provided or can provide an adequate justification to sustain such reforms. Many believe it fails for one or more of four reasons: (1) it cannot adequately defend a set of criteria for attributing inherent value to animals of the strength Regan attributes; (2) it fails to show that being a subject of a life is an adequate criterion of animal rights and human obligations; (3) it rules out all balancing of costs and benefits (so critical to public regulations of human uses of animals); and (4) it confers upon animals too many rights, at the same time stripping humans of some of their rights.[59]

However, some believe that the most important elements in inherentism can be retained through an adequate theory of rights. This leads us to a third type of theory.

Rights Theories and Animal Rights

The language of *rights* derives historically from the need for strong and meaningful protections of citizens in political states against oppression, unequal treatment, intolerance, arbitrary invasion of privacy, and the like. Given this history, many framers of declarations about protections for animals, including Regan, choose rights language as the basic termi-nology. But when such writers appeal to "rights," what precisely are they appealing to?

Rights are justified claims that individuals, groups, and institutions can make upon others or upon society. To have a right is to be in a position to control what others are required to do.[60] Rights give parties a claim based on a system of rules that authorize those parties to affirm, demand, or insist upon what is due to them. If an individual or group possesses a right, others are validly constrained from interfering with the exercise of that right. A moral right, then, is a justified claim validated by moral principles and rules.[61]

Animal Rightists and Animal Welfarists

"Animal rights" is a generic term that, in popular use, refers to a wide range of accounts of how animals should be protected against human misuse and how valid claims to protection can be exercised on behalf of animals. The term "animal rights movement" is a generic label for social movements that seek to protect the interests of animals. However, not every movement that is referred to under the label "animal rights" uses the language of rights or asserts that animals have rights. Social movements centered on protection of the interests of animals have often been said to be divided into two types: (1) Those who, strictly speaking, believe that animals have rights (animal rightists) and (2) those who believe that whether or not animals have rights, humans have obligations to protect the welfare interests of animals (animal welfarists).

Animal rightists are said to endorse strong positions on rights, e.g., declaring that certain animals have a right to a life, a right to an uncontaminated habitat, a right not to be constrained in tight cages or pens, and other comparable rights. Animal welfarists, by contrast, are said to hold more utilitarian and pragmatic perspectives that acknowledge that humans have a duty not to cause avoidable harm to animals. Animal welfarists are also said to be prepared to allow the use of animals for human benefit and to weigh benefits against costs—for example, by not seeking to abolish factory farms, but rather making them decent places for farm animals.

This distinction between animal rightists and animal welfarists is not entirely accu-rate and should be used with great care. The many theories that aim to afford greater protections for animals are best understood as a spectrum of theories lying on a con-tinuum, rather than as neatly dividing into two types. The label "animal rights" has also been a polarizing one. It suggests conflict between "rightists" and "welfarists" even when there is no conflict. It has also been, at the hands of some writers, a way of signi-fying that animal rights theories are a form of extremism, whereas animal welfarism is balanced and reasonable.

To see how unsatisfactory this simple bifurcation into two types of theories is, it is easy to construct a third "type" of theory merely by combining the alleged approaches of animal rights and animal welfarism. One can hold that rights and obligations are correlative; therefore, whenever an animal has a right, some human has an obligation, and whenever a human has an obligation to an animal, the animal has a right. Thus, if a farmer has obligations to feed his cattle and to abstain from using painful electrical prods, then the cattle have rights to be fed and not to have the pain inflicted.

The thesis that there is always a correlativity between obligations and rights is a plau-sible idea widely accepted in both philosophy and law.[62] This correlativity thesis acknowledges that if humans have *obligations* to animals, then animals have all the *rights* that are correlative to these obligations. Thus, if a research investigator has an obligation to animal subjects to feed them and abstain from extremely painful procedures during the conduct of research, then animal subjects have rights to be fed and not to have the pain inflicted. Anyone who recognizes obligations of this sort must recognize correlative rights for animals. From this perspective, a polarization into two fundamentally different types of theory, premised on a difference about rights and obligations, makes little sense.[63]

Opposition to Animal Rights

Many writers on human uses of animals reject both animal rights and any strong animal welfare position. They take human obligations to animals to be either self-imposed obligations or obligations owed only to the owners of animals. The so-called "rights" of animals are not truly rights, in this conception; they are ways of restating various provisions that have been or could be made by humans for the protection of animals. A more appropriate vocabulary, from this perspective, is *charity, stewardship,* and *moral ideal.* In this conception, even the idea of obligations of beneficence toward animals should be stated in terms of kindness, compassion, and generosity; the language of rights is wholly misplaced.

Carl Cohen has defended a robust and influential version of this position. He aims to show "why animals have no rights." He argues that activities of making claims occur only within a community of moral agents who can make claims against one another and are authorized to do so. Since claiming a right occurs only within a community of moral agents authorized to make such claims, rights "are necessarily human; their possessors are persons" with the ability for moral judgment and the ability to exercise moral claims, and animals cannot have rights because they lack these abilities. Cohen concludes that, "in conducting research on animal subjects, therefore, we do not violate their rights, because they have none to violate."[64]

Rights Exercised by Surrogates

A related matter concerns whether a nonhuman animal can have a right despite the fact that the animal is not able to *exercise* the right. A common answer to this question is that a rights holder need not be able to assert rights in order to have them. For example, when infants, the comatose, and mentally disabled individuals are not able to claim their rights, claims can be made for them by legitimate representatives, or surrogates.

At least one of the functions of members of review committees established to protect the interests of research animals could be to see that prevailing policies of protection are properly implemented and that pain and suffering are minimized. If members of these committees have obligations to ensure that the pain and suffering of animals is minimized, then they could also be viewed as established to protect the rights of animals. This matter is further discussed in the section "Alternatives, Government Regulations, and Committee Review" below.

Conclusion

To summarize this section, both rights theories and Kantian-deontological theories sharply contrast with utilitarian theories. For the latter, obligations are fixed entirely by consequences; the obligatory action is the one that produces the best consequences. Kantianism and rights theory take principled exception. Each of these types of theory is a powerful tool for thinking about the issues in the cases and about one's moral commitments. Those who master this theoretical material should find that it gives quality and precision to moral thinking. At the same time, it is important to appreciate the limits of theories. They require thoughtful specification of their principles and cannot be mechanically applied to achieve resolutions in the cases in this book. The values defended in these theories can be and have been turned in very different directions in the attempt to grasp the moral dimensions of the human-nonhuman relation.

THE JUSTIFICATION OF HUMAN USES OF ANIMALS

The centerpiece of moral philosophy has often been thought to be how to justify a moral position. Usually we do not need to deliberate very hard to justify our moral decisions, but occasionally the whole point of moral thinking is to justify or find a failure of justification in some proposed practice, policy, or course of action. Nowhere is this truer than in literature on animals, whether the topic is food production, hunting, sport and recreation, wildlife conservation, medical research, zoo life, or religious sacrifice. Historical practices as well as innovative policies all need justification.

The analysis here will concentrate on the justification of research involving animals, both because of its centrality to the chapters below and because a well-developed literature exists on the subject. However, the points made can be generalized to the many other human uses of animals found in the cases in this book.

The Concept of Justification

The term "justification" has several meanings in English, but in its customary sense, "to justify" is to show to be right, to vindicate, or to furnish adequate grounds for. The objective of justification is to establish one's case by presenting sufficient grounds for action. For example, one might attempt a justification by appealing to preexisting rules, such as those in codes of ethics, to authoritative institutional agreements and practices, or to the moral convictions in which we have the highest confidence and believe to have the lowest level of bias. In each case, appeals are made to the most compelling moral reasons for the proposed course of action.

However, a reason can be a *good* reason without being *sufficient* for justification. We have many good reasons for what we do with animals in biomedical and behavior research, but these reasons are not always sufficient to justify the research. There is always a need to distinguish a reason's relevance to a moral judgment from its *final adequacy* in support of that judgment.

General Justifications for the Use of Animals in Research

Many cases in this volume center on research of some type: biomedical, behavioral, museum collecting, and safety testing for cosmetics (including toxicity testing). At least since the scientific and philosophical writings of Claude Bernard (1813–78), research involving animal subjects has been widely regarded as essential for scientific and medical advances and as morally justifiable.[65] Many believe today that further advances in diabetes, hypertension, cancer, and AIDS research will occur only if animals are involved. Likewise in veterinary schools, advances in the treatment of animals often require that animals are used in research.

However, all research is morally troublesome when subjects are exposed to a significant level of risk. When we present a risk or cause harm, the burden of proof for the action is on the person who initiated it. This simple point about burden of proof leads to questions about justification. Under what conditions, if any, is such research justified? Does it make a difference whether the subjects are human or nonhuman, and, if so, why?

Almost everyone agrees that the general justifications for using both human and animal subjects in research are that benefits to be gained from research are substantial and that the disease, displeasure, and harm that could be expected to result if we did not perform the research would be exceedingly grave. Medical research and veterinary research have produced benefits of the highest importance for humans and animals alike, thereby lending credibility to claims that research is essential.[66] Intact, live animals respond to research interventions in a manner that cannot always be simulated through research techniques that rely on non-animal systems. For example, administering a drug to a rat may produce a complex reaction that affects multiple physiological systems. This response often cannot be understood through computer modeling or the manipulation of cells in tissue culture. Human subjects could be substituted for animal subjects in many cases, but the painful, invasive, and even lethal character of much animal research poses insuperable moral problems for proposals that human subjects be used.[67]

However, the absence of a justification for using human subjects does not by itself justify using animal subjects. If the goals of research cannot be carried out using humans because of the suffering that would be inflicted, the justification for inflicting the same or similar suffering on animals is presumably made more difficult, not somehow facilitated. A complicating problem is that at present we have no shared conception of what counts as a justifiable "harm" and a justifiable "risk" of harm for an animal. If "harm" is defined as any thwarting, defeating, or setting back of a nontrivial interest, then many harms are suffered by animals in biomedical research and elsewhere.[68]

We also lack a shared conception of what counts as a significant benefit. Research in the behavioral sciences that uses animals has had a long history of controversy about whether its results are significant contributions to knowledge. The higher the degree of harm and the more questionable the benefits, the more difficult is the justification of causing harm to animals. Although scientists rightly point out that we often do not see the utility in scientific experiments until some time after their completion, this fact is not sufficient to justify all forms of experimentation. The key question seems to be, when knowledge will be gained but there is no clear application or rationale for its use, should we declare the information trivial, or should we allow experts in science to determine when a line of approach is promising? (See chapters 14 and 15.)

It is also unclear whether research that exceeds some threshold or upper limit of pain, suffering, anxiety, fear, and distress can be justified. In research with human subjects, it is conventional to insist both on thresholds—for example, upper levels of risk, pain, and discomfort—and on a balancing of benefits and potential costs. If the threshold of harm is not exceeded, benefits of the research may justify the risks and costs involved in using humans or animals; but if the threshold is exceeded, the research cannot be justifiably conducted, regardless of its value and potential. For such a threshold to be meaningful in research involving animals, careful guidelines must be prepared for investigators and review committees in planning and evaluating research, including a grading of research procedures as to their noxious, aversive, and painful properties.

The argument against a firm threshold in our use of animals is that any criterion proposed will be too restrictive. It will impede or block some valuable research or some use of animals in educational training, food production, and the like. In particular, setting a threshold might prevent the balancing of risks and benefits in critical areas of clinical research and would therefore cause us to forgo forms of knowledge with vital benefits for humans.

In the end, the main problem seems to be less *whether* we should require a threshold in research with animals (almost everyone thinks that we should) than *how and where* to draw the threshold line. The threshold also may need to be drawn in different places for different species. For example, we now set the threshold of suffering, anxiety, fear, and distress differently for primates than for species "below" primates. A justification for this differential treatment is itself needed. The fact that we already employ the principle that it is justified to vary the threshold in accordance with species differences may not be morally determinative of where the threshold should be set.

The Justification of Research Protocols

The *general* justification of research, usually stated in terms of overall benefit, needs to be revisited for each *particular* research protocol to see if that protocol is justified. From the fact that research is valuable in general, it does not follow that any particular research protocol is warranted. We need a carefully reasoned demonstration that any particular research investigation will significantly contribute to the health, safety, and welfare of future persons (or, in some cases, animals) and that the information obtained will be of sufficient significance that it offsets associated animal pain and suffering.[69]

Pain and Suffering

A careful assessment of types and levels of pain, suffering, and deprivation must be included in any justification. There are imposing empirical problems of measuring how much pain is felt, whether analgesic drugs are adequate for intended analgesia, whether the animal conceives the experience as agony or torment, and the like. For example, researchers need to determine the precise impact of small-diameter holes drilled through the skull, just to the surface of the dura (outermost covering of the brain) of an experimental animal, if the protocol calls for this surgery. They will need to determine what pain and suffering will later be experienced, even if proper anesthesia is used during the surgery and other precautions are taken.

Such questions are at the heart of the ethics and review of animal research. If anything deserves the most careful and detailed scrutiny, it is the effect of such interventions on the animals involved. Surprisingly, little is often reported on this subject in research protocols, at least in any detail, although reassurances are given of the benign character of the intervention, the adequacy of anesthesia and analgesics, and the overall comfort of the animal. The critical matter is that carefully reasoned conclusions be drawn, preferably by an independent assessment that is free of investigator or institutional bias and conflict of interest. The absence of detailed and unbiased evaluations has led in the past to many criticisms that could have been avoided if appropriate review had occurred. (See the cases of review in chapters 12, 13, and 15.)

Mental and Emotional Reactions

Of equal importance as pain and suffering, and directly connected to them, is the impact of the intervention on the *mental* and *emotional* lives of animals. It is often said that during the course of animal research, "indices of psychological well-being" will be monitored. Such indices are required in U.S. Department of Agriculture (USDA) regulations and by the American Psychological Association in its "Guidelines for Ethical Conduct in the Care and Use of Animals."[70] Persons examining justifications offered in defense of research protocols should ask, "What role did information about psychological well-being play in the prior peer review of the research? Were mental states a part of the review process?"

Such evaluation is of the highest importance when reviewing invasive research that places animals in restraints and in unfamiliar surroundings. Many protocols report only the *physiological* effects (on fibers, enzymes, and the like) of interventions, but the mental and emotional effects of the restraints are more pertinent to ethical review. To assume that the *psychological* lives of animals are, were, and will be unaffected would be more than precarious; it would be false.

In some countries, legal requirements compel investigators to categorize the invasiveness of their proposed work, as to the harm—pain, suffering, social deprivation, confinement, etc.—that will befall the animals during the experiment. Even if no such legal requirements exist in a country, this form of evaluation is essential for moral justification.

Conclusion

Scientists commonly obtain new and valuable information from their investigations with animals. Science feeds on incremental new knowledge, and it is an important part of the justification of the research. Even so, every scientific investigation that uses live subjects, human or nonhuman, requires a comprehensive risk-benefit assessment. Threshold levels of permissible harm are also needed. In the simplest terms, the question is, "How much new knowledge beyond that gained in previous investigations will be gained, and does the merit of the new knowledge *justify* the harms or costs to the animals (as well as the costs in dollars, an issue of another sort)?" No list of rules of humane care and treatment will be adequately sensitive to answer this question, and it is a confusion to suppose that research is justified merely by conformity to such rules.

Benefits for Humans and Costs for Animals

A related problem concerns the fairness of how we determine whose risks and benefits are to be balanced. Attempts to resolve problems of either the general justification of research or the justification of particular research protocols through broad risk-benefit and cost-benefit analyses are strategies that demand close scrutiny. Costs to animals can easily be ignored in institutional and public policies when the use of those animals benefits some larger human community. Humans receive the benefits, animals the costs. Animals are subjects or objects of sacrifice; humans are not. (Several cases in this book discuss this problem, and the case of religious sacrifice in chapter 9 presents it in a somewhat novel way.)

Animal welfare proposals about research involving animals have often suggested that the main way to combat this problem is to appoint review committees that are truly impartial. This objective, however, is difficult to achieve. Even under obligatory systems of review, as long as researchers themselves heavily populate the committees, with few neutral parties or animal advocates present, costs to animals are not as likely to be taken as seriously as they would be if a more impartial committee were formed. The practical implication is that a committee with broad representation, including a mandate to weigh the cost of the research to the animals involved, might approve only a small segment of the research that is presently approved.[71]

This problem extends beyond research with animals. There have been active discussions of problems in factory farming and zoos, which are generally designed to maximize efficiency of operation. Some of the most morally troublesome cases of factory farming (see the cases of pigs, veal, and broiler chickens in chapters 2, 3, and 4) have been defended by the way such farming produces the greatest good for the greatest number of people—for example, high-quality broiler chickens at a price every family can afford. But does this form of balancing, even if highly efficient for humans, adequately consider the interests of animals? Can unnecessary suffering be justified by these considerations of economic efficiency?[72]

Cost-benefit analysis is an essential tool of public policy in many areas, but deciding issues of animal welfare through cost-benefit trade-offs is a risky conception of how to formulate public policy. It may be much better to look directly and sympathetically at the circumstance of the animals, while placing a limit on the suffering that is allowable.

ALTERNATIVES, GOVERNMENT REGULATIONS, AND COMMITTEE REVIEW

Many interested in animal research and testing have urged the scientific community to vigorously pursue *alternatives* to the direct use of animals. They have also urged governments and research institutions to provide careful oversight of the work done at research centers.[73]

The Three Rs: Replacement, Reduction, and Refinement

The requirement to seek alternatives entails a search for ways to accomplish scientific goals while reducing the amount of pain and distress to animals. From the beginning, the objective of finding alternatives has been an attempt to promote the humane treatment of animals without compromising legitimate scientific and clinical aims. However, whether both aims can be coherently sustained has never been entirely resolved.

Virtually all analytical treatments of alternatives begin with three components originally presented in an influential treatise by William Russell and Rex Burch: *replacement* of animals with non-animal research methods (e.g., cell lines and computer models), *reduction* in the numbers of animals used in experiments, and *refinement* of experimental techniques to reduce the pain and suffering experienced by experimental animals.[74]

Replacement

"Replacement" refers primarily to the use of dead animals, non-animal models such as computer simulation, or "lower-order" species, whenever consistent with good science. Even the strongest defenders of animal research acknowledge that the *unnecessary* use of animals is morally perilous and creates an obligation that we desist from animal experimentation, as long as alternative methods can be used to accomplish the same result.[75] There is widespread agreement that requirements of humane treatment take precedence over mere preferences that the researcher may have about the need for and use of animals in research. Although proponents of animal research are quick to point out that the day of complete animal replacement is difficult to envision, many support new models that are consistent with scientific accuracy and progress.

Reduction

Reduction refers to the incorporation of techniques and approaches that decrease the number of animals used in research. For example, reduced numbers could be achieved by carefully guided research, as opposed to freewheeling trial and error, by the elimination of an unnecessary repetition of experiments, by the incorporation of statistically well-planned experimental designs, and by limitation to the precise number of animals required to provide statistically significant results. The admonition to reduce sometimes encourages researchers to question standard laboratory procedures and to make animal-use decisions on different bases. It also encourages rethinking how many animals are needed, consistent with obtaining adequate scientific outcomes. (See the cases of cosmetic testing in chapter 13.)

Refinement

The objective of refinement is the reduction of pain or distress by shifting, insofar as maintenance of the scientific integrity of the experiment allows, to a lower category of pain and distress.[76] For example, a design that caused significant distress or discomfort could possibly be refined to produce a lower level of distress and discomfort. Many defenders of animal research acknowledge that investigators have an obligation to subject animals only to *necessary* pain.

Positive response to Russell and Burch's proposal of replacement, reduction, and refinement has gained momentum in recent years, and many now argue that scientists are both morally and legally required to comply with this "Three-Rs" framework.[77] They view the Three Rs as a basic test of justified research involving animals and think that no reasonable person would reject them. However, some scientists and defenders of research worry that a significant body of scientific investigation will be retarded or eliminated by such tests. Others worry about some ethical issues in this framework. For example, what constitutes a member of a "lower" species, and is this judgment merely a matter of cultural or subjective preference? Also, how practical and far reaching are the three Rs? How many animals will actually be replaced, and how much computer modeling and the like can be devised to replace animal models? The scientific community is divided over these issues. Some groups, such as the Society of Toxicology,[78] have openly discussed and even actively promoted the Three Rs as a matter of good ethics in scientific practice; other scientific groups believe that they have no such obligations. A similar split appears in various government agencies.[79] (See, further, the problems presented in chapters 11, 13, and 17.)

Convergence of opinion toward acceptance of the Three Rs among both defenders and critics of animal research will likely take decades, if it ever occurs. Agreement tends to weaken as the precise obligations of researchers and institutions are formulated. It is one thing to say that alternatives are desirable, another to reach the conclusion that research institutions overuse many animals in research.

Some who defend the Three Rs as an ideal are still leery of the model's implementation. They maintain that instead of reducing the total number of animals at the present time, "we should increase it" and that "enlargement in the use of animals is our obligation," as Carl Cohen puts it.[80] Cohen and others believe that the use of animals has already been dangerously reduced in our pursuit of highly desirable goals and that if we do not use animals, then humans will have to be subjected to risks that animals could have borne in their place. This view is attractive to those who believe that too much clinical experimentation with humans occurs prior to scientific animal studies.[81] However, it has proved difficult to document the empirical assumptions in this thesis about the number of animals and the number of humans.[82]

In assessing the role of alternatives in the evaluation of scientific protocols, it should be remembered that there are *three* Rs, not just the first R of replacement. It is easier to cast doubt on the value of replacement if one ignores the options (and the imperatives) of refinement and reduction. Refinement is generally the most feasible option, given the current state of knowledge and scientific investigation.

Animal Welfare Regulations and Committee Review

In 1966 *Life* magazine ran a story titled "Concentration Camps for Dogs" that portrayed various abuses of animals.[83] The ensuing outcry, together with efforts of animal welfarists, led in the United States to the landmark 1966 Laboratory Animal Welfare Act. Provisions about adequate housing, food, cage size and the like were staples of the bill, and these provisions have been expanded over the years by amendments and additional U.S. federal regulations. Also covered were provisions for transportation carriers, the handling of animals, oversight responsibilities, and the like.[84]

The Health Research Extension Act of 1985 is another fundamental law governing research uses of animals in the United States. This act is practically implemented by a National Institutes of Health publication titled *Public Health Service Policy on Humane Care and Use of Laboratory Animals*. This document governs all activities conducted or supported by the U.S. Public Health Service (PHS). PHS policy requires that each institution receiving federal support provide a written assurance that its facilities comply with mandated standards and that it will comply with federal regulations. This assurance establishes a minimum basis for animal welfare provisions at each institution and requires use of its policies as the cornerstone of care at the institution.[85]

Virtually every developed country has seen an evolving set of laws and regulations over roughly the same period as developments in the United States.

Committee Review

PHS policy requires the creation of an Institutional Animal Care and Use Committee (IACUC), which is a mandated oversight committee that includes at least five members, including one veterinarian, one animal investigator, one layperson, and one nonaffiliated public member. This committee is specifically charged with oversight responsibility for ongoing review of animal care and use, facilities inspection, review and approval or disapproval of research protocols involving animals, recommendation of personnel training, and suspension of improper activities.

Review committees in the United States and in many other countries are established to examine protocols to see if they can be improved in various ways, including (as is implicit in current public policy) by reducing, replacing, or refining animal use. These committees serve as gatekeepers determining whether the proposed use of animals is warranted. Since its modest beginnings, a robust and increasingly international system for prior review of research with living subjects has evolved.[86] Universities, government facilities, and many corporations in the pharmaceutical, chemical, and cosmetics industries have such committees, often with veterinarians and other experts on animals involved in deliberations. Other industries—such as circuses, slaughterhouses, and farms—generally do not use ethics committees for purposes of reviewing their practices (though these industries are regulated by governments in some instances). Concerns in these industries center more on having healthy animals, a pragmatic rather than a moral concern.

Each committee is likely to use its local and national standards, but there is a broad consensus internationally on the types of moral rules that should govern human research, and a gradual evolution has occurred toward international guidelines on research with animals. This fact should not be taken to mean that this review is always thorough or adequate. Understandably, the rules are seldom specific, and even whether these committees adequately understand the available rules is a matter of controversy.[87] Inconsistencies in committee deliberations have been noted, as has the lack of information about animal pain and suffering provided in the protocols of investigators and on the basis of which review occurs. The investigator's description of the project may only briefly describe the procedure, and committee approval is sometimes pro forma. Often missing or minimized is a serious assessment of the degree of animal pain or suffering, forms of analgesia, and the effect on animals of the experimental methods used. A search for alternatives is also often not undertaken. (See the case in chapter 15.) The limited empirical evidence about these committees suggests wide variation in how duties are executed and also suggests that a review that is impartial and free of conflict of interest may be more uncommon than common.

Institutions often point out that they have followed proper procedures of review and that all rules have been followed by duly constituted committees. This observation seems generally to be true both in the United States and in most countries with such requirements. However, the deep ethical issue is not a *procedural* one about whether legal requirements have been followed; it is a *substantive* question about the actual standards and work of these committees in discharging their moral responsibilities. (See, for example, chapter 12.)

These committees are given extensive data about proposed scientific investigations. These data show intricate planning, probing scientific hypotheses, and familiarity with the relevant literature. Rarely are the committees given anything comparable in detail by way of *ethics* materials or ethical problems in and defenses of the research. For an adequate ethics review, the ethical reasoning would have to be spelled out, just as the science has been specified. The absence of such searching moral examination has led to widespread suspicion about the quality and worth of the committees' deliberations and conclusions.

Many members of these committees would say that framing the issues in this way holds researchers to an unrealistically high ethical standard. They claim that if the review has been done "by the book," then one's moral responsibilities have been met. "The book" in the United States is, roughly speaking, the U.S. Animal Welfare Act and its implementing regulations,[88] the Council for International Organizations of Medical Sciences (CIOMS), the World Health Organization document on *International Guiding Principles for Biomedical Research Involving Animals,*[89] and the PHS Policy on Humane Care and Use of Laboratory Animals and *Guide for the Care and Use of Laboratory Animals.*

How are we to evaluate the thesis that whenever review occurs in conformity with these guidelines, the review is morally sufficient? There are three potential problems with such a claim: (1) an investigator can follow the procedures and rules in "the book" but can do so in a cursory and perfunctory manner; (2) those doing the review may be poorly trained for the work or have serious conflicts of interest; and (3) even if the experiments under review conform to the book, that fact alone does not make them ethically acceptable, because the experiments may not be consistent with the most appropriate standards articulated in various parts of the profession, the public, and the scholarly literature on the subject. "The book" is not always up to date, comprehensive, or relevant.

For example, neither the CIOMS *International Guiding Principles,* which was never intended as a regulatory set of guidelines, nor the PHS policy is as rigorous and demanding as the Canadian *Guide to the Care and Use of Experimental Animals*[90] or the compact *Australian Code of Practice.*[91] The point is that there are more and less comprehensive guides to review. Some use higher standards than others. Some committees may intentionally allow a high level of harmful activity, such as the acute toxicity test (increasing doses until animal welfare is seriously compromised), whereas other committees will not allow such practices. A middle ground or minimally decent level of requirements has never been identified, but for those who want to take the "moral high ground" in the review of research (as many institutions now say that they wish to do), it is well to remember that there are several candidates for the gold standard.

Outside the United States, the regulation of research and other practices involving animals is in some countries far stricter, but in other countries it is far more lax. Differences in the review of uses of animals understandably derive in part from tradition and in part from diverse conceptions of when animals have interests that must, from a moral point of view, be protected.

Pain and Suffering

Suggestions about replacement and reduction have been minor activities for many review committees, but refinement has been a primary activity for virtually all committees. U.S. federal regulations require minimization of pain, suffering, and distress to an extent consistent with scientific objectives. Researchers with inadequate plans must modify their research design to improve analgesics, tranquilizers, and anesthetics used, as well as methods of euthanasia. Careful committee review considers whether immobilization for the animals is necessary, whether tumor burden in cancer research can be reduced, and the like.

The nature and role of animal pain and suffering has proved difficult for members of these committees to assess and for federal regulations to capture.[92] Suffering is even more difficult than pain, partially because of the breadth of the concept of suffering. The term "suffering" is generally used to include both discomfort and disease, as when animals are kept in unsanitary and crowded conditions that deprive them of freedom of movement. "Discomfort" is itself a broad notion and is often used to refer, for example, to tension, anxiety, stress, exhaustion, and fear.

Different empirical assumptions are at work in current literature about the degree to which animals suffer, including whether they suffer *more* or *less* than humans do. In the scientific literature, there is a tendency to assume that animals have different forms of pain reception and cannot anticipate or remember pain, and therefore suffer less than humans. A contrasting view is that animals suffer more, not less, because they have less understanding of the origin, nature, and meaning of pain. That is, an animal may be a captive of the momentary experience of pain and without the capacity to deal with danger, injury, and the like. What can be processed and put in context by a human may be experienced as terror by a captive animal.[93]

The Definition of "Animal" and the Differential Treatment of Species

The animal welfare community has long hoped to reach legal protections for *all* animals used in research. One of the most controversial aspects of animal-welfare regulations in the United States is that birds, mice, and rats that are specifically bred for research use are not *animals* according to the definition of "animal" in the USDA regulations for the Animal Welfare Act. These species are therefore unprotected by the legislation and by federal regulation. Approximately 85% of research and testing animals belong to these excluded species. The exclusion was introduced to reduce the costs of oversight and USDA inspections, but it has had the effect of leaving many forms of research and even whole facilities both uninspected and unregulated.

The moral issues reach beyond the obvious ones of unprotected animals and the potential unfairness involved in including some species under legal protections while excluding others for no morally relevant reason. There is also a problem of moral coherence in public policy. The PHS policy definition of "animal" (unlike that of USDA regulations) includes all vertebrates. Birds, mice, and rats are therefore included in its protections. The effect is that in institutions not included in PHS coverage (including private industry and colleges not receiving PHS funding), research, testing, and education involving birds, mice, and rats are unregulated—a striking incoherence, and one confined to the United States.[94]

CONCLUSION

This book is not a theoretical work in ethics. It is a book of *cases* involving human-animal relationships. Though the cases in this book occasionally involve some aspect of law or government policy, these are not legal cases, and they should not be evaluated as if law or government should decide them. These cases are all about ethical issues, and they must be evaluated from a moral point of view.

Daniel Callahan and Sissela Bok have suggested that in contemporary ethics, "case studies are employed most effectively when they can readily be used to draw out broader ethical principles and moral rules . . . [that call] the attention of students to the common elements in a variety of cases, and to the implicit problems of ethical theory to which they may point."[95] However, it is difficult to use theory, draw out principles, and find common elements in these discussions, and there are no easy answers to the tough problems presented in these cases. The essence of good reflection on and discussion of the cases is to start without any assumption that one has the right answer to the problem. It is best to think of the process as one of advancing hypotheses and then defending or modifying them. We should not mask how difficult these issues are and how strongly people feel about them. At the same time, we should not forget that moral thinking by reasonable persons has often taken us further down the path of progress than we might at the outset have thought we could go.

Although many hostile partisans do square off in the so-called culture wars, discussions about the proper treatment of animals have been carried on in journals of ethics for many years without bitter partisanship or ill feelings. Many of the participants in opposite camps have become good friends. The authors of the present volume can only hope that the following cases will contribute to this more civil and polite discourse over the human uses of animals.

NOTES

1. See, in general, Richard Sorabji, *Animal Minds and Human Morals: The Origins of the Western Debate* (Ithaca, NY: Cornell University Press, 1993). On the early modern period, see James C. Whorton, "Animal Research, Historical Aspects," *Encyclopedia of Bioethics,* 3rd ed., ed. Stephen Post (New York: Macmillan Reference, 2004).

2. Porphyry, *On Abstinence from Animal Food,* ed. Esme Wynne-Tyson, trans. Thomas Taylor (New York: Barnes & Noble, 1965). See esp. chap. 3.

3. Plutarch, "Whether Land or Sea Animals are Cleverer" and "Beasts are Rational," in *Moralia,* vol. 12, trans. Harold Cherniss and William C. Helmbold, 14 vols. (Cambridge, MA: Harvard University Press, Loeb Library, 1927–69). See esp. pp. 959a–992e.

4. See, in Aristotle's corpus (all in the Loeb Library editions of the Harvard University Press), *Parts of Animals* 641b7–20; *On the Soul* 414a29–415a12, 427b28–428b3, 432a15–434b12; *Politics* 1332b4–5; *Nicomachean Ethics* 1098a2–7; and *Metaphysics* 980b1–981a1.

5. See Lucius Annaeus Seneca, *On Anger (De ira)* 1.3.4–8, in *Moral Essays,* trans. John W. Basore, 3 vols. (Cambridge, MA: Harvard University Press, Loeb Library, 1928–62); and *Epistles* 113.18–20, 124.1, in *Ad Lucilium epistulae morales,* trans. Richard M. Gummere, 3 vols. (Cambridge, MA: Harvard University Press, Loeb Library, 1917–25). See also Cicero, *De finibus* 3.67 (on Chrysippus) and *De finibus bonorum et malorum* 3.67, trans. H. Rackham (Cambridge, MA: Harvard University Press, Loeb Library, 1921). The topic of reason in animals was also discussed by Sextus Empiricus.

6. Pierre Bayle, *The Dictionary Historical and Critical of Mr. Peter Bayle,* ed. and trans. Pierre Des Maizeaux, 2nd ed., 5 vols. (London, 1734–38; fac. New York: Garland, 1984). See esp. "Rorarius" (F–L); "Barbara" (C); and "Pereira" (C–I).

7. See, for example, Ronald Dworkin, *Taking Rights Seriously* (Cambridge, MA: Harvard University Press, 1977); Judith Jarvis Thomson, *The Realm of Rights* (Cambridge, MA: Harvard University Press, 1990); and Ruth Macklin, "Universality of the Nuremberg Code," in *The Nazi Doctors and the Nuremberg Code,* ed. George J. Annas and Michael Grodin (New York: Oxford University Press, 1992), pp. 240–57.

8. William James, "The Stream of Thought," in *The Writings of William James,* ed. John J. McDermott (Chicago: University of Chicago Press, 1977), p. 73. For commentary on James's views, pertinent to ethics and animals, see James M. Albrecht, "What Does Rome Know of Rat and Lizard? Pragmatic Mandates for Considering Animals in Emerson, James, and Dewey," in *Animal Pragmatism,* ed. Erin McKenna and Andrew Light (Bloomington: Indiana University Press, 2004), esp. p. 27.

9. See the relevant passages in *The Philosophical Writings of Descartes,* ed. and trans. John Cottingham, Robert Stoothoff, and Dugald Murdoch, 3 vols. (vol. 3 also trans. Anthony Kenny)

(Cambridge: Cambridge University Press, 1984–91); vol. 1, pp. 5, 99, 141; vol. 2, pp. 88, 96, 128, 161–62, 246, 287–89; and vol. 3, letters to Henry More, pp. 365–66, 374. For a brief, pertinent excerpt, see Descartes, "Animals are Machines," in *Animal Rights and Human Obligations,* 2nd ed., ed. Tom Regan and Peter Singer (Englewood Cliffs, NJ: Prentice Hall, 1989), pp. 17–18 (hereafter, "Regan-Singer").

10. Cottingham et al., vol. 3, p. 366.

11. Anita Guerrini, "The Ethics of Animal Experimentation in Seventeenth-Century England," *Journal of the History of Ideas* 50 (1989): 391–407; Lloyd Stevenson, "Religious Elements in the Background of the British Anti-vivisection Movement," *Yale Journal of Biology and Medicine* 19 (1942): 125–57.

12. David Hume, *An Enquiry concerning Human Understanding,* ed. Tom L. Beauchamp (Oxford: Oxford University Press, 1999), sec. 9, para. 2. Two different editions exist: one is in the Clarendon Hume, and the other is a student edition in Oxford Philosophical Texts.

13. David Hume, *A Treatise of Human Nature,* ed. David Fate Norton and Mary J. Norton (Oxford: Oxford University Press, 2000, 2007), 1.3.16; 2.1.12. Two different editions exist: one is in the Clarendon Hume (2007), and the other is a student edition in Oxford Philosophical Texts (2000).

14. Donald R. Griffin, *Animal Thinking* (Cambridge, MA: Harvard University Press, 1984); Griffin, *Animal Minds: Beyond Cognition to Consciousness,* 2nd ed. (Chicago: University of Chicago Press, 2001).

15. Many of these problems not explored here are examined in Marc Bekoff, Colin Allen, and G. M. Burghardt, eds., *The Cognitive Animal* (Cambridge, MA: MIT Press, 2002); Daniel C. Dennett, *Kinds of Minds: Towards an Understanding of Consciousness* (New York: Basic Books, 1997); Bernard Rollin, *The Unheeded Cry: Animal Consciousness, Animal Pain, and Science* (Oxford: Oxford University Press, 1989; expanded ed., Ames: Iowa State University Press, 1998); Daisie Radner and Michael Radner, *Animal Consciousness* (Buffalo, NY: Prometheus Books, 1989).

16. See Bernard Rollin, "Scientific Ideology, Anthropomorphism, Anecdote, and Ethics," *New Ideas in Psychology* 13 (2000): 109–18; Marian Stamp Dawkins, "Animal Minds and Animal Emotions," *American Zoologist* 40 (2000): 883–88; Marian Stamp Dawkins, *Through Our Eyes Only: The Search for Animal Consciousness* (Oxford: Freeman, 1993); John Webster, *Animal Welfare: A Cool Eye towards Eden* (Oxford: Blackwell Science, 1994), chaps. 2 and 16, for an overview; Dorothy L. Cheney and Robert M. Seyfarth, *How Monkeys See the World: Inside the Mind of Another Species* (Chicago: University of Chicago Press, 1991); Dorothy L. Cheney and Robert M. Seyfarth, "Monkey Responses to Three Different Alarm Calls," *Science* 210 (1980): 801–3.

17. Cf. Griffin's assessment in *Animal Minds,* pp. 245–52.

18. Charles Darwin, *The Descent of Man;* all material quoted and cited from Darwin, unless otherwise noted, is from the selection of this work in *Philosophy and the Human Condition,* 2nd ed., ed. Tom L. Beauchamp, Joel Feinberg, and James M. Smith (Englewood Cliffs, NJ: Prentice-Hall, 1989), pp. 107–10.

19. In *Origin of the Species,* Darwin does not attempt to pinpoint a single ancestral origin of humans and apes, although he does try to trace a general line of descent from a primitive ape "low in the mammalian series."

20. For an engaging explication of Darwin's views, see James Rachels, *Created from Animals: The Moral Implications of Darwinism* (New York: Oxford University Press, 1990).

21. Charles Darwin, *The Expression of the Emotions in Man and Animals* (Chicago: University of Chicago Press, 1965).

22. Various aspects of these questions are discussed in Jeffrey M. Masson and Susan McCarthy, *When Elephants Weep: The Emotional Lives of Animals* (New York: Delacorte Press, 1995), esp. chap. 8; Richard Dawkins, *The Selfish Gene,* 2nd ed. (Oxford: Oxford University Press, 1989); and Rachels, *Created from Animals.*

23. Marc D. Hauser, *Moral Minds: How Nature Designed Our Universal Sense of Right and Wrong* (New York: Ecco/HarperCollins Publishers, 2006); Frans de Waal, *Primates and Philosophers: How Morality Evolved* (Princeton, NJ: Princeton University Press, 2006).

24. See, for example, James C. Whorton, "Animal Research, Historical Aspects," in *Encyclopedia of Bioethics,* 3rd ed., ed. Stephen Post (New York: Macmillan Reference, 2004);

Andrew N. Rowan, *Of Mice, Models, and Men: A Critical Evaluation of Animal Research* (Albany: State University of New York Press, 1984), chaps. 3–4.

25. *Genesis* 1:26. For the practical significance of this and other biblical teachings, see several essays in Tom Regan, ed., *Animal Sacrifices: Religious Perspectives on the Use of Animals in Science* (Philadelphia: Temple University Press, 1986), especially the essays by J. David Bleich and Andrew Lindzey.

26. Cass Sunstein, two essays in *Animals Rights: Current Debates and New Directions,* ed. Sunstein and Martha C. Nussbaum (New York: Oxford University Press, 2004); Gary L. Francione, *Animals, Property, and the Law* (Philadelphia: Temple University Press, 1995), chap. 4; Stephen M. Wise, *Rattling the Cage: Toward Legal Rights for Animals* (Cambridge, MA: Perseus, 2000).

27. Several distinct notions of dignity are distinguished in Lennart Nordenfelt, "The Varieties of Dignity," *Health Care Analysis* 12 (2004): 69–81.

28. For a more complex account of types of theory, see Mary Anne Warren, *Moral Status* (Oxford: Clarendon Press, 1997), esp. chaps. 2–5, 10.

29. Paola Cavalieri and Peter Singer, eds., *The Great Ape Project: Equality beyond Humanity* (New York: St. Martin's Press, 1994); Cavalieri, *The Animal Question: Why Nonhuman Animals Deserve Human Rights* (Oxford: Oxford University Press, 2001), esp. pp. 117–18; *Etica Animali* 8/96 (1996), special issue devoted to the Great Ape Project. The project is composed of an international group of primatologists, psychologists, moral philosophers, and others who promote a United Nations Declaration of Rights for great apes that would confer basic legal rights on chimpanzees, bonobos, gorillas, and orangutans (www.greatapeproject.org; accessed February 23, 2007). On the legal implications of this project in the United States, see Adam Kolber, "The Moral and Legal Standing of Humans and Other Apes," *Stanford Law Review* 54 (October 2001): 163–204. On the looming threat of the extinction of the great apes, see Ian Redmond, "An 11th-Hour Rescue for Great Apes?" *Science* 297 (September 27, 2002): 2203.

30. S. Hurley and M. Nudds, eds., *Rational Animals?* (Oxford: Oxford University Press, 2006); C. Wynne, *Do Animals Think?* (Princeton, NJ: Princeton University Press, 2004).

31. See, as examples, Allen Buchanan and Dan Brock, *Deciding for Others: The Ethics of Surrogate Decision Making* (Cambridge: Cambridge University Press, 1989), pp. 197–99, 261–62; Gerald Dworkin, *The Theory and Practice of Autonomy* (New York: Cambridge University Press, 1988), esp. pp. 15–20; D. Browne, "Do Dolphins Know Their Own Minds?" *Biology and Philosophy* 19 (2004): 633–53; David DeGrazia, "The Moral Status of Animals," *Kennedy Institute of Ethics Journal* 1 (1991): 58.

32. See Ronald A. Lindsay, "Slaves, Embryos, and Nonhuman Animals: Moral Status and the Limitations of Common Morality Theory," *Kennedy Institute of Ethics Journal* 15 (December 2005): 323–46.

33. See David DeGrazia, *Taking Animals Seriously: Mental Life and Moral Status* (New York: Cambridge University Press, 1996).

34. Griffin, *Animal Minds,* esp. p. 248. See also Rosemary Rodd, *Biology, Ethics, and Animals* (Oxford: Clarendon Press, 1990).

35. Donald R. Griffin, *The Question of Animal Awareness: Evolutionary Continuity of Mental Experience* (New York: Rockefeller University Press, 1976); 2nd ed., 1981.

36. Masson and McCarthy, *When Elephants Weep.*

37. Richard Ryder, *Victims of Science: The Use of Animals in Research* (London: David-Poynter, 1975).

38. See Peter Singer, *Animal Liberation,* 2nd ed. (New York: New York Review of Books/Random House, 1990), p. 6.

39. Mary Midgley, *Animals and Why They Matter* (Athens: University of Georgia Press, 1984); Jeffrey Gray, "On the Morality of Speciesism" and "Reply," *Psychologist* 4 (1991): 196–98, 202–3. On how speciesism became a label willingly accepted by some writers and not merely a pejorative term, see Hugh LaFollette and Niall Shanks, "The Origin of Speciesism," *Philosophy* 71 (1996): 41–60.

40. Jeremy Bentham, *The Principles of Morals and Legislation* (New York: Hafner, 1948), chap. 17, sec. 1. See the Bentham selection in Regan-Singer, p. 26. Bentham reasons as follows: "If the being eaten were all, there is very good reason why we should be suffered to eat such of them as we like to eat: we are the better for it, and they are never the worse. They have none of

those long-protracted anticipations of future miserys which we have. The death they suffer in our hands commonly is, and always may be, a speedier, and by that means a less painful one, than that which would await them in the inevitable course of nature. . . . But is there any reason why we should be suffered to torment them? Not any that I can see. Are there any why we should *not* be suffered to torment them? Yes, several."

41. See, for example, Andrew N. Rowan, Martin L. Stephens, Francine Dolins, Adrienne Gleason, and Lori Donley, *Proceedings for Pain Management and Humane Endpoints: Animal Welfare Perspectives on Pain and Distress Management in Research and Testing,* altweb.jhsph. edu/meetings/pain/rowan.htm (accessed February 23, 2007); Marian Stamp Dawkins, *Animal Suffering: The Science of Animal Welfare* (New York: Chapman and Hall, 1980); A. H. Flemming, "Animal Suffering: How it Matters," *Laboratory Animal Science* 37, special issue (January 1987): 140–44; Andrew N. Rowan, "Animal Anxiety and Animal Suffering," *Applied Animal Behaviour Science* 20 (1988): 135–42; and Ryder, *Victims of Science.*

42. Peter Singer, "Comment," *Between the Species* 4, no. 3 (Summer 1988): 203; and "The Significance of Animal Suffering," *Behavioral and Brain Sciences* 13 (1989): 9–12. On underlying claims about preferences, pain, and suffering, see Marian Stamp Dawkins, *Animal Suffering.*

43. Peter Singer, "Animal Research, Philosophical Issues," in *Encyclopedia of Bioethics,* 3rd ed., ed. Stephen Post (New York: Macmillan Reference, 2004).

44. Raymond G. Frey, "Moral Standing, the Value of Lives, and Speciesism," *Between the Species* 4, no. 3 (Summer 1988): 191–201, esp. p. 196. See also his "Animals," in *Oxford Handbook to Practical Ethics,* ed. Hugh LaFollette (New York: Oxford University Press, 2003), pp. 161–87; and "Medicine and the Ethics of Animal Experimentation," *The World and I* (April 1995): 358–67.

45. Raymond G. Frey, "Medicine, Animal Experimentation, and the Moral Problem of Unfortunate Humans," *Social Philosophy and Policy* 13 (1996): 181–211; "Justifying Animal Experimentation: The Starting Point," *Science and Modern Society* 21 (2002): 81–98; "Animals, Science and Morality," *Behavioral and Brain Sciences* 13 (1990): 22; "On the Ethics of Using Animals for Human Transplants," in *Ethical Issues in Biotechnology,* ed. R. Sherlock and J. D. Morrey (Lanham, MD: Rowman and Littlefield, 2002), pp. 291–96.

46. Peter Singer, "Animal Research: Philosophical Perspectives," in *Encyclopedia of Bioethics,* 3rd ed., ed. Stephen Post (New York: Macmillan Reference, 2004). On the problem of reaching coherence in our thinking about animals and humans, see David Thomas, "Laboratory Animals and the Art of Empathy," *Journal of Medical Ethics* 31 (2005): 197–202, and a response ("Pain, Vivisection, and the Value of Life") by Raymond Frey, pp. 202–4, available at www.jmedethics. com (accessed February 22, 2007).

47. See Evelyn B. Pluhar, *Beyond Prejudice: The Moral Significance of Human and Nonhuman Animals* (Durham, NC: Duke University Press, 1995); and Stephen R. L. Clark, *The Moral Status of Animals* (Oxford: Clarendon Press, 1977).

48. Tom Regan, "Animals, Treatment of," in *Encyclopedia of Ethics,* ed. L. C. Becker and C. B. Becker (New York: Garland Publishing, 1992), 1:43.

49. Immanuel Kant, *Foundations of the Metaphysics of Morals,* trans. Lewis White Beck (New York: Macmillan, 1990), p. 46.

50. Ibid. (italics added).

51. For problems with Kant's vision of animals as instruments to our ends, see Mary Midgley, "Persons and Non-Persons," in *In Defense of Animals,* ed. Peter Singer (Oxford: Basil Blackwell, 1985), esp. pp. 56–57; and Alexander Broadie and E. Pybus, "Kant's Treatment of Animals," *Philosophy* 49 (1974): 375–76.

52. Immanuel Kant, "Duties in Regard to Animals," in Regan-Singer, pp. 23–24 (italics added).

53. Immanuel Kant, *Foundations of the Metaphysics of Morals,* pp. 57–58. Kant added that the dignity deriving from this capacity is of a priceless worth that animals do not have: "[Each person] possesses a dignity (an absolute inner worth) whereby he exacts the respect of all other rational beings. . . . The humanity in one's person is the object of the respect which he can require of every other human being." *The Metaphysical Principles of Virtue,* pt. I, trans. James W. Ellington, in Kant, *Ethical Philosophy* (Indianapolis, IN: Hackett Publishing, 1983), pp. 97–98.

54. See Tom Regan, *The Case for Animal Rights* (Berkeley: University of California Press, 1983; rev. ed., 2004), pp. 178, 182–84.

55. Ibid., pp. 236–37; Regan, "Animals, Treatment of," 1:44; and selection in Regan-Singer, p. 111.

56. Tom Regan, *The Case for Animal Rights,* pp. 240, 243, 258–61; Regan, *Empty Cages: Facing the Challenge of Animal Rights* (Lanham, MD: Rowman and Littlefield, 2004), chaps. 3–4.

57. Regan, *The Case for Animal Rights,* pp. 236–37.

58. See Regan's strongly worded conclusion on his website, under "Empty Cages," www.tomregan-animalrights.com/regan_rites2.html (accessed December 12, 2006).

59. For a subtle defense of the intrinsic value of animals, in their own right, that may escape such objections, see Elizabeth Anderson, "Animal Rights and the Values of Nonhuman Life," in Sunstein and Nussbaum, *Animal Rights,* pp. 277–98.

60. Cf. H. L. A. Hart, "Bentham on Legal Rights," in *Oxford Essays in Jurisprudence,* 2nd series, ed. A. W. B. Simpson (Oxford: Oxford University Press, 1973), pp. 171–98.

61. See Joel Feinberg, *Social Philosophy* (Englewood Cliffs, NJ: Prentice-Hall, 1973), p. 67.

62. See David Braybrooke, "The Firm but Untidy Correlativity of Rights and Obligations," *Canadian Journal of Philosophy* 1 (1972): 351–63.

63. Not all uses of the word "obligation" entail correlative rights. For example, we sometimes refer to obligations of charity, and no person can claim another person's charity as a matter of right. In this instance, obligation takes the form of a self-imposed obligation and is not literally a moral (or a legal) obligation. The correlativity relation holds only for moral obligations that everyone similarly situated would have—namely, those required by a system of law or social morality.

64. Carl Cohen, "The Case for the Use of Animals in Research," *New England Journal of Medicine* 315 (1986): 865–70, esp. pp. 865–66; Carl Cohen and Tom Regan, *The Animal Rights Debate* (New York: Rowman and Littlefield, 2001).

65. Claude Bernard, *An Introduction to the Study of Experimental Medicine,* trans. Henry C. Greene (New York: Dover, 1957), pp. 59ff; see also Hugh LaFollette and Niall Shanks, "Animal Experimentation: The Legacy of Claude Bernard," www.stpt.usf.edu/hhl/papers/bernard.htm (accessed February 25, 2007).

66. In the discussion that follows, it is generally assumed that the term "animals" refers exclusively to nonhuman vertebrates—although it is not assumed that the question of research involving invertebrates does not deserve ethical analysis.

67. For several aspects of this problem, see J. A. Smith and K. M. Boyd, eds., *Lives in the Balance: The Ethics of Using Animals in Biomedical Research,* Report of a Working Party of the Institute of Medical Ethics (Oxford: Oxford University Press, 1991).

68. See a debate on this issue involving Andrew Rowan, Neal D. Barnard, Sephen R. Kaufman, Jack Botting, Adrian R. Morrison, and Madhusree Mukerjee, "A Critical Look at Animal Experimentation," *Scientific American* (February 1997): 79–93.

69. See U.S. Congress, Office of Technology Assessment, *Alternatives to Animal Use in Research, Testing, and Education* (Washington: GPO, 1986), www.wws.princeton.edu/ota/disk2/1986/8601/8601.PDF (accessed February 23, 2007); and William Paton, *Man and Mouse: Animals in Medical Research* (Oxford: Oxford University Press, 1984; 2nd ed., 1993).

70. APA, Committee on Animal Research and Ethics, "Guidelines for Ethical Conduct in the Care and Use of Animals" (Washington, DC: APA, 1985, as revised 1993). Currently available as APA Board of Scientific Affairs, Committee on Animal Research and Ethics, "Research with Animals in Psychology," www.apa.org/science/animal2.html (accessed February 15, 2007).

71. See Rebecca Dresser, "Standards for Animal Research: Looking at the Middle," *Journal of Medicine and Philosophy* 13 (1988): 123–43; and Lawrence Finsen, "Institutional Animal Care and Use Committees: A New Set of Clothes for the Emperor?" *Journal of Medicine and Philosophy* 13 (1988): 145–58.

72. For worries about how such questions can be stated and answered fairly, see Jeff McMahan, "Animals," in *A Companion to Applied Ethics,* ed. R. G. Frey and Christopher Wellman (Malden, MA: Blackwell Publishing, 2003), esp. pp. 532ff.

73. See F. Barbara Orlans, *In the Name of Science* (New York: Oxford University Press, 1993), chap. 5 and appendix B.

74. W. M. S. Russell and R. L. Burch, *The Principles of Humane Experimental Technique* (London: Methuen and Company, 1959; repr. Dover Publications and Potters Bar, UK: Universities

Federation for Animal Welfare, 1992); available at altweb.jhsph.edu/publications/humane_exp/het-toc.htm

75. Cohen, "The Case for the Use of Animals in Research," pp. 866, 868.

76. See F. Barbara Orlans, "Research Protocol for Animal Welfare," *Investigative Radiology* 22 (1987): 253–58.

77. See the many articles published in the journal *Alternatives to Laboratory Animals* (as indexed in 2007 by the U.S. National Library of Medicine website). Several prestigious academic institutions in the United States have created centers for the study and development of animal alternatives. Many professional societies, government agencies, private foundations, laboratories, and associations have centers, websites, and the like pertaining to alternatives. See altweb.jhsph.edu/links.htm (accessed February 19, 2007).

78. Society of Toxicology, "Animals in Research," www.toxicology.org/ai/air/air.asp (accessed February 19, 2007).

79. See National Institutes of Health, Office of Animal Laboratory Welfare, grants.nih.gov/grants/olaw/olaw.htm (accessed February 19, 2007); BBC, "Animal Experiments: What are the Alternatives?" www.bbc.co.uk/science/hottopics/animalexperiments/alternatives.shtml (accessed February 19, 2007); Nuffield Council on Bioethics Report, *The Ethics of Research involving Animals,* May 25, 2005, www.nuffieldbioethics.org/fileLibrary/pdf/RIA_Report_FINAL-opt.pdf (accessed February 23, 2007); A. N. Rowan and K. A. Andrutis, "Alternatives: A Socio-Political Commentary from the USA," *ATLA* 18 (1990): 3–10; H. Lansdell, "The Three Rs: A Restrictive and Refutable Rigmarole," *Ethics and Behaviour* 3 (1993), esp. p. 183; and Gary Francione, "Access to Animal Care Committees," *Rutgers Law Review* 43 (1990): 1–14.

80. Cohen, "The Case for the Use of Animals in Research," pp. 868–69.

81. Ibid., p. 869; also see Cohen, "Animal Experimentation Defended," in *The Importance of Animal Experimentation for Safety and Biomedical Research,* ed. S. Garattini and D. W. van Bekkum (Boston: Kluwer Academic, 1990), pp. 7–16, esp. p. 15.

82. The authors of the present volume have searched data bases for a study that would confirm or refute such claims and have not found significant studies on the point.

83. "Concentration Camps for Dogs," *Life,* February 4, 1966, pp. 22–29.

84. Public Law 89–544, 89th Congress, H.R. 13881, August 24, 1966; Animal Welfare Act, as Amended: see Public Law 91–579 (1970), Public Law 94–279 (1976), Public Law 99–198 (1985, Subtitle F—Animal Welfare), and Public Law 101–624 (1990, Section 2503—Protection of Pets), all available at nal.usda.gov/awic/legislat/usdaleg1.htm. See also Animal Welfare Institute, *Animals and their Legal Rights,* 4th ed. (Washington, DC: AWI, 1990).

85. See National Research Council, Commission on Life Sciences, Institute of Laboratory Animal Resources, *Guide for the Care and Use of Laboratory Animals,* rev. ed. (Washington, DC: National Academy Press, 1996; first published 1963), books.nap.edu/readingroom/books/labrats/ (accessed February 23, 2007); and National Institutes of Health, Office of the Director and Office of Laboratory Animal Welfare, *Public Health Service Policy on Humane Care and Use of Laboratory Animals* (Washington, DC: NIH, as revised 2002), grants.nih.gov/grants/olaw/references/phspol.htm (accessed February 23, 2007).

86. R. A. Whitney, Jr., "Animal Care and Use Committees: History and Current National Policies in the United States," *Laboratory Animal Science* 37, spec. suppl. (January 1987): 18–21.

87. Orlans, *In the Name of Science,* chaps. 6–7; Rebecca Dresser, "Review Standards for Animal Research: A Closer Look," *ILAR News* 32, no. 4: 2–7.

88. 7 U.S.C. 2131–59 (1993). Regulations implementing this act are in 9 CFR, subchap. A, pts. 1–3; available at www.aphis.usda.gov/ac/publications/awa/awaindex.html (accessed February 23, 2007).

89. Council for International Organizations of Medical Sciences (CIOMS), World Health Organization, *International Guiding Principles for Biomedical Research Involving Animals,* 1984, www.cioms.ch/1985_texts_of_guidelines.htm (accessed February 23, 2007).

90. Canadian Council on Animal Care, *Guide to the Care and Use of Experimental Animals* (Ottawa: Canadian Council on Animal Care, 1980, 1984); vol. 1, www.ccac.ca/en/CCAC_Programs/Guidelines_Policies/guides/english/toc_v1.htm; vol. 2, www.ccac.ca/en/CCAC_Programs/Guidelines_Policies/guides/english/toc_V2.htm. See also its "Ethics of Animal Investigation"

(revised 1989), www.ccac.ca/en/CCAC_Programs/Guidelines_Policies/policies/ethics.htm (all accessed February 23, 2007).

91. National Health and Medical Research Council, *Australian Code of Practice for the Care and Use of Animals for Scientific Purposes* (revised 1989) (Canberra: Australian Government Publishing Service, 1990); 7th ed., 2004, available at www.nhmrc.gov.au/publications/_files/ea16.pdf (accessed February 23, 2007).

92. On the background and nature of the problem, see Rebecca Dresser, "Assessing Harm and Justification in Animal Research: Federal Policy Opens the Laboratory Door," *Rutgers Law Review* 40 (1988): 723–95; Rollin, *The Unheeded Cry*, chap. 5, esp. pp. 118ff.

93. See Bernard Rollin, "Animal Pain," in Regan-Singer, pp. 60ff.

94. See Orlans, *In the Name of Science*, pp. 58–60.

95. Daniel Callahan and Sissela Bok, *The Teaching of Ethics in Higher Education* (Hastings-on-Hudson, NY: Hastings Center, 1980), p. 69.

PART II

FARM ANIMALS

2

Humane Housing for Hogs

Bacon, pork chops, ham, sausage, hot dogs, bratwurst, tenderloin, ribs, pork roast, pulled-pork sandwiches, and pepperoni pizza: the variety of products that can be made from pig meat runs the gamut. From a McDonald's Egg McMuffin to the most exquisite pork belly on the menu at the world's finest restaurants, products made from pigs are everywhere. Pigs are the largest single source of meat for human beings, accounting for almost 40% of meat consumption worldwide by weight.[1] Each year in the United States, over 100 million pigs are slaughtered,[2] for total cash receipts in excess of $10 billion.[3]

FINDINGS OF THE HUMANE FARMING ASSOCIATION

Most consumers of pig meat have no contact with the animals they eat and little if any knowledge of the conditions under which the animals are raised and slaughtered. The Humane Farming Association (HFA), a nonprofit group interested in animal welfare, has found that the conditions under which pigs are farmed are generally not of high quality. The HFA has obtained video footage of pigs being boiled alive, beaten, and killed without being stunned or otherwise rendered insensitive to pain.[4] One farm the HFA investigated is HKY, a large hog farm located in Wausa, Nebraska. The HFA found that HKY is a representative example of improper care and harms caused by factory farms.

Joe Suing is a former manager of HKY. After he made several requests for help in his attempts to meet legal standards (all ignored), Suing invited representatives from the HFA to visit the farm a few weeks before he quit on February 20, 2004. The visit, which included Andrew Martin of the *Chicago Tribune,* motivated the HFA to petition Nebraska attorney general Jon Bruning to initiate an investigation of the facility. According to HFA chief investigator Gail Eisnitz, "On its face, this evidence documents a pervasive pattern of unconscionable abuse affecting thousands of animals. In addition to unspeakable cruelty, there exists a serious threat to public health because pigs from this filthy, disease-ridden operation are being sold to one of the largest suppliers of pork in the country."[5] As part of their investigation, the HFA obtained videotape depicting neglect of the animals, picture stills, and interviews with employees.

The HFA found that the HKY facility was in violation of Nebraska law. Other findings were that the farm failed to provide basic veterinary care, did not supply adequate amounts of food and water, lacked proper sanitation and ventilation, and was understaffed by unsupervised employees. Pigs suffered from skin infections and abscesses, often exhibiting sores on their backs, shoulders, and heads. They were living in their own waste, being exposed to disease and, in extreme cases, dying of infection. Overcrowding had even resulted in cases of cannibalism, where pigs had eaten each other alive. "You've heard of hog heaven, haven't you?" Robert Baker, an investigator for the HFA, asked reporter Martin as they walked through the facility. "What this is, is hog hell."[6]

HKY was not the first farm to be reviewed by the HFA. In 2001 the organization gave a secret video taken at a John Morrell slaughterhouse in Iowa to *Washington Post* reporter Joby Warrick. (John Morrell is now a division of Smithfield Foods, which is discussed below.) The video showed conscious pigs struggling as they were lowered into boiling water, contrary to the Humane Slaughter Act, which requires that the animals be rendered unconscious first.[7] In April 2001, Warrick published an article in the *Washington Post* detailing these and other violations of the law that had occurred at slaughterhouses across the country.[8] The article sparked a response from members of Congress. Senator Robert Byrd of West Virginia gave a speech on the Senate floor in which he said, "Barbaric treatment of helpless, defenseless creatures must not be tolerated even if these animals are being raised for food. . . . Life must be respected and dealt with humanely in a civilized society."[9]

While critics of the hog industry applaud the work of the HFA and support Senator Byrd's comments, industry analysts argue that these critics have lost sight of the fact that consumers have benefited from changes in the industry over the past several decades. Industry spokespersons note that from 1974 to 1995 the price of pork fell over 40%, while at the same time product quality increased.[10] During this period, the pork industry consolidated. As a result, a few major corporations, such as Smithfield Foods (Smithfield), now dominate the market. These large corporations purchase products from factory-style farms, such as HKY. The market then introduces strong pressures to lower costs.

Industry critics and politicians such as Senator Byrd persist with questions: Despite market pressures, what obligations do human beings have to animals raised for food? Should humans take the animals' natural behaviors into account when deciding how to raise them? Given the natural behaviors and needs of pigs, should farmers be forced to change how they raise pigs for food?

THE CHANGING FACE OF HOG FARMING

Some pig farmers have conscientiously tried to balance their economic needs and market pressures with the welfare of the animals under their care. As an example, consider the story of Jim Weaver, a once independent farmer who attempted to make a decent living while also looking out for the interests of his pigs.[11]

Weaver first began pig farming more than 20 years ago. As with most pig farmers throughout the history of hog farms, Weaver let his pigs roam more or less freely in fenced areas until they were scheduled for slaughter. This system allows the pigs a fairly natural environment, and Weaver, while not an expert in pig biology, understood the curious nature and needs of pigs. He enjoyed watching them run about. Pigs are widely regarded as the most intelligent farm animal. They communicate through vocalizations and can perform complex tasks requiring them to respond differently to gestures and verbal symbols, reflecting their ability to represent stored information abstractly. Pigs are also inquisitive. In one experiment, piglets, given a choice, consistently preferred to play in a pen that they had learned would contain new toys over a pen that had only familiar toys.[12] Their curiosity is also reflected in the large amount of time pigs spend exploring their environment.[13] Weaver's farm, as he appreciated, allowed pigs to express this natural inquisitiveness by interacting with their surroundings.

According to Jim Weaver, raising pigs in free-range conditions with plenty of fresh air, sunlight, and straw brings added benefits because exposure to sunlight controls most disease without antibiotics. Weaver's experience matches that of reports by many Swedish pig farmers. In 1986, Sweden banned the use of subtherapeutic antibiotics at the behest of its farmers, who had wanted to reassure consumers of the safety of their meat and to address related public health issues. At first the pig industry experienced some difficulty adjusting because the ban exposed background levels of disease that had been masked by the antibiotics. In response, Swedish farmers increased the space and straw available for the pigs and waited to wean piglets until five or six weeks, allowing them to develop natural antibodies while spending more time in family units. These steps eliminated the disease problem and also improved the welfare of the pigs.

By allowing pigs to roam (as Weaver did), the farmers promoted healthier sows and piglets. In free-range conditions like those at a Swedish pig farm, sows leave the herd 24 to 48 hours before giving birth in order to build a nest for their litters. The sow remains careful not to crush her piglets when she returns to the nest. She first makes a furrow in front of her with her snout, then carefully lies down with her hindquarters opposite her piglets. If any of them gets caught under her, they squeal, and the sow lifts herself back up to free them. After about 10 to 14 days, the sow brings her piglets back to the main group, and they begin to integrate socially. Piglets experience social interaction during this period, and they are fully integrated into the group by eight weeks. Piglets wean normally when they are between 13 and 17 weeks old. Weaver followed this timeline, intentionally allowing piglets to wean naturally.

Because pigs are omnivorous and, like humans, will eat a wide variety of foods, they can provide a way of recycling unwanted food. Their waste can serve as manure for fields. Weaver had a good source of fertilizer that he could sustain on his small farm without overwhelming sewage concerns or any threat to the environment. Once the pigs were ready for slaughter, Weaver would take them to one of several slaughterhouses that competed for his business.

After Weaver made farming his occupation, vertically integrated companies began to change American pig farming. Vertically integrated companies own and/or control their pigs at all stages of production from birth through finishing, slaughter, processing, and packaging. The largest such company is Smithfield, which raises more than 13 million pigs a year in the United States.[14] Smithfield processes 19 million pigs a year, representing 20% of the market share.[15] Smithfield markets its products under many different brand names, including but not limited to Smithfield, John Morrell, Farmland Foods, Gwaltney, and Stefano.

The pig-farming industry has undergone massive consolidation in the last 50 years. In 1965 there were over 1 million American farms with pigs, but by 2002 that number had decreased to about 75,000.[16] During this period, pig farms became much larger. Between 1988 and 2000, the percentage of pigs raised on farms with fewer than 1,000 pigs fell from 32% to 2%, while the percentage raised on farms with over 5000 pigs rose from 2% to 51%.[17]

Pig farmers like Weaver needed to make adjustments in light of the competitive presence of Smithfield and other mega-producers. According to Weaver, Smithfield's first move was to gain control over all the slaughterhouses in the area. The absence of slaughterhouses that purchase pigs on the spot left farmers with no choice but to grow pigs under contract to Smithfield. In this system, Weaver was forced to raise his pigs in accordance with Smithfield's requirements. Otherwise, he could not keep his farm. He watched as other pig farmers were forced to mortgage their property in order to buy the equipment required by Smithfield. Because the company retains control of the contracted pigs, individual farmers assume all of the risk. Industry critics view this risk assumption as a form of debt peonage.[18]

After attempting to maintain his own style of control over his farm, while also adhering to Smithfield's requirements, Weaver decided to leave the industry. In his opinion, small producers can manage at a subsistence level. However, he believes that these farmers cannot support their families on the small profit margin that their style of production yields.[19] Some industry analysts agree with this assessment.[20]

There are also economic and environmental concerns about waste control on large farms. On his farm Weaver could use the waste as fertilizer. However, factory pig farming has often had the effect of creating waste without adequate sewage treatment facilities.[21] Inadequate waste disposal has led to complaints and lawsuits involving both odor and water pollution. In 1999 the U.S. Environmental Protection Agency (EPA) won a lawsuit against Smithfield for violating the Clean Water Act.[22] Complaints of negative health effects on neighbors of pig farms have increased in recent years. Much of the concern centers on the large open-air cesspools in which waste is stored, because they emit hydrogen sulfide and ammonia, both poisonous gases. Neighbors complain of neurological damage, diarrhea, nosebleeds, earaches, and lung burns.[23] Researchers have found elevated levels of these symptoms among neighbors of pig operations.[24]

THE LIVING CONDITIONS OF PIGS

Weaver, to this day, worries that Smithfield's production system is bad for farmers and the environment, and also terrible for the pigs. Smithfield's factory production processes prevent pigs from engaging in many of their species-typical behaviors. Gestation crates, for example, force sows to hunch down their backs simply to fit in them. Industry-standard crates measure 2 to 2½ feet wide by 7 feet long by 3 feet high, while breeding sows weigh 500 to 600 pounds.[25] The sows cannot walk, turn around, or socialize with other pigs, and many sows develop lesions on their shoulders and backs. Premature mortality rates for sows in intensive confinement operations are high, with estimates ranging from 10 to 20%.

When they are confined in small cages unable to move, socialize, or investigate their surroundings, pigs exhibit many atypical (so-called stereotypic) behaviors including compulsive, repetitive actions such as bar biting, purposeless chewing, and digging and pawing at the floor and walls of the crates for up to 70% of the time. Sows in farrowing stalls—crates used just before birth until the piglets are weaned—exhibit less bonding with their piglets, make fewer vocalizations to their piglets, and are less responsive to the piglets' vocalizations than those who are allowed to move about and build nests. They also have higher stress hormone levels, which can lead to the development of clinical disease. In addition, piglet mortality in crates is high, despite the fact that farrowing crates are supposed to protect them; death rates are estimated at between 4.8% and 18%.

Piglets are taken from their mothers at, on average, between ten and fifteen days of age, and sometimes even as young as five days. The natural weaning age is 13 to 17 weeks, but piglets are separated from their mothers earlier in order to increase the number of piglets produced per sow. Because they are weaned so early, piglets often have not yet learned how to eat and lack the ability to generate their own antibodies, relying instead on maternal antibodies transferred during pregnancy or in the milk. However, piglets need their own antibodies because nurseries and finishing farms are built with perforated floors through which waste drops and sits in liquefied form, predisposing the animals to disease (through stress and tissue damage due to high gas levels).

To address this problem, antibiotics are administered as a standard part of the feed. Extensive subtherapeutic use of antibiotics (not intended to treat infections, but rather to keep the level of infection down) allows farm animals to be raised in otherwise unsustainable density levels on growing and finishing farms. Administering subtherapeutic doses of antibiotics through feed also leads to higher growth rates in animals. In the United States, 93% of pigs receive antibiotics in their diet at some time during the growing and finishing period, and 70% of all antibiotics used are administered to farm animals. Smithfield's policy on antibiotics states that it does not *routinely* administer the same antibiotics used in human medicine to pigs.[26] However, "routine" is defined in the policy as the consistent use over an animal's entire life. Smithfield declined to answer questions (in the writing of this case) regarding the extent to which its pigs receive antibiotics in their diet for nontherapeutic reasons. In 2003, the World Health Organization (WHO) recommended that the use of antibiotics in animal foodstuffs be halted due to concerns that the use of antibiotics in farm animals will result in the evolution of some human pathogens resistant to antibiotics.[27] The United States has declined to follow this recommendation.

Smithfield has for years been criticized by animal protection groups for the way it raises pigs, especially for the 2 × 7-foot gestation crates, which the Animal Welfare Institute calls "steel prisons."[28] On January 25, 2007, Smithfield appeared to yield to its critics: It announced, in what it called a "landmark decision regarding animal management," that it would "phase out" the use of gestation crates in its own factories by

2017.[29] It also announced that it would give its contractors (which supply the majority of its pigs) until 2027 to make the switch. Smithfield made no announcement about whether changes would take place in the 10- and 20-year transition periods. The company denied that animal activists played any role in the decision but acknowledged that some of its best customers, including McDonald's, had expressed concerns about gestation crates. CEO Larry Pope said that Smithfield "worked with our customers" to take this "precedent-setting step" to resolve "the issue of gestation stalls." McDonald's praised the change of policy. However, CEO Niel Dierks of the National Pork Producers Council stated that, despite Smithfield's new policy, the council continues to consider gestation crates humane and suitable for the industry.[30]

SLAUGHTERHOUSE CONDITIONS, OLD AND NEW

When their weight reaches 60 pounds, pigs are moved to a finishing site. These mechanized, indoor, growing-finishing facilities consist of barren pens with concrete slatted floors. The liquefied waste below the pens releases air contaminants that increase mortality due to respiratory disease, and the concrete floors lead to abscesses, arthritis, muscle lesions, scarring of the liver, reduced growth, and porcine stress syndrome (a factor in reduced meat quality).[31] At approximately 5½ months of age the pigs are removed from the finishing pens and taken to slaughter.

Pigs are large enough animals that they are difficult to control and to stun before being bled out, a procedure that kills them. Stunning is required by the Humane Slaughter Act of 1978, which is enforced by the Food Safety and Inspection Service (FSIS) of the U.S. Department of Agriculture (USDA).[32] The speed of large slaughterhouse assembly lines, unlike the small businesses that used to compete for Weaver's pigs, leads to many pigs not being properly stunned and thus being bled out or boiled alive while conscious.

In response to the outrage caused by the previously mentioned *Washington Post* exposé, Congress earmarked funds for the enforcement of humane slaughter practices.[33] In fiscal year 2002 Congress directed the secretary of agriculture to enforce the Humane Slaughter Act with the strictness originally intended.[34] In fiscal year 2003 Congress appropriated additional funds for enforcement and also asked the Government Accountability Office (GAO) to report violations of the Humane Slaughter Act and to recommend solutions. The GAO responded by investigating the FSIS.

The GAO investigation found that little progress had been made and that the Humane Slaughter Act was still not being adequately enforced. The investigation was hindered by incomplete FSIS records, with many inspection reports missing. The GAO found that many inspectors did not know the rules, failed to report violations, and consistently did not note properly the severity of the violations they did report, as required by law. Despite the inadequate records, the USDA had reported to Congress in 2003 that there were "very few" violations of the act. The GAO found that its own more extensive analysis did not support this claim, that enforcement was spotty and uneven between districts, and that plants that had failed to stun animals properly were often not shut down, as is required.

As for Weaver, he returned to the industry only when Niman Ranch opened a new slaughterhouse that enabled him to raise pigs humanely while making a reasonable profit to sustain his business. Weaver sells all of his pigs to Niman Ranch, which slaughters them and sells to Whole Foods Market, Chipotle Mexican Grill, and a number of upscale restaurants.[35] Niman Ranch worked conjointly with the Animal Welfare Institute to develop guidelines that require producers to raise their pigs in free-range conditions without gestation crates, to refrain from using antibiotics, to wean piglets at five weeks of age minimum, and to provide straw for the pigs to chew and manipulate.[36] Weaver is finally happy with how his pigs are both raised and slaughtered. He judges that, at present, raising pigs in free-range conditions is not only good for pigs, but also good for the renewal of rural economies and for the health and safety of farmers.

ETHICAL ISSUES

The Benefits and Costs of Pig Farming

The methods presently used by Smithfield in its factory pig farms prevent pigs from engaging in many species-typical behaviors and cause them various forms of suffering. This type of farming raises questions about whether the benefits derived from its methods of pig production outweigh the costs the methods impose. These costs and benefits can accrue to both humans and animals. Smithfield itself cites many advantages to its vertically integrated business model.[37] From a financial perspective, control over all stages of production makes Smithfield less susceptible to fluctuations in the market. In the past, low pig prices meant a big profit for processors and hard times for farmers, while high prices brought a reverse fortune to farmers. By controlling both farming and processing, Smithfield is able to offer Wall Street investors increased and sustainable earnings stability.

Vertical integration also benefits Smithfield by enabling it to control completely the quality and safety of the product. A profile of every pig is assembled, including its genetic makeup and also data on nutritional and medical regimes. This provides Smithfield with traceability of its products, which could prove valuable in the event of an epidemic disease in humans or in animals. Traceability also aids the development of new pork products by making it possible to discover which pigs have the genes for desirable traits.

Smithfield and some industry analysts maintain that the modern American system of corporate pig production results in benefits to American consumers and to the U.S. economy. According to the USDA, the average price of pork has fallen by 1% a year since 1990, while healthy pork products have been developed, such as Smithfield's Lean Generation™ line, which won the American Heart Association seal of approval. The USDA study also found that vertically integrated companies can create products with the characteristics valued in specific export markets such as Japan, resulting in a 12-fold increase in U.S. exports of pork since 1986. Smithfield claims that its production methods create jobs, especially in distressed areas such as rural North Carolina where many plants are located. Thus benefits to humans may include a cheap, accessible source of protein, tasty food, and jobs. Some of these benefits (primarily in the price of pork) would probably not be realizable if only free-range pork was produced by independent growers.

It has often been pointed out that pigs receive a benefit in factory farms simply by the fact that they owe their lives to the existence of the industry, without which they would never have been born. However, this "benefit" can count as a real benefit only if their lives are on balance worth living. It is not a benefit to be born into a life lived under inhumane conditions that involve extreme suffering to the point of misery. Conditions on some pig farms must be counted as causing misery. These conditions include various forms of fear, tension, stress, anxiety, distress, confinement, ill health, pain, frustration, and even boredom. Of course, assessing the costs to pigs is problematic because the suffering of animals is difficult to calculate, given our lack of access to their inner, subjective experiences. At the same time, the rapidly growing field of animal welfare science is helping to overcome this hurdle.

Smithfield's pig production methods also present risks of harm and costs for humans. These may include the loss of farms and jobs for independent farmers, environmental harms, and reduced effectiveness of antibiotics for sick persons and other animals. Weaver and other critics contend that rather than bringing new jobs to distressed rural communities, the very efficiency that contributes to Smithfield's success may cause job losses. An investigation by reporters in North Carolina concluded that the pig-farming industry relied heavily on convict and migrant labor, rather than local labor, and that few jobs were created in supporting industries because most of the supplies were brought from out of state.[38] Most of the jobs that are created are low-wage, low-skill jobs. Intensive indoor hog farming can also result in health risks for workers, such as respiratory problems and zoonotic diseases such as Salmonellosis.[39]

In 2004, Human Rights Watch issued a report on the meatpacking industry in the United States.[40] It found dangerous and unlawful conditions at plants throughout the United States, including Smithfield facilities such as its Tar Heel, North Carolina, plant, the largest hog-killing facility in the country. The line moves so fast at the Tar Heel plant that it takes only between five and ten minutes after a pig is killed to complete draining, cleaving, organ removal, and the other steps needed before jointing the carcass. Injuries to workers include broken bones, torn tendons, rashes, and swelling, and some appear to have been killed by injuries resulting from inhaling chemical fumes. Some workers have complained that Smithfield often does not provide necessary safety equipment and that when injuries do occur, workers are denied medical treatment and are sometimes fired for being unable to work. Human Rights Watch found many instances in which medical bills remained unpaid, workers' compensation was not provided, and state governments failed to enforce the law.

The most obvious questions raised by these costs and benefits are: If raising pigs for food is justified by its contribution to human health and well-being (cheap pork, creation of jobs, etc.), can we do so in a way that causes less suffering for the animals and humans associated with the industry? Are we morally obligated to change our practices to make life better for pigs and human workers? And to what extent does the suffering of pigs impose moral obligations that society ought to address through more careful regulatory oversight? Finally, to what extent are individuals morally obligated to change their behavior?

Is There a Justification of Suffering?

There is overwhelming evidence of both physical and psychological suffering by pigs on factory farms and in slaughterhouses. This evidence has been collected not only by animal welfare organizations but also by government investigators, such as the GAO study discussed earlier. Is there any justification for causing this suffering? If so, is it a moral justification (animal welfare), or is it perhaps some nonmoral justification (e.g., an economic one)?

Smithfield has offered several justifications for any suffering that might be cau...
by its production practices. The company maintains that it works hard to see that all the
physical needs of the pigs are met. It therefore denies that there is excessive or unwarranted suffering. However, it defines "physical needs" narrowly, tending to equate need
satisfaction with good health. It argues that when sows produce large litters of pigs,
their capacity to produce is proof that the pigs are well maintained and healthy. When
evidence of physical suffering and abuse is presented to the company, it tends to blame
the problem on employee carelessness rather than on corporate policies.

These industry claims must confront two issues. First, physical growth and sexual
maturity do not seem to provide an adequate measure of physical well-being. Such a
standard would seem most odd in determining the welfare of human beings or of our
companion animals. An owner who fed his dog and raised puppies but also allowed disease to develop without treatment would not be paying sufficient attention to the dog's
physical welfare. Second, physical growth (and even physical vigor) and capacity to
reproduce do not prove that an animal is psychologically healthy. An owner who kept
his dog in a small cage and raised its puppies would be ignoring its psychological well-
being. Neither the large producers nor the industry groups they support acknowledge a
duty to take steps to *reduce psychological suffering* in the pigs they raise, because psychological suffering is not included within the scope of welfare considerations.

In the end, the most plausible justification that might be offered for the conditions
found in many factory pig farms is probably not moral, but financial. These farms are
efficient and profitable. From a business perspective, they are competitive and lean.
Many, like Smithfield, are publicly traded companies. Some people, such as the econo-
mist Milton Friedman, have argued that the officers running corporations have only one
moral duty: to maximize shareholder profit within the confines of the law. These farms
have a strong commitment to pursue this duty. But is this their only duty? Are there not
other duties to employees and their families? And if there are duties to them, are there
not also duties to the animals whose lives they control? And what if the law is out of
date and everyone knows it, but legislators have not allocated the time to amend it?

It is interesting that virtually all companies acknowledge that they have a duty to
reduce at least some of the physical suffering that animals raised for food endure, even
if doing so leads to some reduction in profits. According to the Pork Board, an industry
group, "While profits provide an economic incentive for husbandry, livestock producers
have never evaluated animal welfare solely in terms of dollars and cents. Taking proper
care of one's animals has always been understood as an ethical responsibility, as well as
a necessary business practice."[41] But what does this mean, and what should it mean in
actual practice? Also, would it be immoral, morally praiseworthy, or morally neutral for
the officers of Smithfield or any other company to take steps that would reduce the suffering of pigs, knowing that these steps could considerably reduce shareholder profits
and make the company less attractive to investors?

Moral Status and the Intelligence and Social Nature of Pigs

As discussed in the introduction to this volume, if an animal could be shown to have
intelligence, memory, moral capacities, and the like, whether it is or is not human, would
not that consideration be a significant factor in framing our moral obligations to the creature? We would look to see if such a being has capacities of intelligent responsiveness

emotional life, or an organized social life. If it did have such properties,
.t some level would seem assured, whereas if it had no such properties,
vould likely be in question (depending on the precise properties it had).
plications of this viewpoint for pigs?

y complex brain structures, have been shown to be very intelligent, and
have structured social arrangements. It is generally acknowledged that more intelligent
animals may suffer more as a consequence of their intelligence, in part because they are
able to understand what is happening to them and to foresee harms. In addition, animals
with significant cognitive abilities can have those abilities stifled and frustrated, making
it possible for them to suffer in ways less gifted animals cannot. There is evidence that
pigs do exhibit signs of psychological suffering due to boredom and frustration. Pigs
raised in confinement exhibit higher levels of stress hormones, disease, and compulsive
repetitive behaviors than pigs raised in more stimulating environments, and they engage
in destructive behaviors such as tail biting, which are not normally part of the pigs'
behavioral repertoire.

Does the fact that pigs are highly intelligent, social creatures give them a higher
moral status than they have been accorded in the past? Does it impose a moral obligation on us to raise them in conditions that allow them to exercise that intelligence while
socializing with their fellows? Should special provisions be made for the bond between
mothers and their piglets?

Practical Alternatives to Current Practices

What might we do, practically, to alleviate some of these problems? There are a number
of practical alternatives. Some involve legislation that has already been implemented
by the European Union, by individual states in the United States, or by private organizations that raise and market meat in accord with humane standards. From the moral
perspective, it should be asked whether these alternatives are morally required or simply
have the status of moral ideals that some have proposed for the modification of systems
of pig production.

Here are some practical alternatives that have been proposed, and some implemented:

1. We could refrain from eating pork from pigs that have been reared in this way.
Most people eat pork because they enjoy the taste and because doing so is part of culinary tradition. Furthermore, the pig industry provides employment for many people
and is a traditional part of rural life—though the rise of factory farming may already
be eroding these considerations. Nonetheless, we need to ask whether the benefit that
humans derive from eating pigs outweighs the burdens that doing so imposes on the
animals we consume, as well as the costs that other humans incur through direct health
risks, environmental destruction, and the overuse of antibiotics.

Many who believe in animal rights accept vegetarianism as the solution to the problem of animal suffering, because they believe that animals have either a right to life or
a right not to be made to suffer for human benefit. Many others, by contrast, tend to
acknowledge that we should avoid inflicting unnecessary harm on animals, but they
also accept that some minimal level of animal suffering may be necessary for the benefit of humans, such as in the production of food. Either of these two perspectives may
lead one to stop eating pork if one concludes that the harm done to pigs outweighs the
benefits provided by eating them.

2. Consumers could choose to buy only pork that has been produced in accordance with humane standards. Every time we choose to spend our money we are in effect voting with our dollars. Consumers can vote in favor of cheap factory-farmed pig meat and the suffering it entails, or they can purchase only pig meat produced on farms that raise their pigs humanely, thus creating a larger market for such meat. As the humane meat market grows, companies that are seeking to increase their profits will increasingly adopt humane methods of production. The very market forces that have led to problems of suffering by factory-farmed pigs could, theoretically, instead be harnessed to promote their well-being.

This approach suggests that every one of us should consider carefully how we do and do not contribute to the suffering of pigs through our decisions. Factory pig farms do not exist because bad people wish to inflict suffering on pigs; they exist because consumers demand cheap meat products and have so far been unwilling to pay more in order to reduce animal suffering. Each individual consumer faces an ethical decision every time he or she goes to the grocery store or eats at a restaurant. Does the small amount of money saved, or the culinary pleasure enjoyed, justify the conditions that the consumer is paying large pig-producing corporations to inflict on their animals and on other people? Does it make a difference that, in many cases, what is a small profit for farmers could be used to significantly improve the well-being of their animals?

3. The laws of countries and their territories could be changed. The Humane Slaughter Act is the only federal law in the U.S. that is designed to protect the welfare of intensively farmed animals, and it is often violated. The United States has no federal laws protecting pigs during the production phase prior to slaughter. Except for those raised in research institutions, farm animals are exempt from the Animal Welfare Act.[42] Perhaps the United States should follow the European Union and other major meat-producing countries in mandating more humane farming conditions for animals, including pigs.

Attempts to change national laws raise additional ethical questions that need to be considered. Should consumers be forced to pay more in order to reduce animal suffering? Should food be better labeled to empower consumer choice? Should we be concerned that the economic impact of increased costs would fall disproportionately on the less fortunate, who already spend a higher proportion of their income on food? At the same time, we also need to consider the possibility that the current price of pig meat does not capture the actual production cost—i.e., the full scope of the costs of the industry. When pig factories pollute the environment, depress land values, or sicken workers, these costs are often passed on to society at large and are paid in the form of higher taxes, lost productivity from illness, and publicly subsidized health care for workers.

While the United States has generally left pig production standards to the free market, the European Union (EU) has taken a very different approach. In 1997, concerns over the welfare of intensively raised pigs led the Scientific Committee on Animal Health and Animal Welfare to compile a report on the pig industry for the European Commission. This report included a study of pig biology, cognition, and social behaviors and how these relate to the welfare of pigs raised in intensive conditions. In response to the report, some council directives were issued in 2001, requiring European nations to take steps to guarantee pigs an environment corresponding to their needs for social interaction and investigatory behavior.[43] The directives establish minimum space requirements, mandate group housing for most pigs, require the provision of bulky, high fiber foods (such as straw) for pigs to chew on, prohibit weaning prior to 28 days of age, and call for better rules on tail docking and castration to prevent pain.

4. International law could be changed. One major concern expressed by the EU in implementing its humane standards is that these standards could increase costs and enable nations without such protections to take market share from European farmers. This is a serious practical problem, because requiring that *imports* meet the same humane standards as those accepted in a country would be illegal under the rules of the World Trade Organization (WTO). WTO judicial interpretations have held that products cannot be distinguished by their methods of production, only by their nature as a product. These problems posed by WTO point to a larger issue for the industry in general, primarily the fear of a "race-to-the-bottom" phenomenon in which pig production shifts away from areas with stringent environmental, animal welfare, and worker safety requirements in favor of areas with lower standards. Such a shift could force areas with higher standards to lower them or risk losing jobs. This is an old problem of business and social ethics (e.g., concerning the conditions of low-wage workers in so-called sweatshops) that is no less pertinent for ethical issues in the human use of animals.

To conclude, most of the problems encountered in this section on ethical issues telescope to some issue about the benefits and costs of pig farming. We are probably in a primitive stage of understanding how to do a morally responsible cost-benefit analysis of the factory farming of pigs. In the past, most of the envisioned benefits have been for humans, while the harms (costs) were to pigs. But this narrow scope of benefits and costs seems one-sided. Perhaps humans should suffer more of the costs and pigs more of the benefits?

NOTES

1. *Agriculture, Trade, and the Environment: The Pig Sector* (Paris: Organisation for Economic Co-operation and Development, 2003), pp. 23–24.

2. U.S. Department of Agriculture, National Agricultural Statistics Service, *Livestock Slaughter Annual Summary 2003* (USDA, 2004), p. 1, usda.mannlib.cornell.edu/reports/nassr/livestock/pls-bban/.

3. U.S. Department of Agriculture, National Agricultural Statistics Service, *Meat Animals Production, Disposition, and Income Annual Summary 2003* (USDA, 2004), p. 1, usda.mannlib.cornell.edu/reports/nassr/livestock/zma-bb/.

4. Many videos are available on the Humane Farming Association's website (www.hfa.org/). The HFA's investigations are detailed in Gail A. Eisnitz, *Slaughterhouse: The Shocking Story of Greed, Neglect, and Inhumane Treatment Inside the U.S. Meat Industry* (New York: Prometheus Books, 1997).

5. "Nebraska Hog Factory Exposed," Humane Farming Association, www.hfa.org/campaigns/hky.html.

6. "At Some Farms, It's 'Hog Hell,' " Humane Farming Association, www.hfa.org/campaigns/tribarticle.html.

7. Joby Warrick, phone conversation, October 13, 2004. John Morrell & Co. has since been purchased by Smithfield Foods.

8. Joby Warrick, "They Die Piece by Piece: In Overtaxed Plants, Humane Treatment of Cattle Is Often a Lost Battle," *Washington Post,* April 10, 2001, p. A1.

9. U.S. Senate, *Congressional Record,* July 9, 2001.

10. Steve W. Martinez, *Agricultural Economics Report,* No. 777 (USDA, April 1999), pp. 25–26, www.ers.usda.gov/publications/aer777.

11. Jim Weaver is a composite based chiefly on a personal interview with a pig farmer on July 29, 2004. Jim Weaver is not his real name. The farmer requested anonymity due to fear of reprisals.

12. Animal Welfare Institute, *AWI Quarterly* 41, no. 10 (Summer 2002).

13. Report of the Scientific Veterinary Committee of the European Commission, *The Welfare of Intensively Kept Pigs,* September 30, 1997, p. 15, europa.eu.int/comm/food/fs/sc/oldcomm4/out17_en.html.

14. Smithfield Investor Snapshot, June 18, 2005, www.smithfieldfoods.com/Investor/Snapshot/.

15. Smithfield Foods, Inc. *Annual Report 2003,* p. 1, www.smithfieldfoods.com/Upload/SFD_AR2003.pdf (accessed August 29, 2007).

16. Andrew Martin, "Factory Farm Foes Fed Up; Sick of the Foul Odors and Government Inaction, Critics of Huge Swine Operations are Taking Complaints to Court," *Chicago Tribune,* March 24, 2004.

17. John D. Lawrence, Ron Plain, Glenn Grimes, "The Structure of the U.S. Pork Industry," Econ Papers 10149, Iowa State University, Department of Economics, 2002, econpapers.repec.org/paper/isugenres/default20.htm (accessed August 29, 2007).

18. Joby Warrick, "They Die Piece by Piece," p. A1.

19. Personal interview, July 29, 2004.

20. John McGlone and Wilson Pond, *Pig Production: Biological Principles and Applications* (Belmont, CA: Thomson Delmar Learning, 2003), p. 16.

21. Joby Warrick and Pat Stith, "New Studies Show Lagoons are Leaking; Groundwater, Rivers Affected by Waste," *News and Observer* (Raleigh, NC), February 19, 1995.

22. *United States v. Smithfield,* 191 F3d 516 (4th Cir. 1999).

23. Jennifer Lee, "Neighbors of Vast Hog Farms Say Foul Air Endangers Their Health," *New York Times,* May 11, 2003.

24. K. M. Thu, "Public Health Concerns for Neighbors of Large Scale Swine Production Operations," *Journal of Agricultural Safety and Health* 8 (2002): 175–84, esp. p. 180.

25. Bernard Rollin, "Farm Factories: The End of Animal Husbandry," *Christian Century,* December 19, 2001, pp. 26–29.

26. "Animal Welfare: Murphy-Brown Antibiotic Usage Policy," Smithfield Foods, www.smithfieldfoods.com/Enviro/Policies/antibiotics.asp. There is evidence that resistance can be transferred between organisms, and resistance to one antibiotic may mean resistance to that group, which is the worry.

27. World Health Organization, *Impacts of Antimicrobial Growth Promoter Termination in Denmark* (Geneva, Switzerland: World Health Organization, Department of Communicable Diseases, Prevention and Eradication, Collaborating Centre for Antimicrobial Resistance in Foodborne Pathogens, November 2002), pp. 6–9. The antibiotic use under discussion in this paragraph does not preclude the transfer of resistance between organisms in humans and animals.

28. *AWI Quarterly* 56 (Winter 2007): 8.

29. "Smithfield Goods Makes Landmark Decision Regarding Animal Management," Smithfield News Release, January 25, 2007, www.smithfieldfoods.com.

30. Marc Kaufman, "Largest Pork Processor to Phase Out Crates," *Washington Post,* January 26, 2007, p. A6.

31. Iowa State University, *Iowa Concentrated Feeding Operations Air Quality Study Final Report* (Ames, IA: Environmental Health Sciences Research Center, 2002), pp. 115–20.

32. Government Accounting Office (GAO), *Humane Methods of Slaughter,* GAO 04–247. See also Food Safety and Inspection Service website for key facts about the Humane Slaughter Act; www.fsis.usda.gov/factsheets/key_facts_humane_slaughter/index.asp.

33. Public Law 107–20, 115 Stat. 155, 164 (2001). See also GAO, "Humane Methods of Slaughter," pp. 2–3.

34. Farm Security and Rural Investment Act of 2002, Public Law 107–171, Section 10305 116, Stat. 134.

35. Peter Slevin, "Pork is Finding Its Niche: Farmers of 'Free-Range' Hogs Ride Surge in Demand," *Washington Post,* November 21, 2004, p. A3.

36. See Niman Ranch's description of its pigs at www.nimanranch.com/.

37. From Smithfield's *2001 Annual Report,* available at www.smithfieldfoods.com/Understand/Vertical/.

38. Joby Warrick and Pat Stith, "North Carolina's Booming Hog Industry Is Generating Jobs and Tax Revenue. But Some Residents Say the Cost is too High. The Smell of Money," *News and Observer* (Raleigh, NC), February 24, 1995. The investigation focused on Murphy-Brown, now a division of Smithfield.

39. Iowa State University, *Iowa Concentrated Feeding Operations Air Quality Study Final Report*. See www.extension.iastate.edu/airquality/reports.html (accessed August 12, 2007).

40. Human Rights Watch, *Blood, Sweat, and Fear: Workers' Rights in U.S. Meat and Poultry Plants* (New York: Human Rights Watch, 2004), www.hrw.org/reports/2005/usa0105/usa0105.pdf.

41. Paul B. Thompson, *Swine Care Handbook*, preface, www.porkboard.org/docs/swinecarehandbook.pdf (accessed June 18, 2005).

42. Phone interview with Gail Eisnitz, chief investigator, Humane Farming Association, November 22, 2004.

43. Council Directives 2001/88/EC (October 23, 2001) and 2001/93/EC (November 9, 2001).

3

Veal Crates and Human Palates

On February 1, 1995, Coventry Airport in the United Kingdom was alive with animal welfare campaigners protesting the transport of very young calves to Europe to be reared for veal. The animal protesters were of all ages and backgrounds, even old-age pensioners. Some watched animal rights protester Jill Phipps try to block the path of a large transport truck by running alongside it and finally cutting in front of the truck and raising her hands. To their horror, she slipped and was crushed to death as the wheels ran over her chest and stomach. Just before her death she had said in an interview, "We will continue even if someone gets hurt. Someone will eventually be hurt."[1] This 31-year-old mother became a martyr for her cause. Representatives of many animal rights and animal welfare organizations attended her funeral some weeks later. The movie star and veteran animal rights campaigner Brigitte Bardot flew from France to attend the ceremony.

The issue of veal crates has perhaps caught the attention of more persons than any other animal welfare issue in recent times. According to a senior police officer, on the force for more than 37 years, the protests in the United Kingdom were at a new level. He had never seen so many people, from such diverse backgrounds, unite on an issue. It had brought together "vegans [strict vegetarians] and villagers, grandmothers and mothers, animal rights and pensioners in a campaign of civil unrest."[2] Many of the protestors had never been involved in a public demonstration before. Why were so many people so concerned about these calves? And why, many years later, are the issues still largely unresolved?

THE VEAL TRADE AND METHODS OF PRODUCTION

Veal calves are on the market as a by-product of the dairy industry, which supplies consumables such as milk, cheese, cream, butter, ice cream, and yogurt. For cows to produce milk they have to become pregnant. Shortly after birth, calves are separated from the cows so that all the milk produced by the cows can be taken and used by the farmer. Typically, calves either feed once from the cow or they are artificially fed so that they receive antibody-rich colostrum, the milk produced by the cow for a few days after she gives birth to protect the calf from disease. Calves can absorb antibodies from this milk only during the first 12 hours of life.[3]

Not all calves are sold to produce beef or veal, but most are. Some dairy calves are genetically unsuitable for beef or veal production. This is because dairy calves have been selected genetically for milk yield and milk quality, not for fast growth rates or lean meat. The genetically unsuitable calves may be killed after a week or two and used to make processed meats such as "veal and ham" pies. While some dairy calves grow to replace dairy cows that have to be culled, the majority of dairy calves are used in some form of meat production through traditional forms of beef farming. But there is also a significant trade in the production of veal, and it is this production that has raised so much concern about animal welfare.

There are approximately 20 veal producers in the United Kingdom. They kill some 5,000 calves a year. Because little veal is consumed in the United Kingdom, there is virtually no home market for these animals. Calves from the United Kingdom, often less than two weeks of age, are exported to be reared for veal in Europe, primarily in France and Holland. In France they raise "veau sous mare,"[4] which is a niche market for calves kept with their mother on her milk until they are slaughtered. This market comprises about 12% of veal production and commands a premium price of 18% more than ordinary veal. The United Kingdom imports a small amount of "European" veal for gourmet restaurants, and some of this veal may have come originally from U.K.-born calves. In the United States the leading producers of veal are the Amish and the Mennonites, whose production accounts for as much as 45% of national production and 60–70% in the eastern states.[5]

The traditional way of keeping these newly born animals for the production of veal has been in small, individual wooden crates with slatted floors with no bedding kept in the dark,[6] though it is now illegal to keep them in complete darkness in Europe. In the United States some 800,000 calves enter this special-fed veal system every year and may be kept on a tether of 2 to 3 feet (with no back to their crate or stall).[7] They are fed twice daily on an exclusively liquid diet of milk replacer. They gain between 2 and 3.5 pounds per day for some 16 to 24 weeks, after which they are killed at around 400–500 pounds.[8] Keeping calves in crates and/or on tethers prevents them from licking and sucking each other and from expending energy on natural activities. Keeping them in the dark and feeding them a milk-only diet has been thought essential to produce the coveted pale white meat.

Welfare concerns about this system are that the crates are so small that, as the animals grow, they cannot turn around or lie down naturally with their legs out sideways or adopt a normal sleeping position. They are unable to carry out natural patterns of behavior such as walking, running, grooming, and playing with other animals. They cannot make social contact even though they may be able to hear and smell, and they often lie with their rumps touching their next-door neighbor. That is all the interaction that is possible between the animals. The exclusive feeding of milk that is low in iron for such a long time causes the animals to develop the white flesh as well as an anemia rarely found in normally fed calves.

Because the animals are not permitted access to roughage such as straw, grass or hay, their gut (rumen) fails to grow normally. In order to obtain roughage, the calves, if permitted, "overgroom" themselves and eat their coats, resulting in hair balls and chronic indigestion. Moreover, fully grown calves may suffer from heat stress because of the intensive conditions and poor ventilation. The incidence of infectious disease is often high and can be exacerbated if calves do not receive sufficient colostrum at the right time. Any subsequent disease then has to be controlled by the administration of antibiotics.

During the first three weeks of life, up to 5% of animals in veal units die from infection.[9] Within the first six weeks, 10% may develop enteric disease (diarrhea) and over 55% will contract some respiratory disease; 21% have been found to have injuries such as abraded and swollen knees and hocks.[10] Animals frequently show stereotypic behaviors such as crate licking, tongue rolling, and excessive grooming. If they are able to make contact with the animal in the adjacent crate, they often suck each other's mouths and tongues. These sorts of behavior are often associated with stressful housing conditions and indicate that animals are not adapting to their environment.

Since 1990, the use of veal crates in the United Kingdom has been prohibited by government regulation, which requires that animals must have room to turn around, must have adequate iron to maintain full health and vigor, and, after 14 days, must have access to roughage to allow their gut to develop normally.[11] In practice, the regulation has led to calves being kept in groups on straw bedding, providing them with room to carry out natural behavior patterns and to have social contact. Similar legislation was subsequently proposed in the United States Congress as an amendment to the Animal Welfare Act, but it was not enacted into law.[12] More recently in the state of New Jersey a similar bill was enacted.[13]

THE PROTESTS

The campaign against the export of live animals, mainly sheep and calves from the United Kingdom to Europe, started in February 1994 but ended a few years later due to the ban on exports to Europe—a ban put into effect first because of bovine spongiform encephalopathy, or mad cow disease, and later because of foot (hoof) and mouth disease. In 2006 exports restarted, but the scale of protest has not been the same as it was around and just after 1994. The protests were originally motivated by animals being taken on long journeys, sometimes several days, without breaks for feeding, watering, and resting, a practice in violation of European laws and guidelines.[14] Animal "detectives," usually Royal Society for the Prevention of Cruelty to Animals (RSPCA) inspectors, followed the trucks and recorded the suffering of these animals on videos, including heat stress, dehydration, food deprivation, and death.[15] Some of the animals were also being slaughtered inhumanely, again in breach of European laws. Animal welfare campaigners called for meat animals to be exported "on the hook and not on the hoof." In 1995, U.K. laws were tightened and heavy fines were introduced for such illegal journeys (up to 1,000 pounds sterling—$1,900 U.S.—per animal). If several hundred animals were carried at one time, the total fine could be substantial.[16] In addition to transport and slaughter, various other aspects of the export trade were denounced as offensive, such as veal production in crates and the exportation of live lambs from the United Kingdom that would be killed only a few hours after arriving in France so they could be labeled and sold as "French lamb."

For these reasons, the export trade attracted publicity. Minor demonstrations began at ports. The larger ferry operators stopped taking live exports for fear of losing trade, which led to expanded publicity, followed by independent ferry operators attempting to pick up the animal trade from the minor ports. Public reports of these events shocked the British public. Protests against the export of animals took place at seaports all over the country. Ferry operators refused to carry farm animals. Exporters subsequently made their own arrangements for sea transport, but boarding the ships still required port access, which was successfully blocked by the protesters. Because the exporters were unable to use the seaports, they commissioned private companies to fly animals to Europe, but the protesters followed them to the airports.[17]

Some violence has occurred during these protests, but violence has been condemned by both the campaigning organizations and the majority of protesters.[18] The protests became well-organized picket lines, and it was claimed that the organizers could muster a vigil of around 200 persons on ordinary days, with up to 2,000 on days when an export was likely to take place.

Several countries condemned the veal crate system, but calf exports continued to increase while lamb exports decreased. Alan Clark, former U.K. government minister for defense, warned that the government and others involved could not continue to flout public opinion without expecting some form of backlash.

THE INTERESTED PARTIES

For farmers in the United Kingdom, the live animal export trade is claimed to be worth £200 million ($300 million U.S.). It processes 2.5 million lambs and calves a year. In 1993, approximately 500,000 calves were exported to Europe,[19] worth £92 million.[20] Around 90% of French and 80% of Dutch veal production was kept in crates.[21] Because so little veal is consumed in the United Kingdom and the crating system of producing white flesh has been banned, many purebred dairy calves are worth relatively little, and more money can be made if they are sent to market where they may be bought by foreign buyers or exporters who send them to Europe. The view of the U.K. National Farmers' Union is that as long as the veal trade is legal, it should be permitted to continue.

Dutch and U.S. farmers have aggressively disputed the claim that veal crates cause harm to the animals.[22] In the United States, until very recently, farmers have had their way. Prior to the election on November 7, 2006, no state in the United States banned veal crates. However, on that day Arizona voters passed an initiative called the Humane Treatment for Farm Animals Act that made Arizona the first state to prohibit veal crates (and also the second state to prohibit the confinement of breeding pigs in gestation crates; see chapter 2 on the factory farming of pigs).[23] Arizonans and many others see a broad range of harms. Rearing calves in the absence of their mother is thought to be psychologically stressful for both mother and calf due to the natural instinct of bonding. This bond can be established very quickly, even after only a few minutes, and calves are often kept with their mothers for at least 24 hours to allow them to take in colostrum.[24] Calves in a normal environment suckle for about a year, and the weaning process is prolonged. Alternative strategies for weaning are being developed, therefore, in order to minimize the distress caused by the current practice of abrupt removal.[25]

Some dairy farmers appear to be changing their breeding system to produce calves more suitable for the British beef market, rather than for European veal production.[26] Other farmers have capitalized on the welfare sensitivities of the general public by agreeing to produce veal in a welfare-friendly way. They have secured contracts with large supermarkets that advertise as calf-friendly. They have also restricted transport time to less than one hour to slaughterhouses, where the animals are killed immediately.[27]

Exporters and haulers have fought to retain their legal trade despite ferry companies and airlines banning live animals on their boats and airplanes. Port authorities claim that by law they have to take any cargo and have no other option but to accept live animals for export.[28] Exporters (probably fewer than 20 people in the United Kingdom are involved) have, under these conditions, commissioned their own boats and airplanes. As a result, some known individuals and their families have been personally attacked and harassed. There is evidence that some haulers are guilty of atrocities, but part of the problem stems from a need for better training of haulers and improvements in the design and standards of their trucks.[29]

The veterinary profession finds itself in a dilemma because a government veterinarian must sign a certificate stating that the animals are fit for travel prior to transport. By refusing to sign such certificates, government veterinarians could prevent all exports of live animals. Veterinarians have been under pressure from within their own ranks, as well as from outside bodies, not to sign certificates.[30] The chief veterinary officer has stated, however, that government veterinarians cannot refuse to sign an export certificate on grounds of conscience if the conditions for the certificate are in order, that is, if the animals are fit for travel and comply with disease control regulations.[31] The professional oath for veterinarians commits them "to ensure the welfare of animals committed to their care." Veterinarians are thus caught in a situation of being able to prevent the cruelties of long-distance transport and veal production while, as a consequence, having to resign from their positions as government employees.

Governments in Europe and the United Kingdom have responded in a variety of ways to these problems. For example, the United Kingdom has banned practices in veal production that promote poor welfare and has tightened national standards of animal transport.[32] Possibly as a result of the demonstrations, the U.K. government has also commissioned a research project (at a cost of £30,000 sterling; $45,000 U.S.) to demonstrate that quality veal can be produced profitably and humanely.[33] The government has been under considerable pressure to ban the export of calves, but it insists that it cannot do so because of the single-market trade agreement within the European Union (EU). The United Kingdom believes that the way to move forward is to raise standards throughout member states in the EU, and the EU has begun to do so as a result of pressure from both nongovernmental organizations (NGOs) and governments. Since January 1, 2007, no calf has been allowed to be kept in single crates or stalls or to be tethered.[34]

A major concern in any large country, however, is how to implement legislation and monitor standards fairly and effectively.[35] The transport of live animals has caused considerable furor, with little agreement among member states on journey times, rest, feed, and watering intervals. The EU Commission has heeded scientific advice on these issues, and new rules on transport came into force in 2007, including provisions such as the restriction of transport of calves less than ten days of age.[36]

Farmers claim that many of these calves are worth little because of their conformation and genetic makeup. If they did not send the calves to market, their only other option would be to kill the animals at birth. The organization Compassion in World Farming (CIWF) disputes that the poor conformation of some dairy calves prevents them from being raised for beef, because 40% of the beef sold in the United Kingdom is sold as minced meat used in meat pies, making quality of conformation irrelevant. They argue that farmers simply want to make "a few pennies more" and are choosing to sell to the highest bidder, which is likely to be the heavily subsidized continental veal producer.[37] CIWF maintains that U.K. dairy farmers are disadvantaging their beef counterparts, as well as slaughterhouse owners, by obtaining such high prices for their calves. They claim that this strategy prevents beef farmers from buying and rearing home-grown calves.

The public in the United Kingdom consumes little veal, both because veal is expensive and because many citizens consider such consumption unethical. Veal consumption in France averages 5.6 kg per head of population, Italy 4.0 kg, and United States 0.68 kg, compared with 0.1 kg in Britain.[38] The increase in public concern has been heightened by media coverage that presents the sight of the large baleful eyes of calves poking their heads out between the bars of the trucks held up at the ports. These scenes have engendered empathic public responses and have encouraged some people to protest against the live animal export and veal trades.

The protesters range from those who have never been in a demonstration before and who have been shocked by what they have recently learned about the veal and export trades, to those who are frequently involved in protests against various misuses and abuses of animals. The protests have also attracted some who are committed to violence and who use any demonstration or crowd-gathering event for their own ends.[39]

The U.K. police are in a difficult position because they are legally bound to enforce what is lawful. At one port, the police introduced a restriction that exports could take place only on two consecutive days of the week in order to reduce the costs of police protection, but in a major court action by a livestock transport company, a judge ruled that this restriction is unlawful.[40] The police can be sued in Britain for compensation for the loss of trade.

Retailers in the United Kingdom, including many supermarkets, now claim to sell only British veal, which accounts for one-third of that consumed, the rest coming from Europe and being sold through other outlets, presumably to the restaurant trade. Some supermarkets have contracted with farms to produce veal in a welfare-friendly way. However, these changes, together with relabeling the veal as "baby beef" or "lightweight rose beef," do not seem to have changed the public's views.

Several professions have been affected by these developments. Gourmet restaurants frequently serve veal, which is described in the Larousse Gastronomique as "pale meat, smelling of milk, with satiny white fat." Julia Child has similar tastes: "Pick veal by its color, pale creamy pink about the shade of raw chicken thigh. Some cuts of the dark pink or reddish so-called free-range veal may be tender, but in my opinion, it neither looks nor tastes like veal. It should be called calf."[41] Milk-substitute manufacturers have also been affected. One manufacturer (Volac) has withdrawn from supplying veal farmers with milk powder: "British people don't like it and it will never lose its reputation for cruelty whatever the welfare standards are."[42]

ETHICAL ISSUES

Animal Rearing Systems: Cruel or Welfare Friendly?

Many methods of farm animal husbandry, particularly those that involve confinement or intensive systems, continue to raise concerns. An analytical approach by which to assess welfare was first put forward in the United Kingdom by the Brambell Committee in 1965. It proposed that animals should have the freedom to stand up, lie down, turn around, groom themselves, and stretch their limbs. This was developed into the "Five Freedoms" by the U.K. Farm Animal Welfare Council:[43]

1. Freedom from thirst, hunger, and malnutrition
2. Freedom from discomfort
3. Freedom from pain, injury, and disease
4. Freedom to express normal behavior
5. Freedom from fear and distress

These Five Freedoms are goals by which to evaluate a particular system of husbandry. In effect it is an ethical framework for analysis of cases. It does not mean that a particular system is or must be completely free from the mentioned harm(s), but only that some systems are better at avoiding, mitigating, or alleviating a specific harm than are other systems of husbandry. The Five Freedoms strategy also implies that, with good management, an owner of animals can and should minimize any fear, discomfort, and the like that might be caused by that system of husbandry.

The veal crate system fails to meet these goals, particularly the fourth, second, and first. If loading, transport, and unloading of calves is also taken into account, then fear and distress will also be incurred, contravening the fifth goal.

Many participants in these discussions have pointed out that alternative, more welfare-friendly husbandry systems can be practically put in place. For example, it is possible to rear animals in groups that provide them with social contact and to supply the space for them to display many of the natural behaviors that they would display in fields. The provision of higher levels of iron could prevent the animals from becoming anemic, but the flesh would be pink, not white. No evidence indicates that keeping these animals in the dark causes their meat to be white, which means that natural daylight can be provided without cost to farmers (and, by and large, it now is provided in the United Kingdom). The provision of straw allows for normal physiological development of the rumen without affecting meat quality other than its color. The provision of dry food, rather than an exclusively liquid diet, can help meet the physiological needs of the animals, but it also makes the system slightly less profitable.

An important ethical question that arises, in light of cost-benefit analyses of implementing alternative husbandry systems, is this: Under what conditions, if any, should farmers be permitted to sacrifice animal welfare for personal gain? Farmers receive substantial agricultural subsidies from the public purse, without which they would not be able to survive. Does this support oblige them to be responsive to public opinion about animal welfare? Should the government require that they be even more responsive?

Should the government subsidize these forms of responsiveness? Do farmers and government officials have a moral responsibility to use or allow only welfare-friendly alternatives? If the public will not buy the welfare-friendly product and will instead buy cheaper, less welfare-friendly alternatives, then welfare-friendly farmers will not survive (or perhaps will survive less well). What responsibilities, if any, does the general public have in making purchases?

Another important question is whether farmers have a stronger obligation to protect animals than do other members of society. It could be suggested that farmers are society's stewards of animals. If they fail to meet either *society's* (reasonable) expectations of animal welfare or *general moral standards* of appropriate care, then they not only undermine their guardian status, but they also set in place a resistance to eating meat and other animal products. They also leave many moral problems unaddressed.

Do Veterinarians Have Special Responsibilities?

Veterinarians subscribe to an oath stating that they are obliged to protect animals. As a result of this commitment and their professional training, society accords veterinarians special privileges and assigns them certain responsibilities, though any wording that states those responsibilities is very general and in need of specification. What, precisely, are veterinarians entrusted to do in caring for and protecting animals in the present case? By not signing certificates of fitness for animals to travel, U.K. veterinarians would not be committing an illegal act, but would they endanger their government positions? Is it *social* responsibilities that are at stake, or rather *personal* responsibilities that derive from the moral obligations and ideals of veterinarians?

Perhaps it is a matter of conscientious objection, which has had an honorable tradition in Western moral and political thinking. Moral conflicts of conscience sometimes emerge because people regard as unethical some role obligation or official order that descends from a hierarchical structure of authority. In many cases, such as the refusal to sign a certificate, the individual need not rebuke others or obstruct them from performing an act, but only says, "Not through me will this be done." Occasionally this situation arises when a veterinarian refuses to perform a procedure requested by an owner, customer, or institution. Even if a veterinarian wishes not to comply with a request to perform a legal act, it may still be right to respect the conscientious conviction. The veterinarian is then free to withdraw from the circumstance.

In some situations, however, the question is not whether the veterinarian has a *right* to refuse involvement, but rather a *duty* to refuse involvement. Which, if either, best characterizes the present case? In the United States, the American Veterinary Medical Association (AVMA) at its 2006 annual meeting rejected a resolution from the Farm Sanctuary proposing that veterinarians place "a higher priority on animal welfare when required to choose between animal welfare and economic considerations."[44] Instead they passed a resolution that supports the "responsible use of animals for human purposes." In that context, they chose to place human enterprises above the welfare interests of animals.[45] Under this resolution, it appears to be acceptable that calves can be tethered, constrained so that they cannot make social contact, etc. However, the exact wording of the resolution is cautious and rather difficult to interpret.

The following is the paragraph at the AVMA website (as this case goes to press):

[Resolution 8] The AVMA affirms that the responsible use of animals for human purposes such as companionship, food, fiber, education, exhibition, and research conducted for the benefit of humans and other animals is consistent with the principles of the Veterinarian's Oath. These principles include the protection of animal health, the relief of animal suffering, the conservation of animal resources, the promotion of public health, and the advancement of medical knowledge.

The resolution mentions nothing about *excluding* psychological concerns and other considerations of "animal health," and it does not claim that the "responsible" use of animals can include tethering them. At the same time, the AVMA also does not state that a veterinarian must *include* such considerations in assessing the health and welfare of animals. The AVMA, it appears, leaves these moral questions open; the veterinarian may do as he or she sees fit.

Moral Coherence and Social Solidarity

Veal crates were banned in the United Kingdom in 1990. The method was considered unacceptable on grounds that it caused avoidable animal suffering. Questions of moral coherence arise when a country bans a product for ethical reasons and yet permits importation of the same product from another country. Furthermore, retailers and restaurant owners in the United Kingdom are permitted to sell veal, the public is allowed to purchase it, farmers and exporters can provide animals for its production, and haulers are able to transport it long distances. They are all part of a society that, in one part of its official public policy, has deemed veal crates to be cruel and unacceptable, and yet, in another part of its public policy, allows the trade with full knowledge of what happens to the animals.[46]

This problem of moral coherence arose in a dramatic fashion in Britain in a celebrated case of the U.K. Minister of Agriculture and his wife. They jointly owned a farm that raised and sold cattle. The minister's wife was producing and recommending veal recipes, while her husband served as the minister of state and was responsible for ensuring that veal crates and other banned conditions were not used in the United Kingdom. While both husband and wife could be said to have maintained their moral integrity by each remaining faithful to their individual moral views, many in Britain sensed that the minister had an untenable conflict of interest, especially in light of the fact that he and his wife had a beef cattle farm that exported their cattle to continental Europe.[47]

The Ethics of Gourmet Writers and Chefs

A related moral issue concerns whether gourmet recipe writers and chefs have a responsibility to encourage people not to eat animal products that are produced inhumanely. In some parts of Southeast Asia, dogs are strung up off the ground and beaten in order to tenderize the flesh before they are killed and consumed, snakes are skinned alive, and cats are immersed in cauldrons of boiling water to kill them, rather like lobsters. Would it be acceptable for gourmet writers to produce recipes specifying that these ingredients make for the best dishes? If it is morally evil to kill animals in these ways, would it be a *comparable* moral evil to recommend use of meats killed in this way, or to supply such meat to restaurants? Are these truly comparable events? If not, how do we delineate the boundary between an unacceptable and an acceptable use of farm animals and related forms of animal supply?

In a dialogue between top chefs Julia Child and Paul Prudhomme, Child recalls that male calves "in the old days" were disposed of by being left in a ditch to die, but they now can survive and are raised as veal.[48] She implies that today's practices in raising veal are acceptable because they upgrade a worse bygone practice. Is this a valid line of argument, or is it fallacious? Prudhomme and Child go on to discuss the famous "Bambi syndrome." They lament false depictions in which fantasy animals are elevated to the same status and value as human beings.

There is no doubt that cartoons and Disney movies depict animals unrealistically, but does the fact of fantasy in this realm provide any basis for saying that animals have no moral status or value or, if some value, much less value? Prudhomme states, "I would love that person to be really hungry and put in the same place [location] as that animal and still think of it as something they can't touch. They'd take out a knife, cut its throat, and eat it very quickly." This claim is bold, because it suggests that even the strongest defenders of animal rights would so behave. Setting aside this question of what such persons *would* do, what does Prudhomme's claim show *morally?* Hungry people have been known to eat other humans at such time. Is this a valid test of value or yet another challenge to moral coherence, or some other sort of moral problem?

Do Some Animals Have Higher Moral Status Than Calves?

In order to prevent the export of unwanted horses to continental Europe to be killed for meat, the U.K. government permits only horses over a certain monetary value to be exported. The value is high enough to make the trade uneconomic. This special treatment of horses raises questions of whether and why horses are morally different from other species, such as cattle and sheep. Many in the public appear to hold horses in high esteem and attribute higher moral status to them than to beef cattle. Is it because of our closer relationships with some animals on specific kinds of farms (notably horse farms)? Horses have always been seen as noble creatures, even in ancient literature, and we commonly interact with them more intimately than with other farm animals such as cattle—often in very different settings and for different purposes. Does this general outlook justify making horses a special case with increased protection? Is this the same kind of problem we have in conferring higher status on primates (see the introduction, pp. 16–18, and chapter 10) or a different problem? What should we say about cats and dogs? Why should the life of a calf be less worthy of protection than the life of a puppy?

How Far Can Protesters Legitimately Go?

Protesters who feel that some lawful activity is morally wrong have several options (beyond becoming vegetarians or vegans).[49] They can make their views known by attempting to rationally persuade others to change practices. For example, they can communicate their concerns and argue their case to the public, to governments, and to producers. In one recent case in the United Kingdom, protestors dug up a grave and removed the bones of a relative of a farmer who had supplied animals for research. They targeted others in the village with whom the farmer had only indirect connections.[50] These tactics seem extreme and unwarranted, but when protesters feel ignored or believe their protests have failed, they often consider themselves helpless in the face of what they believe to be deep moral wrongs. They may regard forceful protests as their only recourse. In the case of the export of veal calves, many with no particular axe to grind feel strongly about the moral wrongness of the practice.

Although there was some violence by a small number of persons (damaging trucks and harassing police), the picket lines in the United Kingdom were generally peaceful. Civil disobedience can be nonviolent and has been used in many social movements to achieve change after other efforts have failed. But, again, where are the limits of non-violent protest to be drawn? Lying down in front of trucks to try to prevent them moving forward had a tragic consequence in the veal protests and may, like many tactics, be questioned as a morally justified form of protest. But how does one draw the line between a justified and an unjustified strategy of protest?

NOTES

1. "Calf Protest Victim Was Sacrificed to a Vile Trade," *Daily Telegraph*, August 16, 1995, p. 5.

2. At Brightlingsea, 30 people, including a 78-year-old woman, were arrested for willful obstruction of the highway; *Daily Telegraph*, February 11, 1995, and February 19, 1995.

3. See South Dakota State University, "Special Fed Veal," issued October 19, 2004, ars. sdstate.edu/animaliss/veal.html (accessed August 24, 2007).

4. See Pays de Abers, Les Viandes: Le veau. Date not given. www.cadour.net/cuisine/veau. htm (accessed August 24, 2007).

5. See "Better Cuisine, Topics: Veal," www.vealusa.com/What_is_Veal/history.html; Fur Commission USA Press Release of January 26, 2003; Teresa Platt, "Amish Veal Producers Threatened by NJ Politicos: Consequences for All Livestock Farmers?" www.furcommission. com/news/newsF05z.htm#Anchor-49575 (both accessed August 24, 2007).

6. J. Webster, C. Saville, and D. Welchman, *Improved Husbandry Systems for Veal Calves* (Bristol, UK: Department of Animal Husbandry, University of Bristol School of Veterinary Science, 1986).

7. See South Dakota State University, "Special Fed Veal," October 19, 2004, ars.sdstate. edu/animaliss/veal.html (accessed August 24, 2007).

8. Calves at pasture, when fed a natural diet, gain 1.8–2 pounds per day.

9. Royal Society for the Prevention of Cruelty to Animals, Farm Animals Information Leaflet on Veal Production (Horsham, UK: RSPCA, April 1995).

10. A. J. F. Webster, C. Saville, B. M. Church, A. Gnanasakthy, and R. Moss, "Some Effects of Different Rearing Systems on Health, Cleanliness and Injury in Calves," *British Veterinary Journal* 141 (1985): 472.

11. In the United Kingdom, the Welfare of Calves Regulations 1987 (SI 2021) came into force on January 1, 1990, and is now embodied in Schedule 2 to the Welfare of Livestock Regulations of 1994.

12. HR 263: "To amend the Animal Welfare Act to require humane living conditions for calves raised for the production of veal." Introduced January 4, 1996, by Andrew Jacobs (D-IN) in the 104th Congress.

13. See M. L. Westendorf, "LookSmart," August 2004, findarticles.com/p/articles/mi_qa4035/is_200408/ai_n9455196; S1478 (accessed August 24, 2007).

14. The RSPCA has archival evidence in-house according to a Compassion in World Farming briefing, "The Export of Live Animals," February 4, 1994.

15. Compassion in World Farming video, "For a Few Pennies More." Available from CIWF, Charles House, 5a Charles Street, Petersfield, Hampshire, GU32 3EH, United Kingdom.

16. The U.K. Welfare of Animals during Transport Order (1995), made under the Animal Health Act of 1981.

17. Phoenix Aviation tried to open an "air bridge" for live exports to Europe from Bournemouth, but the local authority refused them a license. One of their planes crashed on December 21, 1994, killing five members of the crew; see the *Independent* 5 (January 1995) and *Daily Telegraph*, February 9, 1995. In 2006 the airport authority in Doncaster was targeted and as a consequence has refused to handle live animals for export.

18. Truck windscreens have been smashed and haulers have had themselves and their homes and their families threatened with attack; see the *Daily Telegraph*, February 3, 1995 ("Mob Stones Country Home of Veal Flights Manager"); February 9, 1995 ("Death Note for Son of Flight Boss"); and February 21, 1995 ("Animal Export Chief Quits over Threats to His Family"). The *Guardian* ("Veal Protest at Waldegrave's Farm after Minister Gets Razors in Post," on January 16, 1995) reported that the minister of agriculture had received razors in the mail.

19. RSPCA Farm Animals Information Leaflet on Veal Production. Of the 0.4 million calves, 192,000 went to France, 177,000 to Holland, and 46,000 to Belgium and Luxembourg.

20. See Trade and Environment Database, UK Veal Exports, November 1, 1997, www.american.edu/TED/VEAL.HTM (accessed August 24, 2007).

21. G. C. Barling, *Welfare of Calves: Lawfulness of Export Restrictions* (London: Berwin, 1995), p. 4; "Editorial Comment," *Veterinary Record*, April 8, 1995, p. 338.

22. A spokeswoman for the Dutch Landbouwschap Farmers organization said there was no evidence that rearing the calves in crates harmed the animals' welfare; "The Science of Veal Calf Welfare and Nutrition: Executive Summary," January 10, 1995, www.vealusa.com/Media/vealsci.pdf (accessed August 24, 2007).

23. "Election '06: Animals Win in Arizona and Michigan," November 7, 2006, community.hsus.org/ct/up1ktWF1wRjj/ (accessed August 24, 2007); 62% of the voters and 11 out of 15 Arizona counties supported the measure.

24. F. C. Flower and D. M. Weary, "Effects of Early Separation on the Dairy Cow and Calf: Separation at One Day and Two Weeks after Birth," *Applied Animal Behavior Science* 70 (2001): 275–84.

25. D. B. Haley, W. Bailey, and J. M. Stookey, "The Effects of Weaning Beef Calves in Two Stages on Their Behavior and Growth Rate," *Journal of Animal Science* 83 (2005): 2205–14.

26. David Brown, "Calf Protests Open up Bull Market for British Beef Stock," *Daily Telegraph* (February 11, 1995) reported that pedigree beef bulls were fetching record prices.

27. Katy Brown, "Veal, the Facts You Should Know," *Country Living* (April 1995): 45–46.

28. The Harbors, Docks and Piers Act (1847) on one interpretation compels a port to accept any lawful cargo.

29. The RSPCA found that, on average, nine out of ten trucks exceed maximum journey times. One consignment supposedly destined for Holland ended up in Greece two and a half days later with 400 of 600 animals dead; David Nicholson-Lord, "Green Lobby with Power to Pluck at Heartstrings," *Independent*, January 5, 1995.

30. Joyce D'Silva, "Veterinarians and Animal Transport," *Veterinary Record*, April 8, 1995, p. 371.

31. Anon., "Welfare of Animals during Transport," *Veterinary Record*, March 25, 1995, p. 282; Neil King, "Veterinary Certification for Livestock Export," *Veterinary Record*, June 3, 1995, p. 571.

32. United Kingdom, Welfare of Calves Regulations 1987 (Statutory Instrument 2021).

33. Demonstration unit at ADAS Research Center, Rosemaund, Hereford. See David Brown, "Humane Veal Unit Has Beds of Straw and Room to Move," *Daily Telegraph*, May 24, 1995, and Toby Harndon, "Kinder Veal Farming Could Cut Calf Exports," July 21, 1995.

34. See EU Council Directive, November 19, 1991, on laying down minimum standards for the protection of calves, europa.eu.int/eur-lex/en/consleg/pdf/1991/en_1991L0629_do_001.pdf (accessed August 24, 2007).

35. There has been a string of cases "uncovered" by the RSPCA after following U.K. haulers. For example, on January 6, 1995, three British firms that export live calves were found guilty of animal cruelty. The prosecution claimed that calves were packed into trucks for 37 hours without food, water, or rest for a journey of 1,100 miles to southwest France (Reuters report, January 7, 1995, London). For Compassion in World Farming videos and cases, see Agscene 118 (Summer 1995): 3–8, and "The Case against the Veal Crate 2001." Detailed study of scientific evidence

given in the EU's SVC report on veal calves (1995) that led to legislative reform and ban (1997) on veal crates in EU from 2007. Written for US and other countries where veal crates still legal. Includes alternative systems used in Netherlands, Italy and France," www.ciwf.org/publications/veal.html (accessed August 24, 2007).

36. See UK Department for Food, Environment and Rural Affairs (defra), "Animal Welfare: Implementation of EU Welfare in Transport Regulation," (EC) No 1/2005-Main Requirements, www.defra.gov.uk/animalh/welfare/farmed/transport/eu-treg_detail.htm (accessed August 24, 2007).

37. *Agscene* reported on a Meat and Livestock Commission conference in April 1995: "The Case against the Veal Crate 2001" (as above note 35).

38. *Independent,* "A Heavy Diet of Hypocrisy," January 13, 1995, quoting UK National Farmers' Union figures.

39. James Ehrlichman, "Rent-a-Mob Fear Drives Away Farm Campaigners," *Guardian,* January 5, 1995; "Protests Continue as Live Exports Resume," *Veterinary Record,* April 29, 1995, p. 427.

40. Terence Shaw, "Police Curb on Animal Export Was Unlawful," *Daily Telegraph,* July 27, 1995.

41. Julia Child, *The Way to Cook* (New York: Alfred A. Knopf, 1995), p. 207.

42. Katy Brown, "Veal, the Facts You Should Know," *Country Living* (April 1995), pp. 45–46.

43. Farm Animal Welfare Council, *Second Report on Priorities for Research and Development in Farm Animal Welfare* (London: Ministry of Agriculture Fisheries and Food, Tolworth, 1993).

44. See American Veterinary Medical Association (June 2005), www.avma.org/issues/policy/animal_welfare/veal_calf.asp (accessed August 24, 2007).

45. See American Veterinary Medical Association (June 2005)—now removed online because later Congress proceedings are reported at www.avma.org/convention/news/monday02.asp and www.avma.org/onlnews/javma/jun06/060615c.asp.

46. D. B. Morton, "Ethics of Farm Animal Exports," *Veterinary Record,* March 11, 1995, p. 252. A similar situation applies to drugs that are developed in other countries using animals in research models that are banned in the United Kingdom (e.g., models of learned helplessness and the development of antidepressants).

47. Trade and Environment Database, UK Veal Exports, November 1, 1997, www.american.edu/TED/VEAL.HTM (accessed August 24, 2007).

48. *Modern Maturity* (Winter 1994), as quoted in *Animals' Agenda* 15, no. 4, p. 13.

49. See en.wikipedia.org/wiki/Vegan (accessed August 24, 2007).

50. Nicola Woodcock, "Animal Rights Grave-Robbers Are Given 12 Years Each," *The Times* (London), May 12, 2006, provides a summary.

4

What Is a Chicken Worth?

"This must constitute, in both magnitude and severity, the single most severe, systematic example of man's inhumanity to another sentient animal."[1] So said John Webster, emeritus professor of animal husbandry at the University of Bristol's Veterinary School. He was referring, rather surprisingly, to broiler chickens. In reaching this conclusion, he noted that in the United Kingdom alone, one-quarter of the heavy strains of these animals are in chronic pain for at least one-third of their six-week lives; only 10% are able to walk normally; up to 6% die during rearing; 4% have chronic arthritis; 3% break their bones; and 2 million die during transport each year. In 2003, some 9.1 billion of these animals were eaten in the United States,[2] 3.5 billion in the European Union,[3] and 840 million in the United Kingdom.[4]

THE BROILER CHICKEN INDUSTRY

In less than 50 years, the broiler chicken—so named because of the way it is cooked—has become one of the most common animals consumed in human diets. The poultry meat sector is a significant employer (40,000 to 50,000 jobs in the United Kingdom alone) as well as a major consumer of cereals, soy, and meat, bone, and fish meals. These birds are reared intensively, in large numbers and at relatively low cost, and they provide a ready source of palatable tender meat for many people.[5] It takes less than seven weeks to complete the growth process from chick to table-ready product, and farming methods have become heavily engineered and automated to help meet the birds' physiological requirements, as well as to facilitate their catching, transport, and slaughter.

Some 10,000 to 50,000 (sometimes as high as 100,000) day-old chicks are reared in windowless sheds on a litter of wood shavings, chopped straw, or shredded newspaper. A farmer (sometimes referred to as the producer or grower) might have responsibility for several sheds. The birds are maintained under near-continuous low-level lighting for 23, even 24 hours a day in order to discourage the birds from becoming overactive, which would lead to aggression and divert energy consumed in the diet away from body growth. Unlike chickens kept in cages for egg production, broiler chickens display little cannibalism or feather pecking. The litter is gradually "replaced" by feces, and the original shed floor is difficult to see after two to three weeks. In areas of water spillage, or if the ventilation is inadequate, the floor can become damp and smelly, which can, in turn, lead to skin lesions.[6] The surface of the litter can also become hard and cause contact dermatitis such as hock burns and breast blisters as the birds lie down.

Ventilation is provided by means of louvers and automated fans in the roof and sides of the building, though some farmers may have heat exchange or evaporative cooling systems. The ventilation controls ambient temperature and humidity by way of regu-lating airflow, which also helps to avoid the buildup of irritant and toxic gases such as carbon dioxide and ammonia from the litter. In cold weather the ventilation rate is reduced, sometimes leading to a buildup of these gases (particularly ammonia) and causing damp litter. High outside temperatures can also have important consequences, because the ventilation system has to cope with the hot weather in addition to the heat the birds themselves produce.

The heat produced by the birds increases substantially as they get heavier, and there-fore a spell of hot weather at the end of their commercial growth period can be ruinous.[7] In hot weather, surplus heat has to be removed or the birds will grow more slowly or even die of heat stress and high humidity.[8] If the ventilation fails—e.g., during a power failure—tens of thousands of birds can die overnight.[9] In hot, dry climates, such as parts of the Middle East, the provision of adequate humidity to prevent the birds from dying of dehydration is a major problem.

The birds have been intensively bred and almost exclusively selected for rapid growth, food conversion rate, high appetite, and breast muscle volume, though this is changing for the selection of more robust and disease-resistant animals. They are provided with a nutritionally balanced, high-protein, high-energy diet, which accounts for about 70% of the cost of production. Water and food are always available throughout the shed in specific feeding areas. Various dietary formulations are given to the birds, depending on their age. Initially, they are fed a high protein "starter" diet, which is later followed by a lower protein "grower" diet. Both diets contain growth promoters, as well as antibiotics and antiparasite drugs to prevent clinical infections.[10] For the last five days or so they are given a "finisher" diet free of chemical additives.

In Europe there is a space allowance of 0.5 square feet (450 sq cm) per bird at the outset of stocking, but toward the end of the production time, when the birds have sig-nificantly increased in size and weight by some 25-fold, this space becomes extremely small. The floor becomes "carpeted" with birds. In the United States and the United Kingdom, the maximum recommended stocking density is around seven pounds of bird mass for every square foot, which is approximately equivalent to a space allowance of one bird on a single sheet of legal-size paper.[11]

The birds are put through the system on an all-in/all-out policy. That is, the birds are all started at the same time and, after a predetermined length of time has passed or a sufficient number of birds has reached the finishing weight, the batch is considered ready to go to slaughter. The sheds are then thoroughly cleaned and disinfected in order to minimize the risk of cross infection between batches. Rates of disease due to infection are generally low because animals are routinely given vaccines and treated with other preventive measures.

The food is removed for several hours before teams of catchers come in and load the birds into crates, which are then packed onto open trucks. The birds are unloaded at the processing factory and shackled by their legs onto a moving conveyer belt. Once on the conveyer belt, the birds' heads are dipped into a water bath, at which point they are stunned instantaneously by an electric current passing between the shackles and their heads. They then pass through a mechanical neck cutter where their throats are cut so that they bleed to death before passing through a scalding water tank, which facilitates plucking. The carcass is then eviscerated (the chance of fecal contamination of the plant due to intestinal perforation during evisceration is reduced by the removal of food before transport) and inspected for public health reasons. The carcass is dressed, cooled, and packed according to the retailer's requirements.

HEALTH AND WELFARE CONSIDERATIONS

There are practical difficulties in the production methods described above that make it difficult to ensure normal good farming husbandry practices, such as daily inspection and killing of birds that are irretrievably sick. This problem is exacerbated by the large number of birds per stockperson, the low lighting levels, and the high density of stocking, all of which make adequate inspection difficult, if not impossible.[12]

Problems of Leg Weakness and Lameness

Daily inspection to cull sick and moribund birds is important because many develop a lameness or "leg weakness," which can sometimes be severe enough to cause death because the animals are not able to reach food and water. It is thought that the leg weakness is partly due to the disparity in growth between the muscle tissue and the skeletal frame needed to support the weight of the body and muscular activity, particularly in the last two weeks of their lives.

S. C. Kestin and coworkers (as well as others) have carried out surveys of leg weakness in birds reared under normal commercial conditions.[13] They scored the birds for lameness and found that only one-tenth of the birds walked normally. The rest (90%) had detectable gait abnormalities. Gait was scored on a scale from zero to five; a score of zero represented no detectable abnormality, the bird being dexterous and agile. At the other end of the scale, a bird with a score of five was incapable of sustained walking, though it might be able to stand. Locomotion in score-five birds could be achieved only with the assistance of wings or by crawling on their shanks. Between normal and severely abnormal gaits, a score of three was given when a bird had an obvious gait defect, which might comprise a limp, a jerky or unsteady strut, or a marked splaying of one leg as it moved. Such birds often preferred to squat when not made to move, and their maneuverability, acceleration, and speed were adversely affected by their gait defect. (Overall, several studies show that 26%–30% of birds had gait scores of three or above at some point during their lifetime.)[14]

When the behavioral patterns of these birds were examined, it was found that broiler chickens without any leg weakness spent 80% of their time lying down. This figure increased to 88% in moderately lame birds, which also spent 40% less time walking. Further studies showed that unaffected, normal gait birds made 70 visits to the feeders for a total of 67 minutes a day, whereas gait score-three birds made only 32 visits but for the same length of time. Other work has shown that analgesic drugs can reverse some of these observations and increase the number of visits to the feeders by score-three or higher birds, indicating that these birds may be in pain.[15]

Lameness is important not only because of the pain involved, but also because the birds may not be able to feed properly, stunting their growth. One study showed that when the birds were allowed to live longer, to 85 days of age, in order to breed, 20% of males and 16% of females died.[16] Studies of the causes and pathology of leg weakness indicate that it is a complex disease with three main causes. The cartilage from which the drumstick bone (tibia) grows and develops may be malformed (tibial dyschondroplasia); there may be a septic arthritis; or the Achilles tendon of the main muscle in the drumstick may become displaced from the hock or ankle bone. In humans and other animals, all of these conditions are likely to cause pain, either directly or indirectly, which suggests that many of these animals are constantly in some pain. Every year hundreds of millions of birds in the United States would be in this condition.

The genetic make-up of these birds has inevitably exacerbated their leg problems through their selection for appetite and fast body muscle growth, coupled with a highly nutritious and energy-rich diet. The lack of space for exercise during the latter part of their rearing could also contribute to leg weakness, as exercise can promote strength and proper bone development. Alternatively, even if there were sufficient space, the birds might not be able to use it because of their leg and respiratory problems. Many birds with severe leg weakness can die of dehydration or be trampled by others as they become exhausted trying to reach the food and water stations, which are raised off the ground to avoid contamination.

Given these problems, many now believe that good-practice standards should be formulated that require twice-daily inspections to cull severely affected birds.

Lung, Heart, and Contact-Dermatitis Problems

Leg weakness is not the only problem for these birds.[17] They also suffer from lung infections and heart disease (1%), leading to congestive heart failure and an accumulation of fluids in the abdomen (ascites).[18] Other birds develop blisters over the breast as well as hock "burns" or "scalds" due to the close contact with the damp litter when they squat, which is more likely to occur when birds suffer from leg weakness.[19] One survey showed that 29% of birds had hock burns.[20] These superficial skin lesions are likely to be uncomfortable, even painful, and they may be likened to grazes or wet eczema on humans. The mortality of birds in the sheds before they are taken to the slaughterhouse increases with age, but typically may be 6%. The difficulties faced by the birds do not end, however, when they are removed from the environment of the sheds.

Problems in Catching, Transport, and Slaughter

Catchers of chickens are charged with "depopulating" sheds that contain tens of thousands of animals.[21] The litter, dust, darkness, and high levels of ammonia make it an arduous and unpleasant task for both humans and birds. The birds are "harvested" early in the morning, as fast as possible, because it appears less stressful for the birds, and also to ensure that the processing plants be kept busy during the day. They process birds at the rate of 5,000 to 10,000 per hour. Usually four birds are held in each hand by the feet (and sometimes wings, although this method is illegal in some countries).[22] This method has several disadvantages for the animals. The birds may be frightened by being handled roughly, by being carried upside down,[23] or by hearing the noise of other birds trying to escape.[24] If the animals are already in pain from the leg disorders described above, then this handling will compound any suffering. Legs are often inadvertently broken during catching.

The birds are then packed into crates from which they are removed at the processing factory. There is risk of injury during procedures at both locations, arising from inept handling that can lead to bruising and bone fractures. Studies have shown that 3% of birds have broken bones before they are stunned.[25] Between 0.19% and 0.42% of birds arrive dead at the processing factory. The deaths are due to preexisting pathology (25%), catching and transportation injuries (35%), or stress and suffocation (40%), with the proportions varying throughout the year. Some of the birds included in the study had more than one injury; 51% had died from congestive or acute heart failure; and 35% showed evidence of trauma such as dislocated and fractured hips, dislocated necks, ruptured livers, crushed heads, and intraperitoneal hemorrhage.

These injuries are not essential to the production process. Catching can be made more humane, and there can be significant differences in mortality rates between different teams of catchers.[26] If birds are removed from the crates one at a time, with the catcher holding two legs instead of one, fractures are less common (4.6% vs. 13.8%).[27] Mechanical harvesters, driven through the broiler house, have been designed to catch the birds using a sweeping system. The harvester has a retractable boom and sweeper arms fitted with rotating, foam-rubber paddles that move the birds onto an inclined conveyor and transfer them into a crate behind the harvester.[28] These machines appear to frighten the birds less than human contact,[29] and they have lower injury rates.[30]

During transport, the control of ventilation and temperature inside the carrying crates on the trucks is minimal, and birds are often exposed to outdoor elements. The animals may suffer not only from thermal stress, but also from noise, vibration, and motion stress, depending on the design of the truck, the route, and the skill of the driver.[31] It is difficult to maintain standards for transport at all times in a journey because temperatures and ventilation rates at standstill (for example, while loading and during traffic delays) are different from those when the vehicle is in motion.[32]

Finally, slaughter presents a controversial part of the process. Death is achieved by an electrically induced stoppage of the heart followed by bleeding. If insufficiently high currents are passed when the birds are being electrically stunned, they may recover consciousness before they die from loss of blood. There is a tendency in the industry to use a current that is too low, because a high electric current may cause a downgrading of the carcass due to hemorrhages in the breast muscles. Surveys have shown that the currents necessary to achieve cardiac arrest are not always reached and that if, in addition, the automatic neck cutters operate ineffectively, a small proportion of animals may still be conscious when they enter the scalding tank on the automated line.[33]

Processing plants sometimes employ people to ensure effective stunning and neck cutting so that only dead animals enter the scalding water tank. Advances have recently been made in the development of gas stunning and killing methods known as controlled atmosphere stunning. This method has several advantages even though it is not as rapid as the electrical methods. First, birds need not be removed from their crates at the processing plant, and they can be killed *in situ*. This avoids the problems and pain of shackling, failures of stunning, failures to bleed out properly, and entry into the scald tank while still alive. However, the gas used, carbon dioxide, is aversive to the animals until they become unconscious, and thus may cause the birds pain and distress. Consequently, better gas mixtures are being researched using inert gases such as argon, from which the animals would die from a shortage of oxygen. Early studies show little aversion in birds to these new gases. Experimental birds even seem to voluntarily enter such gas mixtures.[34]

Problems in the Production of Breeding Birds

Birds kept for breeding have to be reared to sexual maturity to produce eggs for future generations of broilers.[35] Only about 1% of the birds eaten are sexually mature. Selection of the breeding stock is for genetic lines that grow fast, convert food into muscle efficiently, and develop muscles in the right places (breast, thigh). However, the lifespan of most of these broiler birds, given unrestricted feed, would rarely be long enough for them to reach sexual maturity, due to the leg weaknesses and other diseases mentioned earlier.[36]

To mitigate this problem and keep these breeders alive and fertile, they are fed only a quarter to a half of their normal intake for their 60-week production life. This restriction appears to cause them to display behaviors such as abnormal preening and pecking at inanimate objects, presumably in an effort to satisfy their hunger drive. It has been suggested that these birds are in a constant state of hunger because of their restricted rations. Male breeding birds may have their toes removed, and both sexes may have their beaks trimmed, which has been shown to cause acute and chronic pain.[37] It is now being advocated that these breeding birds be caged in order to overcome poor breeding and fertility rates. This caging would restrict their ability to carry out natural behaviors such as dust bathing and wing flapping.[38]

These modern problems of efficient production can be compared with the systems of production 30 years ago, when chickens such as these grew at half the rate and relatively few were lost. The birds then took 86 days to reach five pounds, compared with 42 days today. The average flock size was closer to 1,500 birds, compared with 20,000 today. Husbandry and killing were not as mechanized, and poultry production was part of family farming. Moreover, chicken meat 25 years ago cost $3.75/lb., whereas currently it costs $0.46/lb. The industry "improvements" that have occurred over the past 30 years have led to increased production and consumption. Chicken is now widely regarded as a cheap, highly palatable, and healthy meat. These improvements for human producers and consumers have also meant higher animal death rates and animal suffering.

ETHICAL ISSUES

Several questions arise about the ethics of current practices in the treatment of broiler chickens. If these animals are to be used as sources of protein, can it be done at a lower cost to them, and, if so, are we morally obligated to reduce the suffering to a minimal level, even though it may mean consumers will have to pay more? Surveys show that the public's support of standards for improving animal welfare is strong, but this support often does not translate into shopping activities. Moreover, retailers try to persuade and even pressure farmers to produce meat ever more cheaply, which requires farmers to cut their costs further. Farmers claim that such cost cutting prevents them from being able to support animal welfare even if they wanted to. In a global market, retailers can also obtain chicken from countries where wages are lower and the climate is more appropriate to chicken production. Because of the concern that meat is being outsourced from areas that may not have high standards of care for the animals, farm and food assurance programs are being set up, together with food labeling schemes, that will inform consumers about welfare issues and about the country of origin.[39] However, even if the goal of having well-informed consumers is reached, this achievement will likely not resolve the most difficult ethical questions about cost-effective production processes and about the pain and suffering of farm animals.

Death Rates, Disease Levels, and Pain and Suffering

The death rates and noninfectious disease levels found in the broiler chicken industry are not tolerated in any other area of farming. In other parts of the food industry, the farmer would take remedial action, such as calling a veterinarian when a dairy cow is lame. Does our current legal tolerance of the situation in the broiler chicken industry arise from ignorance of what is happening on farms, the small size of the animal, the low margin of profit, or the low moral standing of chickens relative to other farm animals?

Clearly we need to *justify* any treatment of animals that causes suffering by taking account of their interests (utility from the animal's perspective) and not merely their utility as food (utility from the human perspective). We also have a moral obligation to prevent avoidable and unnecessary suffering in animals, even if the fulfillment of that obligation has the consequence of losing benefits for humans.[40] These obligations need not be interpreted as requiring that animals not be used as food sources, but they do suggest that practices in the chicken industry may need considerable rethinking.

A basic consideration is whether these birds suffer and feel pain. There is considerable physiological and behavioral evidence that they do, and no evidence that chickens are not able to experience pain. Chickens are also able to experience mental states such as fear, anxiety, hunger, thirst, discomfort, and distress.[41] Their sentience is beyond reasonable dispute. But what level of moral status do they obtain from being sentient, and is this the only way they gain moral standing?

Intelligence and Moral Status

Perhaps chickens deserve some level of moral status more from their intelligence than their sentience. Current evidence suggests that many species of birds display impressive signs of intelligence that, were humans aware of it, might deeply affect how we view these birds. Consider, for example, the particularly well-researched work of Irene Pepperberg with Alex the African Grey parrot.[42] Alex has demonstrated that he has the ability to count; to identify shapes, colors, and objects; and even to use words to express what he wants. He is able to identify objects that are presented in different shapes (for example, paper), link novel shapes and colors, and even identify shades of color correctly. Through these actions, Alex shows that he is able to make new, previously unlearned connections, confirming that he is not simply learning by rote. More remarkably, he apparently uses words like "no" to express feelings of annoyance, displeasure, and noncooperation, rather than his "native language" of a squawk or a screech. Experiments on other species of birds have also shown that they exhibit various forms of intelligence, including the ability to make tools using new materials and techniques—a form of intelligence extremely rare even in mammals.[43]

The data on intelligence in birds also suggests that their cognitive abilities may function to increase their suffering. It is generally acknowledged that animals with highly developed central nervous systems experience additional suffering as a consequence of their advanced mental abilities. For example, higher mental abilities may enable some animals to anticipate what may happen to them based on their earlier experiences, or they may have their desires frustrated. This anticipation and accompanying mental frustration may enhance the level of suffering they experience (in comparison with animals lacking in these capacities).

If chickens do experience not only pain but fear, distress, frustration, and other emotions, together with intelligent awareness of their circumstances, are we justified in treating them differently from other farm animals, such as sheep and cattle, which to date have not been shown to have quite such advanced capacities? If chickens are able to understand and suffer in these ways, ought we to be farming them in the ways currently practiced?

Desensitization

Perhaps it is the vast scale on which chickens are reared that desensitizes producers, veterinarians, and many others connected with the trade. This desensitization presents its own ethical issues. The care of a small group of animals is easy compared with the care of tens or hundreds of thousands of animals. The same problem may occur in the treatment of some humans in prisoner-of-war camps, or in schools or universities, or in the lives of busy physicians, veterinarians, and politicians. But can a lack of care be justified merely by the difficulties of caring for a creature in a large population? This would be an outrageous thesis if the population were human. Does moral consistency require that we take the same position with chickens that we take with humans?

Duties of care are normally understood in ethics as extending to all as much as to one, which is plainly impossible with broiler chickens as they are reared today. This is both a substantial problem of ethics and a massive practical problem in chicken farming. This problem of the practical care of large numbers of chickens may suggest that a compromise is in order. For example, perhaps we should allow industrial farming techniques but require more humane provisions of handling, slaughter, and care. In this way, the industry could be retained and its ethics substantially improved.

Desensitization with respect to broiler chickens may also be caused by the size of the animal. The bigger an animal, the more we tend to take notice of it. This may be because large animals show more obvious signs of pain, such as louder noises, and cause more damage to the surroundings when trying to escape pain. Humans may find it easier to relate to, and to recognize signs of pain in, the larger animals, particularly in mammals who live in close proximity to humans or who seem human-like. We may also not observe that small animals feel pain because we do not see the ways in which they are limited in their abilities to respond to painful situations. These animals may struggle but be relatively powerless to respond to their circumstance. They also may cry out in ultrasound frequencies that we are unable to hear, or they may freeze (remain immobile), which we then interpret as "not feeling any fear or pain." We may not recognize when small animals are afraid, distressed, or in some form of pain. Finally, small animals may find things painful that we cannot conceive as being so, such as high-frequency sounds, odors, and low or high temperatures. Humans also may not recognize in many cases what causes suffering in animals.[44]

Is it because these animals appear to be so different from our fellow humans and other mammals that we find it difficult to identify (empathize) with their suffering? If this were so, we would more likely be able to identify signs of pain in animals that look like us (for example, the great apes—gorillas, orangutans, chimpanzees) or to whom we are closely connected socially. There is evidence that many humans do find it much easier to identify with these animals. Josephine Donovan has suggested that women may, on the whole, be better at empathizing with them and detecting signs of suffering in them because of their caring nature or responsibilities, and that empathy should be seen as a valid tool of insight, which it currently is not in the case of animal welfare research.[45]

Finally, in the laws of some countries, primates, dogs, and cats are given special protection beyond that afforded to other mammals, whereas other animals are not deemed worthy of moral consideration at all, even though they might be remarkably similar to domesticated dogs and cats (e.g., wolves, coyotes, foxes, and feral cats).[46] These laws, like most moral norms regarding animals, are likely riddled with inconsistencies.

Practical Questions and Alternatives

To many interested in the ethics of the human uses of animals, the most pressing and urgent questions are practical ones: What might be done to eliminate or to alleviate some of the problems mentioned above? The following are some possibilities worthy of discussion. Many of these possible courses of action arise from questions about alternatives and the obligation to seek alternatives that are found elsewhere in this volume (see the introduction, pp. 32–34). Some of these alternatives have been implemented in various legal jurisdictions. From the moral perspective, it is worth asking whether these alternatives are morally required or simply have the status of moral ideals that some have proposed for our consideration.

1. We could stop eating chicken. Undoubtedly, in a short time this would decrease animal suffering. Not eating chicken raises the issue of whether people should become vegetarians or simply eat more welfare-friendly meat products. Most of us eat meat because of tradition and cost considerations and because it adds to our pleasures in life. But is the human benefit outweighed by the cost to the animals?

Believers in animal rights often accept either vegetarianism or veganism as a way forward because they believe that animals have a right to a life (or some comparable right) and should not be caused to suffer in any way, independent of considerations of utility for humans. Animal welfarists, on the other hand, tend to be utilitarians. They acknowledge that humans have a duty not to cause animals avoidable harm, but many animal welfarists are prepared to use animals for human benefit. They accept that some level of suffering may be necessary to produce food for humans, and they do not consider animal life to be sacrosanct. From both of these perspectives, one might find a justification for not eating animals such as chickens. The animal rights advocate believes that chickens should never be killed, whereas some animal welfarists believe that the harms done to the chickens are not outweighed by the benefits of eating chicken.

2. Codes of practice could be introduced (as has happened in some countries, including Canada, New Zealand, the United Kingdom, Sweden, and soon the EU) to help ensure good farming practices and enforce animal welfare standards.[47] This would help increase practices such as a backup power supply, minimum ventilation rates, maximum stocking densities, training of stockpersons, minimum inspection regimens, proper stunning currents, and so on. In addition, animal welfare targets—for example, acceptable levels of dermatitis, mortality, lameness, fractures, ineffective killings, minimum space allowance, and enrichment (say, with perches)—could be given forms of priority over agricultural productivity targets so that breeders, farmers, catchers, and processors would be penalized if they exceeded the established limits placed on pain and suffering.[48] Self-auditing could also be encouraged so that producers will assess their own performance based on score ratings for relevant criteria.[49]

It is also possible to feed the chickens less. The weight gain would then not be so rapid, and the disparity between body weight and skeletal growth not so great. This strategy could reduce leg problems by as much as 50%, but the financial profit per bird would also be reduced. In addition, since the birds have been bred for appetite, reductions of food would probably make the birds chronically hungry. Perches could be provided for the birds that would increase exercise and strengthen their legs for as long as they were motivated to get on and off the perches, but this maneuver might also increase breast blisters from perching. In addition, periods of darkness could be provided, which has been shown to improve skeletal strength. Perhaps most important is that breeders could select for birds that have strong legs and incorporate other health and welfare criteria into their selection programs, as is now starting to occur in some breeding locations.

Crating systems for transporting the birds to the slaughterhouse could be improved with larger openings in the crates so that it is easier to pack and unpack the birds. By increasing the size of the crates themselves, the birds could be killed by exposure to lethal concentrations of natural gases (for example, carbon dioxide or argon) while inside the crates, rather than being removed from the crates and killed by electrocution and bleeding. This strategy would eliminate the stresses and pain associated with unpacking and shackling. Teams of catchers could be paid a "welfare bonus" based on low fracture and bruising rates.

3. The public could pay more for chicken so that broilers could be reared more humanely and still be profitable. The public could be educated about production methods and the suffering of the animals, and chicken products could be labeled to indicate the system of production. If consumers were not prepared to pay more, or not that much more, then other avenues might have to be explored, such as lower profits for producers, processors, or retailers. Some retailers have found a premium market in the production of foods that help animals to maintain higher levels of welfare, but the market currently is relatively small.[50]

It is widely appreciated that animal welfare is itself becoming a factor in the market. Many consumers are attracted to these products, and more retailers are advertising their products as animal friendly (for example, free-range eggs and chicken). But there is concern that these advertisements may be misleading and could become little more than a war of words, misrepresentation, and mislabeling by advertisers and marketing managers. The Royal Society for the Prevention of Cruelty to Animals in the United Kingdom has recently launched Freedom Foods, a program in which farmers can register (providing they meet certain husbandry standards and their methods of production meet certain criteria) that entitles them to use the RSPCA label.[51] This provides the farmer with a niche market and a premium price in that market.

4. National laws could be changed. In the United States, poultry is sometimes exempt under state laws regarding animal cruelty because the birds are not considered "animals." In Europe, all farmed animals were once classified as insentient commodities such as vegetables and fruit, although it was recognized that there was a significant moral difference between sentient animals and objects that do not have the ability to experience pain and pleasure. Today animals are recognized as sentient beings, requiring that their sentience be taken into account when making regulations.[52]

5. International agreements and laws could be changed. We live in an increasingly global market, and the General Agreement on Tariffs and Trade (GATT) promotes world trade. If a country were to ban the importation of goods from another country on the basis of the method of producing those goods, it would be acting illegally and would (in principle) be penalized. The implication is that if stricter laws were introduced within a country to protect the well-being of animals, then cheaper, lower-level-of-welfare chicken imports would undercut welfare-friendly, home-produced products. This public policy could be disastrous, rather than helpful, to the interests of animals. But how far is the World Trade Organization (the controller of GATT) prepared to take the argument that methods of production are morally neutral and irrelevant? More important to ethical debate, how far should such organizations exert controls?

Finally, it is appropriate to finish this case study with a quotation from the same Professor John Webster with whom we began:

> Personally, I almost never eat broiler chicken unless it is of a light, slow growing strain, free range and usually corn fed. By so doing, I can eat smaller portions of a better tasting bird. . . . By such means I satisfy the needs of my conscience, my health (by eating relatively less meat and more vegetables) and my palate. To this consumer, this chicken has real added value.

NOTES

1. John Webster, *Animal Welfare: A Cool Eye towards Eden* (Oxford: Blackwell Science, 1995), p. 156.

2. See U.S. Poultry and Egg Association (Tucker, GA), www.poultryegg.org/Economic Info/ (accessed August 15, 2007).

3. See Ahmed ElAmin, "EU Broiler Production, Consumption Forecast to Rebound," e-news in foodindustry.com, www.cee-foodindustry.com/news/ng.asp?id=70260-avian-influenza-broiler-broiler (accessed September 1, 2006).

4. See British Poultry Council, www.poultry.uk.com/stats/Stats_2004/2004/chick_1.pdf (accessed August 15, 2007).

5. See European Commission, Health and Consumer Protection Directorate-General, Directorate B, Scientific Health Opinions, Unit B3, Management of Scientific Committees II, Report of the Scientific Committee on Animal Health and Animal Welfare, "The Welfare of Chickens Kept for Meat Production (Broilers)," Adopted March 21, 2000, chap. 5. ec.europa. eu/food/fs/sc/scah/out39_en.pdf (accessed August 15, 2007).

6. Farm Animal Welfare Council, *Report on the Welfare of Broiler Chickens* (Tolworth, UK: FAWC, 1992), p. 9. Available from MAFF/FAWC, Tolworth Tower, Surbiton, Surrey, KT6 7DX, United Kingdom.

7. In addition, feed intake falls by about 1.5% for every degree centigrade rise above normal temperatures (around 21 degrees Celsius, or 70 degrees Fahrenheit); the higher the temperature, the greater the depression of food intake.

8. Each bird produces 8W; if the shed has 40,000 birds then 320KW has to be removed at ambient temperatures such as 32 degrees Celsius, or 90 degrees Fahrenheit.

9. In some countries there is a legal requirement for there to be standby generators or high-temperature alarm systems.

10. In the European Union, the incorporation of antibiotics into animal feed has been banned since January 2006, unless it is for therapeutic reasons; see europa.eu.int/rapid/pressReleasesAction. do?reference=IP/05/1687&format=HTML&aged=0&language=EN&guiLanguage=en (accessed August 15, 2007).

11. Farm Animal Welfare Council, *Report on the Welfare of Broiler Chickens,* gives 34 kg/sq meter, which is about 750 sq cm per 2.5-kg bird (0.8 square feet per 5.5-pound bird).

12. One man in charge of four sheds each with 40,000 birds spending four hours day on inspection would need to check 11 birds per second, and no blinks. It is recommended that birds be inspected at least twice a day; sometimes they are inspected more frequently. Scanning of birds achieves a minimum level of inspection, but it is not sufficient to pick up all sick animals.

13. S. C. Kestin, T. G. Knowles, A. E. Tinch, and N. G. Gregory, "Prevalence of Leg Weakness in Broiler Chickens and Its Relationship with Genotype," *Veterinary Record* 131 (1992): 190–94. Kestin has extended his work on leg weakness to some 21 flocks, and basically similar results are being obtained. See S. C. Kestin, G. Su, and P. Sorensen, "Different Commercial Broiler Crosses Have Different Susceptibilities to Leg Weakness," *Poultry Science* 78 (1999): 1085–90; and K. S. Vestergaard and G.S. Sanotra, "Relationships between Leg Disorders and Changes in Behaviour of Broiler Chickens," *Veterinary Record* 144 (1999): 205–9.

14. G. S. Sanotra, "Recording of Current Leg Strength in Broilers," *Dyrenes Beskyttelese* (Danish Animal Welfare Society, 1999).

15. D. McGeown, T. C. Danbury, A. E. Waterman-Pearson, and S. C. Kestin, "Effect of Carpofen on Lameness in Broiler Chickens," *Veterinary Record* 144 (1999): 668–71.

16. P. Hunton, "The Broiler Industry: 34 Years of Progress," *Poultry International* 34 (July 1995): 28, 30.

17. See European Commission, Health and Consumer Protection Directorate-General, "The Welfare of Chickens Kept for Meat Production (Broilers)," chap. 6. ec.europa.eu/food/fs/sc/scah/ out39_en.pdf (accessed August 15, 2007).

18. B. H. Thorp and M. H. Maxwell, "Health Problems in Broiler Production," in *Proceedings of the 4th European Symposium on Poultry Welfare,* ed. C. J. Savory and B. O. Hughes (Wheathampstead, Hertfordshire, UK: Universities Federation for Animal Welfare, 1993), pp. 208–18.

19. See Farm Animal Welfare Council, *Report on the Welfare of Broiler Chickens,* p. 9. Channel 4 TV in the United Kingdom found that 82% of supermarket birds suffered from hock burn; see cityhippy.blogspot.com/2005/07/news-supermarket-secrets.html (accessed August 15, 2007).

20. N. G. Gregory and S. D. Austin, "Causes of Trauma in Broilers Arriving Dead at Poultry Processing Plants," *Veterinary Record* 131 (1992): 501–3; C. Ekstrand and T. E. Carpenter, "Spatial Aspects of Foot-Pad Dermatitis in Swedish Broilers," *Acta Veterinaria Scandinavica* 39 (1998): 273–80 (found a range of 0%–100%).

21. M. A. Mitchell and P. J. Kettlewell, "Catching and Transport of Broiler Chickens," in Savory and Hughes, *Proceedings of the 4th European Symposium on Poultry Welfare,* pp. 219–29.

22. P. A. Bayliss and M. H. Hinton, "Transportation of Broilers with Specific Reference to Mortality Rates," *Applied Animal Behavioral Science* 28 (1990): 93–118.

23. G. Kannan and J. A. Mench have found that carrying birds upright stresses them less; "Influence of Different Handling Methods and Crating Periods on Plasma Corticosterone Concentrations in Broilers," *British Poultry Science* 37 (1996): 21–31.

24. P. J. Cashman, C. J. Nicol, and R. B. Jones, "Effects of Transportation on the Tonic Immobility Fear Reactions of Broilers," *British Poultry Science* 30 (1989): 211–21.

25. N. G. Gregory and L. J. Wilkins, "Broken Bones in Chickens: Effect of Stunning and Processing in Broilers," *British Poultry Science* 31 (1990): 53–58.

26. P. A. Bayliss and M. H. Hinton, "Transportation of Broilers with Specific Reference to Mortality Rates."

27. N. G. Gregory, L. J. Wilkins, D. M. Alvey, and S. A. Tucker, "Effect of Catching Method and Lighting Intensity on the Prevalence of Broken Bones and on the Ease of Handling of End-of-Lay Hens," *Veterinary Record* 132 (Feb. 6, 1993): 127–29.

28. Bayliss and Hinton, "Transportation of Broilers with Specific Reference to Mortality Rates."

29. I. J. H. Duncan, G. S. Slee, P. Kettlewell, P. Berry, and A. J. Carlisle, "Comparison of the Stressfulness of Harvesting Broiler Chickens by Machine and by Hand," *British Poultry Science* 27 (1985): 109–14.

30. J. F. Gracey, *Meat Hygiene,* 8th ed. (London: Balliere Tindall, 1986), pp. 455–57.

31. C. J. Nicol, A. Blakeborough, and G. B. Scott, "Aversiveness of Motion and Noise to Broiler Chickens," *British Poultry Science* 32 (1991): 249–60.

32. P. D. Warriss, E. A. Bevis, S. N. Brown, and J. E. Edwards, "Longer Journeys to Processing Plants Are Associated with Higher Mortality in Broiler Chickens," *British Poultry Science* 33 (1992): 201–6.

33. For example, if only one carotid artery is cut instead of two, it takes 2 minutes for a bird to die (the alternative being 1.5 minutes when both are cut).

34. See European Food Safety Authority, "Opinion adopted by the AHAW Panel on the 15th of June 2004." Publication Date: July 6, 2004; Updated: October 11, 2004. www.efsa.europa. eu/en/science/ahaw/ahaw_opinions/495.html (accessed August 15, 2007).

35. See European Commission, Health and Consumer Protection Directorate-General, "The Welfare of Chickens Kept for Meat Production (Broilers)," chap. 9. ec.europa.eu/food/fs/sc/scah/out39_en.pdf (accessed August 15, 2007).

36. Hunton, "The Broiler Industry: Thirty-Four Years of Progress."

37. M. J. Gentle, "Neuroma Formation Following Partial Beak Amputation (Beak Trimming) in the Chicken," *Research in Veterinary Science* 41 (1986): 383–85. Infrared beak treatment looks to be a promising alternative.

38. J. A. Mench, "Animal Welfare and Management Issues Associated with the Use of Artificial Insemination for Broiler Breeders," in *Proceedings of the First International Symposium on the Artificial Insemination of Poultry,* ed. M. R. Bakst and G. J. Wishart (Savoy, IL: Poultry Science Association, 1995).

39. *Report of the Farm Animal Welfare Council (2006) on Welfare Labelling.* Available from the Farm Animal Welfare Council, Area 511, 1A Page Street, London SW1P 4PQ, United Kingdom; see also www.fawc.org.uk.

40. D. B. Morton, "Is Unnecessary Suffering Avoidable?" *Veterinary Record* 133 (1993): 304.

41. P. N. Grigor, B. O. Hughes, and M. C. Appleby, "Effects of Regular Handling and Exposure to an Outside Area on Subsequent Fearfulness and Dispersal in Domestic Hens," *Applied Animal Behaviour Science* 44 (1995): 47–55; J. H. Duncan and J. A. Mench, "Behavior as an Indicator of Welfare in Various Systems," in Savory and Hughes, *Proceedings of the 4th European Symposium on Poultry Welfare,* 69–80.

42. See the review of Pepperberg's work with Alex and other evidence in Marion Stamp Dawkins, *Through Our Eyes Only? The Search for Animal Consciousness* (Oxford: W. H. Freeman Spektrum, 1993), pp. 119–27, www.alexfoundation.org/irene.htm.

43. A. A. S. Weir, J. Chappell, and A. Kacelnik, "Shaping of Hooks in New Caledonian Crows," *Science* 297 (2002): 981; D. J. Povinelli, *Folk Physics for Apes: A Chimpanzee's Theory of How the World Works* (Oxford: University Press, 2000); J. Chappell and A. Kacelnik, "Selection of Tool Diameter by New Caledonian Crows, *Corvus moneduloides,*" *Animal Cognition* 7 (2004): 121–27.

44. This has been the subject of other investigations. D. B. Morton and P. H. M. Griffiths, "Guidelines on the Recognition of Pain, Distress, and Discomfort in Experimental Animals and an Hypothesis for Assessment," *Veterinary Record* 116 (1985): 431–36.

45. Josephine Donovan, "Attention to Suffering: A Feminist Caring Ethic for the Treatment of Animals," *Journal of Social Philosophy* 27 (1996): 81–102.

46. In the United Kingdom, the Animals (Scientific Procedures) Act, 1986 London, HMSO 182, requires special justification for experiments involving dogs, cats, primates, and horses. In the United States, the Animal Welfare Act (1966 and 1990) governing research does not cover experiments on rats, mice, or birds. See also F. B. Orlans, *In the Name of Science* (New York: Oxford University Press, 1993), pp. 58–60.

47. See Department for Environment, Food and Rural Affairs, U.K Government (1993), www.defra.gov.uk/animalh/welfare/farmed/meatchks/meatchkscode.pdf; Animal Welfare Information Center, United States Department of Agriculture, Agricultural Research Service National Agricultural Library (Beltsville, MD), www.nal.usda.gov/awic/legislat/internat.htm; and National Animal Welfare Advisory Committee, *Broiler Chickens: Fully Housed, Code of Welfare 2003* (issued under the Animal Welfare Act 1999), July 25, 2003 (Wellington, New Zealand), www.biosecurity.govt.nz/files/animal-welfare/codes/broiler-chickens/broiler-chickens.pdf (all accessed August 15, 2007).

48. In some countries, the levels of disease found at abattoirs determine permitted stocking densities on farms.

49. The Foundation for Animal Care, Saskatchewan Inc. produces such a leaflet, titled *Broiler Management Review*.

50. "Waitrose Aims for High Chicken Welfare," *Grocer* 12 (August 2006).

51. See Royal Society for the Prevention of Cruelty to Animals (Horsham, West Sussex, UK), www.rspca.org.uk/servlet/Satellite?pagename=RSPCA/RSPCARedirect&pg=AboutUs and www.rspca.org.uk/servlet/Satellite?pagename=RSPCA/RSPCARedirect&pg=welfarestandards &marker=1&articleId=1121442811407 (both accessed August 15, 2007).

52. See European Biomedical Research Association, "EU Constitution Incorporates Animal Welfare Provisions: The New Constitution for the European Union Includes an Annex on the Welfare of Animals," *EBRA Bulletin* (2004), www.ebra.org/ebrabulletin-eu-constitution-incorporates-animal-welfare-provisions_142.htm (accessed August 15, 2007).

PART III

ANIMALS FOR ENTERTAINMENT

5

The Sport of Rooster Fighting

A young teacher in the midst of a separation from his common-law wife and reflecting on deep questions about his own recent conversion to Christianity was offered the opportunity to rest at a friend's villa in Italy. He invited a small group of his students to accompany him to the villa to continue their work. He held daily seminar discussions that ranged widely. The core focus was on the works of the Latin poet Virgil, especially the meaning of evil and cruelty in a world presumably created by a benevolent God.

One morning, as the group was proceeding to its place of study, members observed two barnyard roosters spoiling for a fight. They stopped and watched with fascination as the fight commenced and took a violent turn. They remained absolutely transfixed by the encounter until it was settled. Later, the teacher reflected on the nature of the episode's fascination and its relationship to the larger question of the place of cruelty and pain in the world. Some of the questions he raised and discussed with his students included:

1. What was it about the fight that gripped their attention and kept them from proceeding to their study?
2. Why do roosters fight with one another for supremacy in the first place?
3. Were the fights a part of the natural order of things or something ugly and outside nature's and God's plans?
4. Should they have intervened to stop the conflict, or were they right to let it take its own course?

5. Could it be that there was an inherent dignity and beauty in the "haughtiness" and the potentially deadly skill of the victor and the "bedraggled," plucked, and bloody look of the vanquished?
6. Do the courage and pride observed in the winner actually require cowed submission for meaning and existence?

After reflection, the teacher proposed that their interest was part of the natural human curiosity, just as the fight was a part of the natural behavior of the roosters. He likened the cockfight to the place of pimps, prostitutes, and executioners in civil society. All have in common a distasteful moral appearance when looked at in isolation. However, when viewed from the context of the larger fabric of the needs of society as a whole, their usefulness in promoting and maintaining the characteristics of a well-ordered society becomes clear. For example, while the executioner kills, he does so as part of a system of criminal control; and prostitutes may help to prevent the danger involved in the expression of uncontrolled lust. Analogously, though the cockfight involves fear, submissiveness, injury, and pain, its presence serves to reveal the higher nature and importance of attributes like courage and pride. Perhaps both the fight between the roosters and the observation of it by humans also serve to reduce the level of aggression respectively in chicken groups and human societies. The teacher concluded that they had been right not to intervene.[1]

Questions and perspectives similar to these have continued to dominate the thinking of defenders of the modern cockfight. But do these comments, written approximately 1,620 years ago by the philosopher-theologian Saint Augustine, still apply to the types of arranged cockfights that take place in many parts of the world? Here we will look specifically at one location: Tommy's Place in Hobbs, New Mexico.

COCKFIGHTING AT TOMMY'S PLACE

Tommy's Place is a typical example of a cockfighting "pit" in one of the two states in the United States where the practice or "sport" of cockfighting remained legal until very recently (the other being Louisiana).[2] The club was housed in a metal building about the size of a junior high school gymnasium located in a sparsely populated desert community near the road that runs between Hobbs, New Mexico, and Denver City, Texas. The pit was not hidden away and stood in clear view just a few yards off the shoulder of the highway.

The historical path of cockfighting that leads to Tommy's Place is a long one. The earliest archeological evidence of the activity was found in the Indian subcontinent in the Indus River valley in modern-day Pakistan.[3] The indications are that the jungle fowl was domesticated for the purpose of fighting around 2,700 years ago, before its use for food.[4] Cockfighting made its way to China from India and then to the peninsula of Indochina. The gamecock was revered by the ancient Babylonians, Syrians, Greeks, and Romans, appearing on artistic images and coins. The sport was active in most of Europe, excluding Germany and Scandinavia. England was the center of activity until the nineteenth century. Indeed, the practice of pitting one animal against another for entertainment was quite common in England. For example, bull, bear, and ape baiting was practiced there from at least the fourteenth century. At first these contests were limited to the elite levels of society for the purpose of training mastiff dogs, which served the function of protecting the household. Only later, in the mid-sixteenth century, were the practices commercialized as sport for the masses. Some have argued that these spectacles were more popular with the public than the theater.[5] The British and Spanish spread the practice to their colonies and into the United States. It remains popular in Mexico, Haiti, the Dominican Republic, Thailand, and the Philippines.

Although illegal in the United States, cockfighting remains popular, and the image of the gamecock as a brave, fearless fighter has been used as the collegiate mascot of the University of South Carolina and Jacksonville State University.

Three openly published magazines (*Grit and Steel, The Game Cock,* and *The Feathered Warrior*) for a long time have devoted their content to the world of cockfighting, and they sell thousands of subscriptions. Their content includes articles on training, breeding, nutrition, ways to get around some laws, advertisements that promote the sale of gamecocks, and the dates of important contests. The sport is particularly popular with Louisiana Cajuns, Delta Blacks, Mexican Americans, and rural whites. However, contests take place in large urban centers from New York City to Los Angeles with participants that cut across all ethnic, social, and economic categories.

On most Friday and Saturday nights between the months of November and the middle of August, while the sport was still legal, cockfighting "derbies" were held at Tommy's Place. They involved dozens of matches each night that went on to early the next morning. In a derby, "cockers" or "galleros" entered a predetermined number of roosters for a specified fee. If there were 20 cockers involved, each entering the 4 required roosters, there would be a possibility of 40 fights that night. At the end of the night the cocker with the greatest number of victories was the winner and got the pot. Derbies were the most popular type of contest.

On "good nights" at Tommy's Place, attendance was about 200 or more patrons, adult men and women, cock owners, handlers, and preteen and teenage youth of both genders. Male attendees tended to outnumber females about ten to one, and most were ethnic Hispanics. Judging from the dress of the attendees and the vintage of the cars and trucks in the parking lot, there was a cross section of economic strata present, with most appearing to be from moderate to poor financial backgrounds. The license plates indicated attendance from the surrounding states of Texas and Oklahoma.

On entering the club on a derby night, one first encountered a familiar southwestern snack bar with a noncommercial-looking kitchen with a menu of green chili hamburgers, burritos, and soft drinks. While no alcoholic beverages could be purchased in the club, patrons were permitted to bring them in as long as they were kept in soft plastic containers. Those wishing to enter roosters into the derby had to pay the admission fee, show evidence of membership in the New Mexico Game Bird Association, and pay the derby entrance fee.

Off to one side of the business area of the club was a recessed nook with one chest-high shelf divided into two compartments. Each compartment contained a set of balance scales where the roosters were weighed prior to being matched with opponents. Roosters who were matched differed in weight by no more than one to two ounces. Handlers cradled the roosters in one arm as they approached the scales. The birds, totally habituated to handling, readily jumped up on the scales and remained still during the process. Once weighed, the roosters were tagged with their weight and the identification of their blindly matched opponent. They were placed into out-of-view wire holding cages where they remained until their match was called.

The roosters were large, confident, and beautiful birds at least two years of age, weighing about five pounds. They crowed frequently and held a "haughty" upright posture. Their colors varied according to their genetic pedigrees and included many shades of grey, black, red, and blue. Their heads are smooth because their combs and waddles had been trimmed, or "dubbed," eliminating the possibility that an opponent could grab them during a fight. This surgical procedure, which requires a careful technique, is done without anesthesia and requires a full 30 days to fully heal.

Behind the scales area was a small room where a man sat at a table with a sharpening wheel and containers of metal polish. Here the gaffs or knives that would be fitted over the bird's trimmed natural spurs were skillfully honed before the competition. Knives are large, flat, tapered fishhook-shaped steel blades. They have an inside cutting surface and a sharp point. The actual dimensions vary depending on the rules of the club. At Tommy's Place, they were approximately one and one-half inches in length. The blades were sharpened until the man was able to shave the hair on the back of his hand and leave small nicks on his thumbnail with the slightest touch. Gaffs are 1.25 to 2.75-inch-long blades closer to the shape of slightly bent ice picks or miniature bayonets. The weapons were tied to the natural heel spurs that had been trimmed to a standard length. Competitions used either gaffs or knives.

Proponents maintain that the use of knives and gaffs began as a way to improve the fairness of the fights between roosters. The size of the natural heel spur varies greatly from rooster to rooster, giving those with larger spurs an advantage in a "bare heel" fight. The concern for fairness was illustrated in 1993, when the U.S. Patent Office issued a patent for an artificial spur for cockfighting. The designers contended that the spur was a sufficiently important technical advance that it deserved patent protection. The device was durable, exhibited superior fighting effectiveness, and, most important, reduced the likelihood of cheating by facilitating the identification of illegal spur alterations.[6] Dr. Francine Bradley of the University of California and others argue that since the wounds inflicted by the gaff or knife are clean cuts, they are more amenable to medical treatment than wounds inflicted by the roosters' natural spurs, and therefore advance the welfare of the animals.[7]

Historically, the use of gaffs and knives derives from different sources of influence. Gaffs are said to be of British colonial origin and are favored in the northeastern United States, and knives are from Spanish influence via Mexico and are popular in the southwest.[8] Gaffs inflict puncture wounds, and fights are known at times to go for an hour or more. On the other hand, knives, or "slashers," cut larger and deeper wounds, and the fights tend to end much more quickly. Their increased lethality also adds an additional amount of uncertainty to the outcome of a fight because an underdog can sometimes "get lucky."

In the center of Tommy's Place, two facing tiers of stadium seats were positioned on either side of three square fighting pits. Each pit was composed of four roughly 15-foot sides completely enclosed by 9-foot-high chain link fencing. The floors of the pits were level and covered with raked red dirt. Near the back wall of the building there were a group of three smaller pits called "drag pits." These pits were used when fights in the main pits "dragged" on for long periods without a clear winner. If the fights were being conducted under so-called Mexican rules, the drag pits were not used because the matches were stopped after 15 minutes if no winner emerged before then.

The Fight

Once the weighing and matchmaking was complete and the birds have been fitted with their weapons, the patrons settled into their seats and the referee entered the main pit. The referee in cockfighting is a very important official. He starts and stops the action, calls fouls, imposes sanctions, and declares the winner if necessary. Tradition requires that no one argue with the referee's directions or judgments. Next, the handlers entered the pit, each cradling his rooster in one arm and stroking him gently with his free hand. Some handlers were the owners of the bird while others had been hired for the purpose. Wagers were offered between the handlers and owners and the audience and among members of the audience. "I'll take 20 on the red one!" "Who will cover 40 on the grey?" The bets were finalized with subtle nods.

Once the bets were settled, the referee inspected the birds and removed the scabbards from the blades, wiping the bare steel with his fingers. This move is to ensure that no irritants or poisons have been applied to the blades. In some venues the handlers are required to lick the blades between their own lips to ensure that they are free of substances. When directed to "bill" the roosters, the handlers, still cradling their roosters, approached each other in what looked like a rhythmic dance where they dipped toward each other, allowing the birds to peck at one another's heads. This procedure is intended to prime the birds and get them "hot" and ready to fight. The handlers then moved to a point approximately eight feet apart, and on the command "pit," they dropped their roosters to the floor.

The roosters took little time before they initiated their attacks. Some "broke high," jumping at their opponent, while others parried, ducked, and counterattacked. The collisions were fast and hard and were not random. The percussive pounding of wings was accompanied by the "cracking" sounds of steel on steel and steel on bone. The actual kicks were so fast that for the inexperienced observer, the form and accuracy could only be inferred from the effect they had on the birds' behavior and appearance. Fatigued birds with bloodstained feathers quickly replaced the initially strutting and confident roosters. The opponents sometimes sat passively before the initiation of another encounter.

Inevitably, the attacks resulted in the blades becoming hung up in the bodies of the birds, making further attacks impossible. At these times, by calling "handle," the referee stopped the action and instructed the handlers to disengage the weapons. Once the birds were detached from one another, a brief 15-second rest period began during which the handlers worked to refresh or revive their birds like a corner man in a boxing match. The handler blew on the rooster's head and under its back feathers or took the rooster's entire head into his mouth, removing the accumulated blood from the bird's throat with a mouth-to-beak sucking maneuver, and then spat the fluid on the floor of the pit. After the rest period, the referee signaled "get ready," and the handlers placed their birds facing each other. On the command "pit," the birds were released to fight again. During the fights the spectators shouted encouragement to their chosen bird, imploring the bird to "shoot" (i.e., attack), "kill," or "finish off" his opponent.

A fight can end in less than a minute if a fatal blow is struck to the neck, head, or deep in the chest. Or it may continue in paroxysms of fighting, exhaustion, and the rest periods called by the referee. If one bird fails to continue the fight, the handler of the fighting bird asks the referee for a "count." If the nonfighting bird fails to reengage during the next several minutes, the fighting bird "with count" is the winner. A bird that has count but dies during a rest period will be pitted one more time. If the previously nonfighting bird now attacks the carcass, it becomes the winner. If it fails to resume the fight, the dead bird is declared the winner. In summary, a rooster may lose a fight in three ways: die, run away, or fail to fight. However, the rules are such that it is hard for any bird to just walk away or stop fighting, because every attempt is made to get the fight going again by the use of the count, rest period, and repeated pitting procedures.

The eventual outcome is hard to predict because bloody and exhausted birds may stage unlikely comebacks, and dominant-appearing birds may suddenly collapse. These kinds of changes in fortune express the "gameness" that cockers admire. Many fights conclude with both birds bleeding heavily and one simply dying before the other.

THE CREATION OF A BATTLE COCK

Proponents deny that the sport is just the crude act of bloodthirsty humans who simply put two aggressive birds together to see who kills whom. They emphasize that the sport is complex and requires skill, specialized knowledge, and a 24/7 commitment. Again, as one proponent put it, "This sport is not about killing, it is about winning." The complexity is reflected in the conversations that take place between cockers as they stand around waiting for the start of the derby. At these times, the conversations at Tommy's Place center not only on the outcomes of past fights and the night's opponents, but on in-depth comparisons of the many approaches to raising successful fighters. They discuss the various breeds, diets, and training regimens, all of which are intended to capture, motivate, or create the set of behavioral characteristics that cockers admire.

These characteristics include:

1. Gameness: The character of having a "no-quit" attitude even during long uphill fights where a bird has been injured early. Birds with this characteristic are referred to as having "bottom." As one cocker put it, "Let's face it, you need to have a rooster who can take some steel and continue fighting."
2. Cutting ability: The level of accuracy possessed by a rooster as it delivers a blow with the gaff or knife. Also included in this characteristic is the tendency of a rooster to deliver multiple leg strokes during a single attack.
3. Power: The strength of a rooster and the force with which an attack is made; also the ability to control the tempo of a fight by forcefully moving an opponent around the pit.
4. Aggression: The level of desire to fight when given the opportunity. The characteristic is determined by how long it takes a rooster to get "hot."
5. Intelligence: The ability of a rooster to fight strategically: adjusting its battle plan, probing for weaknesses, and attacking when openings present themselves.
6. Fighting style: The typical approach that a rooster takes during a fight. Some are characterized as "flyers" and others as "grounders," which define their preferred method of attack.

The Development of Fighting Skills

Breeding

Hundreds of established breeds of gamecocks are known to possess some combination of desirable fighting characteristics from which a cocker can choose. Some of the better-established strains are named after the well-known breeders who developed them. For example, Kelsos are named after Walter Kelso and Sweaters after Sweater McGinnis. These particular breeders carry great historical significance in American cockfighting and are held in absolute awe by proponents. Other breeds carry the name of their primary feather color (e.g., Clarets, Bonanza Blacks) or their location of origin (e.g., Texas Tool Pusher Blues). Local breeders may buy "trios" (one rooster, two hens) of their preferred breeds and then try to inbreed or "fix" a successful phenotype, or they may cross breed established lines in an attempt to improve the mix of winning characteristics. The crosses can be quite simple, as in a basic two-way cross, or quite complex, as in rotational crosses that involve a sequence of mating with three different bloodlines. The serious breeder needs to know a great deal about genetics and must have the organizational skills to maintain the complex record system for making the necessary behavioral outcome evaluations.

Nutrition and Housing

All the breeding credentials will be of little consequence unless the roosters develop properly. During the two-plus years that a rooster is growing, and before it can be entered into an official fight, serious cockers are extremely careful about nutrition and health. Unlike the mash that a common chicken would be fed, fighting cocks are provided special diets composed of seed, meat, fruit, vegetables, milk and other "secret" supplements that are carefully prepared and fed to the roosters each day.

Once the roosters reach one year of age, they are no longer housed in groups but are tethered on a long cord outdoors, a safe distance away from other similarly housed roosters. Each bird has access to a small doghouse-like structure that can be used when the weather is bad. Here the roosters are able to eat insects and develop strength while being exposed to the elements. Particular care is taken to keep the animals free of disease, worms, and lice. Cockers also point out that they must be attentive to the rooster's mental health during development. They firmly believe that if the birds are overly stressed or traumatized in some way, they can be ruined before ever making it to the pit. One cocker said simply, "Happier birds are more successful birds."

Pre-fight Training

A well-bred and well-fed bird is not yet ready to be entered into a derby. For weeks before any scheduled event, roosters participate in a regimen designed to increase their stamina, strength, and fighting ability. To develop aerobic endurance, some owners will force roosters to run long distances by jogging behind them, or put them on specially constructed treadmills. Others house two roosters across from one another in two long, narrow cages. In this situation the natural aggressiveness encourages the birds continually to chase one another back and forth along the length of the cage, doing a form of wind sprints. This might go on for as long as four hours per day. Strength exercises include requiring a bird to right itself by repeatedly placing it on its back and placing the rooster's front toes on the edge of a table while holding its body slightly below the flat surface. This move gets the bird to pull itself up to the level of the table like a chin-up. In addition to these kinds of strength exercises, roosters are massaged and participate in controlled sparring with other roosters. Sparring is done without knives or gaffs and with their natural heel spurs covered. There is no formal proscription against the use of stimulants, blood clotting medications, and other performance-enhancing drugs *before* a fight, but they cannot be used *during* the process of a fight.

ETHICAL AND LEGAL ISSUES

Federal Law and State Law

The U.S. Congress first addressed the issue of animal fighting by adding a number of amendments to the Animal Welfare Act in 1976. The amendments restricted animal fighting indirectly by making the interstate and international movement of animals for the purpose of participation in an animal fight illegal. The amendments state:

> (a) It shall be unlawful for any person to knowingly sponsor or exhibit an animal in any animal fighting venture to which any animal was moved in interstate or foreign commerce.
> (b) It shall be unlawful for any person to knowingly sell, buy, transport, or deliver to another person or receive from another person for purposes of transportation, in interstate or foreign commerce, any dog or other animal for purposes of having the dog or other animal participate in an animal fighting venture.
> (c) It shall be unlawful for any person to knowingly use the mail service of the United States Postal Service or any interstate instrumentality for purposes of promoting or in any other manner furthering an animal fighting venture except as performed outside the limits of the States of the United States.
> (d) Notwithstanding the provisions of subsection (a), (b), or (c) of this section, the activities prohibited by such subsections shall be unlawful with respect to fighting ventures involving live birds only if the fight is to take place in a State where it would be in violation of the laws thereof.
> (e) Any person who violates subsection (a), (b), or (c) shall be fined not more than $5,000 or imprisoned for not more than 1 year, or both, for each such violation.[9]

These amendments did not make breeding, raising, and training of game fowl illegal as long as the birds were transported to states and foreign countries where cockfighting was still legal. Violations were punished at the misdemeanor level.

In 2002, Congress added language to the Farm Bill that prohibited the interstate and international transport of game fowl for the purpose of fighting, regardless of the local legal status of the sport. Left unchanged was the misdemeanor level of punishment. Opponents have argued that misdemeanor punishment is an insufficient deterrent given the large amounts of money in the sport.[10] For example, the purchase of a breeding trio alone may cost several thousand dollars, and the amount of money wagered at large derbies can reach tens of thousands of dollars.[11] Opponents believe that raising the level of punishment to that of a felony will be more effective. This change is the focus of several current legislative initiatives.[12]

All the state laws that limit cockfighting base the restrictions on the claim that intentionally causing an animal to participate in a fight with another animal for the purpose of entertainment or monetary gain is a form of "extreme animal cruelty." However, in evaluating the strength of state restrictions on cockfighting, it is necessary to consider the level of sanction (i.e., felony, misdemeanor) associated with the various components of the practice of cockfighting. The components are:

1. Participating directly in the fight as a pit owner, handler, or referee.
2. Having possession of cocks for the purpose of fighting.

3. Having possession of the implements for fighting, such as knives and gaffs.
4. Being a spectator at a cockfight.

Viewing the laws as a whole, it is accurate to say that all states and the District of Columbia have some form of legal restriction on the practice of cockfighting, while it remains legal in the American possessions of Samoa, Guam, Puerto Rico, and the Virgin Islands. This summary suggests that there is a strong consensus against cock-fighting in the United States. However, a finer analysis of the statutes, considering the components listed above, provides a less clear picture. When the components are considered, we find:

1. Direct fight participation: 35 states and the District of Columbia (Washington, DC) consider it a felony, 15 a misdemeanor.
2. Possession of cocks for fighting: 27 states (and, in addition, Washington, DC) consider it a felony, 7 a misdemeanor, and 16 make possession legal.
3. Possession of fighting implements: 6 states consider it a felony, 5 a misdemeanor, and 39 (and, in addition, Washington, DC) legal.
4. Being a spectator at a cockfight: 12 states consider it a felony, 29 (and, in addition, Washington, DC) a misdemeanor, and 9 legal.

Considering the components as a set, we find that only three states have strict felony penalties for all four forms of participation (Colorado, Florida, and Michigan), and eight states have felony provisions for direct participation, possessing cocks, and being a spectator, while having no sanction for owning gaffs and knives (Connecticut, Nebraska , New Hampshire, New Jersey, Pennsylvania, Rhode Island, Vermont, and Washington).[13] In other words, only 12 states have closed the major avenues of support (i.e. direct involvement, possessing cocks, and being a spectator) for cockfighting. States with legal sanctions for direct participation, while ignoring breeding (possession), ownership of weapons, and spectator involvement, seem to invite violation. For example, assume that the local sheriff shows up at cockfight with only the legal ability to arrest those directly involved. Given warning, those who are directly involved need only leave the pit area and mix with the crowd of spectators. This move would leave only the pit owner vulnerable to arrest. Six states fit into this category: Alabama, Arkansas, Georgia, Hawaii, Mississippi, and Texas. This structure of law sends a mixed message to the cockfighting community.

Virtually each week newspapers from across the United States report arrests and confiscation of birds, money, and fighting paraphernalia from illegal cockfighting operations. It could be argued that this indicates that the laws are a failure, much as prohibition was in the 1920s, and ought to be repealed. Recall that the "noble" purpose of the eighteenth amendment was to reduce crime and poverty and to improve the economy and the overall health of the nation. Instead, the law was found to be unenforceable and resulted in increased alcohol consumption and crime. Do we have a similar situation with anti-cockfighting laws? It is conceivable that the laws simply encourage cock-fighters to move their operations further from the public eye and make criminals out of people who enjoy the spectacle.

Another concern is whether the laws reduce the incentive of game breeders from reporting the presence of dangerous avian diseases that they observe in their flocks and that have the potential to affect the food supply and human health. For example, in 2002 there was an outbreak of exotic Newcastle disease in the state of California. The disease is caused by a respiratory virus that spreads rapidly and produces a high mortality rate.

Many health officials believed that the disease entered the United States from Mexico by the illegal movement of game fowl for the purpose of underground cockfighting. This presumption was strengthened by the finding that two of the first three index cases of the disease were in game fowl. Fortunately, a number of game fowl breeders brought their concerns about the presence of the disease to the state authorities, helping to limit the extent of the outbreak among chickens raised for human consumption. As it was, it cost the USDA $200 million to control the outbreak.[14]

Another concern involves the specter of avian influenza, which has been shown to spread to both birds and humans in Asia at venues like cockfights.[15] The fear is that as the sanctions for involvement in cockfighting get stiffer, the likelihood of participants reporting relevant diseases will diminish. Would state or federal regulation of the sport be a useful alternative to the elaboration of highly restrictive laws?

Is Cockfighting Cruel?

The ethical foundation of the laws restricting cockfighting are based on the contention that intentionally causing a gamecock to participate in a fight with another gamecock is an example of extreme cruelty similar to maliciously injuring, mutilating, poisoning, or needlessly causing the death of an animal. Certainly, causing an animal to fight another animal increases the probability of acute and chronic physical pain, psychological suffering, and the likelihood of a painful death. That this is unethical rests on the assumption that animals have moral standing and value that is independent of their usefulness to humans. That is, animals have access to some of the protections afforded by ethics, by virtue of the fact that they are capable of experiencing pain and pleasure. This position holds that animals are not merely objects owned by humans who can do with them as they please.

Defenders of cockfighting take issue with the cruelty categorization. They maintain that no human can make a cockfight. Rather, fighting is something that the bird does naturally when faced with another cock in its territory. Putting game cocks in a pit merely provides the opportunity for two cocks to fight but does not formally cause the fight. Some believe that putting a cock in the pit is a form of chicken self-actualization. In the pit the rooster is playing out its destiny; if it dies in this pursuit, it is an honorable death even if there is pain involved. Thus the experience of pain is not seen as a setback of the animal's welfare, but part of the fate that awaits it. This point of view is similar to St. Augustine's analysis of whether he should have interfered in the fight that he came across in the barnyard. Both perspectives emphasize respecting the natural propensities of the birds.

But does this appeal to naturalness hold? Gamecocks are not barnyard roosters or jungle fowl living in the wild. Gamecocks have been purposely bred, conditioned, trained, and armed to be lethal fighters. The rules of the cockfight require that the birds continually be pushed back into the fight by their handlers. Gamecocks have no options but to fight. In St. Augustine's example, the roosters were fighting for territory that mattered in their everyday lives. In the pit, the roosters fight for the entertainment of the spectators in a novel environment armed in ways unrelated to their natural lives.

Issues of Pain in Chickens

During the 2007 New Mexico state legislature debate on Senate bill 10, which proposed to ban cockfighting, an "expert" witness, who was identified as a pain management specialist, testified that fighting cocks do not feel pain. Because they do not feel pain, they cannot suffer, and thus the application of the concept of extreme cruelty is inappropriate and misguided. These birds are doing what they want to do and are doing so free of pain.

However, research has shown that chickens have a wide distribution of pain receptors throughout the body and that they respond to injury to the beak, ankle joints, mouth, and comb and from feather pulling. Chickens also show various coping behaviors that are used to minimize the experience of pain. These behaviors include active escape, passive motionless squatting, and sitting with a drooped posture. One review of current data on perception in chickens concluded that any pain treatment accorded mammals should also be provided to birds.[16] During a fight, the cocks often sit motionless for periods of time between attacks. These findings suggest that at these times the bird may be both exhausted and attempting to reduce his experience of pain brought on by the accumulation of fight-induced injuries.

Interestingly, arguments concluding that there is no pain are not typically made by cockfighters. If the birds were incapable of feeling pain and suffering, their gameness, tenacity, and courage during the fight would be called into question. This would reduce the fight to a contest between robots and would cease to have the meaning that it is accorded.

Justification by Tradition and Problems of Moral Relativism

Arguments from tradition set aside the ethical relevance of cruelty and animal welfare. They rest justification of the "sport" on the claim that because it has been practiced by certain nationalities and ethnic groups for hundreds of years, it has become a part of the package of practices that constitute those cultures. Over the years cockfighting has developed into a revered practice that is passed down with pride to children by family members or by nonfamilial elders.[17] In this argument, the traditions of a culture determine its ethical standards governing permissible uses of animals. This approach also asserts that respect for or tolerance of the cultural group requires a position of nonintervention by the majority culture in which it is embedded.

This argument from tradition is based on the notion that issues of right and wrong are in the end based on the traditions of a culture and that there is no way to base a judgment that one set of cultural practices is ethically superior to another. The problem is that this cultural relativist position has hidden dangers. First, the position seems to eliminate the need for people to reflect on the ethical justification of their own behavior. They have only to accept what has been acceptable in the past. Second, this position seems to be a form of ethical relativism asserting that whatever a culture thinks is right or wrong really is right or wrong, at least for the members of that culture. There is no criterion independent of a culture for determining whether a practice is right or wrong. This view is inconsistent with many of our most cherished moral beliefs, which raises suspicion about it. No general theory of morality is likely to convince us that a belief is acceptable merely because others believe in it strongly enough to embed it in their culture. At least some moral views seem relatively more enlightened, no matter how great the variability of beliefs. The idea that practices such as slavery cannot be evaluated across cultures by some common standard seems morally outrageous and unacceptable, not morally enlightened. It is one thing to suggest that such beliefs might be *excused* but another to suggest that they are *right* and a legitimate source of moral beliefs.

"The United States Is a Cockfighting Country"

In a variant of the argument from tradition, proponents assert that the United States is at its historical heart a cockfighting country. As proof, they point out that great founding fathers such as George Washington, Thomas Jefferson, and Benjamin Franklin were involved in the sport. They remind the public that Andrew Jackson held cockfights on the lawn of the White House while he was president and that Abraham Lincoln got the nickname "Honest Abe" not from his principled practice of law but from his work as a cockfight referee.[18] They point to the example of people like the great revolutionary war soldier Thomas Sumter, who was proud to adopt the *nom de guerre* "The Game Cock."[19] They tell the story that the gamecock lost out to the bald eagle for a place on the Great Seal of the United States by one vote in the Continental Congress in 1782.

The desired implication of this evidence is that the founding fathers approved of cockfighting during their lifetimes and would offer the same favorable arguments if they were alive today. In addition, if the founders did offer their support, their status as founders alone would render any attempt to challenge their reasons superfluous. In other words, the critics of cockfighting are the real deviants.

But even if this argument is entirely true to the historical facts, what does the argument prove about acceptable practices, if anything?

What Is at Stake during a Cockfight?

The short answer to this question is money and prestige. However, other writers have suggested that deeper issues need also to be considered.

The Balinese Cockfight

While attempting to study the Balinese culture in the late 1950s, the anthropologist Clifford Geertz unexpectedly got caught in a police raid on an illegal cockfight. When the police arrived, he ran for cover like the rest of the spectators. His presence at the cockfight led to a level of acceptance by the community that had up until that time eluded him. Over time, he came to see cockfighting as a "text" that revealed some of the rich and complex dynamics of Balinese culture.[20] He thought that the fighting cock was not just an instrument necessary to create a gambling enterprise. Instead, it was a host and symbol of its owner's personality, masculinity, and sexuality, a kind of "detachable penis." He learned that "Sabung," the word for a fighting cock, carried many masculine meanings such as "hero," "champion," "lady-killer," "tough guy," and "bachelor." He found that a man's character was often metaphorically described in terms of the behavior of a fighting cock. For example, a man hopelessly mired in a difficult personal conflict from which he was unable to extricate himself was seen as behaving like a dying cock making one last attempt to strike his opponent in a wild hope for escape. This identification with the cock was not, however, part of a more general glorification and respect for animals. In fact, the Balinese deplore the human expression of animal-like behaviors and treat most other domestic animals with "phobic cruelty." He found that cockfights played a spiritual function and could be understood as a form of blood sacrifice necessary to appease the feared dark forces and ghosts of hell.

His research revealed that the system of betting on cockfights involved two different functions. One was typical wagering that took place between individuals, each of whose goal was to outsmart his opponent and take his money. The second and more important function involved the creation of betting alliances between the two groups who backed the different cocks in a match. In the formation of these alliances, crucial status concerns were expressed and played out between members of the village hierarchy. It was the mutual experience of the brief episodes of humiliation in loss and rising status in winning that helped bind the members of the alliances together. Although large sums of money were wagered by the alliances, great care was taken by the officials to match the cocks so evenly that in the long run no one lost or won much in the way of hard money.

Mexican American Cockfighting

In a similar analysis of the tradition of Mexican American cockfighting, Jerry Garcia looked carefully into the meaning and purpose of being a "Gallero." Like Geertz, he found that participation in the sport is male dominated and full of sexual metaphors that are ultimately grounded in the concept of Mexican "macho." He illustrates the complicated meaning of macho by quoting a poem by Rick Najera from the collection *The Pain of Macho:* "See, a macho has no questions. A macho is self-assured. He has no doubt. When I say macho, I see my grandfather, a man: good, kind, gentle, and strong. He was a macho. He raised fighting cocks."[21] He points out that cockfighting came with the Spanish occupation of Latin America and the Caribbean and was well entrenched as a favorite gambling sport in Mexico by the nineteenth century. When the Mexican American War ended in 1848 and the new boundary of the United States came to incorporate parts of northern Mexico, cockfighting *de facto* became a part of the southwestern culture. Garcia sees the continued involvement of a portion of Mexican men in cockfighting as a way of keeping an important element of their Mexican identity in tact. That the sport is considered deviant by the majority Anglo culture actually adds to its importance as a symbol. Participation in the sport also made it possible for socially marginalized Mexican men to gain a degree of economic and social status among their fellow galleros. Finally, Garcia interprets involvement in cockfighting as a statement that says, "We will not totally assimilate. We will stay ourselves." He calls this "resistance masculinity."

While both of these authors identify gambling as an important part of cockfighting, they see the social and self-preservation aspects of the sport carrying the most important weight. Their analyses bring up the question of whether in cases like these it is appropriate for sentient animals, battling to the death with manmade weapons, to play this part in the men's lives. But are there no alternatives to the expression of these concerns other than using the lives of animals? Are we here again encountering arguments that reduce to the argument from tradition?

Condemning the Condemners, or Achieving Consistency in Ethics

Defenders point out that many who criticize their sport fail to take up the ethical case against dangerous human sports (e.g., boxing and extreme fighting), eat factory-farmed chicken, drink to excess, and bet illegally on the Super Bowl.[22] The approach assumes that if people who criticize cockfighting can be found to be ethically inconsistent, their arguments need not be considered.

The Impact on Observers and Participants

Models of Virtue

Just as the Greek general Themistocles required that his troops observe cockfights in order to stimulate the virtues of courage and tenacity as they prepared to take on the Persian forces,[23] may not modern humans also benefit from observing these models? Watching the struggle between two roosters can provide a method for "tempering nerves for the daily struggle, and learning how to carry on upright in the constant mill of life."[24] Given that the struggle is one of life and death, the experience might also serve as an important reminder of the impermanence of life and the importance of living in the present. Mary Midgely has even suggested that observing such agonistic encounters may have a cathartic effect on a human's pent-up anger, thereby preventing its damaging expression toward humans and other animals.[25]

Promotion of Family Values

Since maintaining a serious breeding and training operation involves an enormous amount of work, such enterprises frequently become family-operated businesses. This situation provides the opportunity for family members to learn about cooperation, dependability, and trust. Children learn about caring for animals, animal medicine and nutrition, genetics, and development.

Mistreatment of Animals and Humans

Philosophers such as Immanuel Kant have argued that humans have no direct ethical duties to animals, but they allow that we have indirect ones. Kant was concerned that if humans treated animals badly, these cruel acts might generalize to their treatment of humans. Indeed, there is a great deal of research that strongly suggests that cruel treatment of animals is correlated with cruel treatment of humans. For example, it is now virtually axiomatic that if adults abuse animals in the home, there is a strong chance that any children present are also at risk.[26] From the developmental perspective, it is also well known that adults who are extremely aggressive to other adults, including serial murderers, have childhood histories of animal abuse.[27]

In summary, arguments in favor of cockfighting emphasize the warrant of tradition, the denial of cruelty, and the ethical inconsistency of critics. Supporters see benefits accruing to personal pride, family cohesion, the value of commitment, the local economy, and the development of grit in facing the reality of a cruel and hard life. They are not moved by the motivation to reduce the amount of pain and suffering in the world by finding alternative paths to these kinds of important benefits. On the other hand, critics emphasize the ethical importance of the degree of pain experienced by the birds and the societal dangers inherent in learning to become indifferent or to derive pleasure from live violence. They tend to diminish the importance of traditions and the deeper motivations and meanings espoused by supporters and see instead a prurient fascination in death and a desire to gamble.

AT THE END OF THE NIGHT

At the end of a night of cockfighting at Tommy's Place, the floors of the pits are stained with blood and full of loose feathers. The air smells of stale tobacco smoke, a hint of marijuana, sweat, and beer. Some people's sense of pride and prestige has been briefly sustained or elevated, while others feel diminished. A fair amount of money has changed hands. Some children have participated meaningfully in an activity that their family values, and they share a close bonded feeling with them. Other children wonder why a rooster for which they cared for two years had to die. They promise themselves not to get so close to an animal again. Many feel that they have proudly spent the night close to their roots. They have watched roosters exemplify the daring and strength that they value in humans as well. There have been surprises, laughs, arguments, and disappointments, a slice of real life. Some roosters have won their fights and will survive for another opportunity, maybe as a breeder. Others have lost and died from blood loss and shock and are stuffed in trash cans in the parking lot, where the rustling sounds suggest that all are not dead yet. Some new spectators leave the club elated and interested in returning or maybe even participating themselves. Others leave devoted to the idea of stopping what they just saw from happening again. Two cockers who had been following the debates in the New Mexico legislature agreed that it looked like the cockfighting ban would pass. As they said goodnight to each other, they shook hands, winked, and said, "See you underground."

NOTES

1. St. Augustine, *Divine Providence and the Problem of Evil: A Translation of St. Augustine's De Ordine,* trans. Robert P. Russell (New York: Cosmopolitan Science and Art Service, 1942), pp. 49–53.

2. After the writing of this case, cockfighting became illegal in New Mexico (on June 15, 2007) and banned in Louisiana as of August 2008.

3. R. J. Snow, *Blood, Sweat, and Feathers: The History and Sport of Cockfighting* (Bethlehem, PA: Twiddling Pencil Publishers, 2004), pp. 21–50.

4. M. Visser, *Much Depends on Dinner* (Toronto: McClelland and Stewart Limited, 1986), pp. 125–29.

5. O. Brownstein, "The Popularity of Baiting in England before 1600: A Study in Social and Theatrical History," *Educational Theatre Journal* 21, no. 3 (1969): 237.

6. J. J. Roman and N. M. Carotene, "Artificial Spur for Cockfighting," patent no. 5219396, issued June 15, 1993.

7. F. A. Bradley, "Oral Testimony on H.R. 817 to the Subcommittee on Crime, Terrorism, and Homeland Security, Committee on the Judiciary, House of Representatives," May 18, 2006, p. 40.

8. J. Garcia, "The Measure of a Cock: Mexican Cockfighting, Culture, and Masculinity," in *I Am Atzlan: The Personal Essay in Chicano Studies*, ed. Chon A. Noriega and Wendy Belcher (Los Angeles: UCLA Chicano Studies Research Center, 2004), pp. 109–38.

9. Animal Welfare Act (7 USC, 2155).

10. W. Paccele, "Oral Testimony on H.R. 137 to the Subcommittee on Crime, Terrorism, and Homeland Security, Committee on the Judiciary, House of Representatives," February 6, 2007.

11. "144 Charged in Raid: $40,000 in Cash Seized in Cockfighting Bust," *Knoxville News Sentinel,* June 13, 2005, p. A1.

12. U.S. House bill H.R. 137, The Animal Fighting Prohibition Enforcement Act, which felonized crimes related to animal fighting ventures, was signed into law by President George Bush on May 3, 2007.

13. Humane Society of the United States, Fact Sheet, "Cockfighting: State Laws" updated November 2006.

14. R. S. Nolan, "Emergency Declared: Exotic Newcastle Disease Found in Commercial Poultry Farms," *Journal of the American Veterinary Medical Association* 229, no. 4 (2003): 411.

15. M. Specter, "Nature's Bioterrorist," *New Yorker,* February 28, 2005, pp. 50–61.

16. M. J. Gentle, "Attentional Shifts Alter Pain Perception in the Chicken," *Animal Welfare* 10 (2001): S187–S194.

17. Garcia, "The Measure of a Cock."

18. H. McCaghy and A. G. Neal, "The Fraternity of Cockfighters: Ethical Embellishments of an Illegal Sport," *Journal of Popular Culture* 8, no. 3 (1973): 564.

19. K.G. Heider, "The Game Cock, the Swamp Fox, and the Wizard Owl: The Development of Good Form in an American Totemic Set," *Journal of American Folklore* 93, no. 367 (1980): 1–22.

20. C. Geertz, "Deep Play: Notes on the Balinese Cockfight," *Daedalus: Journal of the American Academy of Arts and Sciences* 101, no. 1 (1972): 1–37; reprinted in A. Dundes, *The Cockfight: A Casebook* (Madison: University of Wisconsin, 1994), pp. 94–132.

21. Garcia, "The Measure of a Cock."

22. McCaghy and Neal, "The Fraternity of Cockfighters," pp. 557–69.

23. M. Visser, *Much Depends on Dinner* (Toronto: McClelland and Stewart Limited, 1986), p. 126.

24. McCaghy and Neal, "The Fraternity of Cockfighters," p. 561.

25. M. Midgely, *Animals and Why They Matter* (Athens: University of Georgia, 1983).

26. R. Lockwood and F. Ascione, *Cruelty to Animals and Interpersonal Violence: Readings in Research and Application* (West Lafayette: Purdue University Press, 1998).

27. J. Wright and C. Hensley, "From Animal Cruelty to Serial Murder: Applying the Graduation Hypothesis," *International Journal of Offender Therapy and Comparative Criminology* 47, no. 1 (2003): 71–88.

6

Winky and Wanda at the Detroit Zoo

Winky, an Asian elephant, resided in the Detroit Zoological Institute for 14 years. Wanda, on loan from the San Antonio Zoo, lived with her for eight years. Their one-acre yard was about half the area of a professional soccer field.[1] This outdoor area included trees, toys, and a pool. Inside the barn, they had heated floors for the days when the Michigan winters made it unpleasant for them to be outside. They received food, baths, pedicures, and expert medical care. In return, Winky and Wanda had only to wander through the yard, occasionally tossing dust on their backs to protect against insects and sunburn.

Suddenly, in May 2004, the Detroit Zoo announced that it would be sending Winky and Wanda away and discontinuing the elephant exhibit permanently.[2] At first glance, this news was unremarkable. Several zoos had closed elephant exhibits in previous years, causing little stir outside their local areas. Some zoos had decided that maintaining elephant exhibits caused too great a financial burden. Others were persuaded to relinquish their elephants by public pressure from the media or from protesters. The Detroit Zoo's decision, however, was indeed remarkable, because it was motivated fundamentally by moral concerns with implications for many zoos.[3] According to Dr. Ron Kagan, a biologist and the director of the Detroit Zoo, "The quality of life for the [elephants] is not adequate and is different from other animals."[4] Over several years, he and his staff observed that the elephants' health was deteriorating in ways that would not likely have occurred in the wild. Kagan believed that the Detroit Zoo lacked the facilities to care properly for elephants.

The Detroit Zoo's announcement received national media coverage and public debate.[5] Kagan wanted to send the elephants to a sanctuary rather than to another zoo. Although many places call themselves sanctuaries or zoos, Kagan was referring specifically to institutions that meet demanding criteria—high-level zoos and sanctuaries, so to speak. The sanctuaries he had in mind have hundreds of acres of land for roaming, keep other elephants in stable herds, and are located in climates better suited to elephants than Detroit—that is, more akin to their natural geographic habitats. In referring to "zoos," Kagan meant specifically zoos approved by the American Zoo and Aquarium Association (AZA), a national organization responsible for accrediting animal care facilities.

Since the Detroit Zoo is a member of the AZA, Kagan and his staff first needed to obtain permission to send Winky and Wanda to a non-AZA sanctuary. Detroit's request was denied. The AZA directed instead that the two elephants be transferred to the Columbus Zoo and Aquarium.[6] In an unusual move, the Detroit staff decided to appeal the decision and ask the AZA to reconsider. Kagan's insistence that the elephants should be sent to a sanctuary prompted several questions. Can other AZA-accredited zoos, let alone unaccredited ones, adequately provide for elephants? Should elephants, as an endangered species, be kept in zoos at all? How important is climate in deciding which animals should be kept in a zoo? Are there many animals kept in zoos that ought not to be there?

THE HISTORICAL AND CONTEMPORARY BACKGROUND

From Exhibition to Conservation

The first animal exhibitions began to appear in North America in the mid-1800s. The major goal of many was profit. Two historians describe the circumstances: "Zoos vied with one another to present the public with the greatest possible variety of species, despite conditions of severe confinement. . . . Animals were objects; species protection was not on the agenda."[7] Early facilities were more like sideshows in which many animals were trained to dress up in costumes and perform tricks.[8]

The first Detroit Zoo was of this generation, born in 1883 when a collection of animals was purchased from a bankrupt traveling circus and euphemistically called a "zoological garden." Financially, this garden had little backing and closed down in a year. Not until 1928 did the second Detroit Zoo emerge (continuous down to today). At the opening ceremonies, the mayor of Detroit had the misfortune of wandering into an area where a polar bear was kept and ran into the bear. The mayor had no idea that polar bears were ferocious and could easily kill him. Little was known about wild animals at the time, even by many people who purchased and housed them. More than 120,000 people flowed through the gates of the Detroit Zoo on opening day. The zoo proved to be immensely popular, especially with children. By 1933, Paulina the Elephant was giving small children rides on her back in the zoo, without parental accompaniment. Paulina was also used by contractors to do hard construction labor when new facilities were needed for the zoo. In a great paradox of history, political activists during the Great Depression publicly complained about the zoo. They objected that while many citizens of Detroit were starving, idle and useless animals lived in the lap of luxury at the zoo.[9]

In this same period, beginning in 1924, the American Association of Zoological Parks and Aquariums established the objective of helping zoos to trade animals and information. This group evolved into the modern AZA. By the 1970s, good evidence had emerged that humans were impinging on and even destroying many wild-animal habitats.[10] When it became apparent that many species were disappearing in the wild, some zoos started to style themselves as modern "Noah's arks."[11] They envisioned preserving animals in captivity to guard against their extinction in the wild.[12] Zoos knew that they could accomplish this mission of preservation only by cooperation with other zoos, so the AZA started to set standards for zoo management and to coordinate efforts to maintain captive animal populations in the United States.

AZA Zoos

As zoos evolved, they found that they needed to address the question, "What is a zoo?" A simple dictionary definition is "a collection of living animals, usually for public display."[13] However, a host of organizations fall under this definition—from the Smithsonian National Zoological Park to a gas station that keeps tigers in roadside cages.[14] In this case study, the word "zoo" will be used to refer exclusively to institutions accredited by the AZA. Accreditation requires conformity with a host of requirements for the care and housing of the zoo's animals.[15] Only about 150 zoos and 65 related facilities in the United States qualify for this status,[16] which represents less than 6% of the U.S. Department of Agriculture's (USDA) licensed animal exhibition sites in the United States.[17] It is unknown how many unlicensed exhibitors exist. Many, though not all, USDA licensed exhibitors have husbandry procedures that would be considered unacceptable by the AZA.

The AZA is a nonprofit organization that sets standards for professional zoos in the United States. These standards address many aspects of animal care and research on animals, from basic husbandry to habitat design to scientific research. The AZA engages in activities such as breeding captive animals, lobbying governments to create protected national parks, and maintaining other plants and animals that keep ecosystems stable. All AZA organizations are required to participate in some breeding and conservation programs, but the precise level of involvement in breeding and conservation differs from zoo to zoo.

Some zoo professionals have concluded that elephants—as well as other endangered species—cannot be saved entirely through captive breeding programs. As Dale Jamieson notes, "If we are serious about preserving wild nature we must preserve the land, and not pretend that we can bring nature indoors."[18] In order to successfully save, protect, and properly care for wild animals, zoos have now modified their approach to conservation to be more holistic. Michael Hutchins puts it this way:

> Outstanding institutions will execute their conservation mission through a broad spectrum of activities, including public education, scientific research, development of relevant technologies, professional training and technology transfer, conservation planning, nature travel programmes, captive breeding for reintroduction, ecological restoration, the direct support of national parks and equivalent reserves, and fundraising to support these activities.[19]

Zoos have diversified their activities and methods of conservation by focusing resources on protecting wild habitats as well as maintaining captive animals.

Zoos now also place a special emphasis on enhancing the welfare of the individual animals in their care. The animals are provided with well-planned habitats and diets, as well as specialized veterinary care. All AZA accredited zoos have veterinarians on call 24 hours a day, every day of the year. Spurred by the 1985 animal welfare law, which was the first U.S. law to address the psychological well-being of captive animals, they have also provided the animals with "environmental-enrichment" programs that improve an otherwise barren, unstimulating environment by providing objects and "furniture" with which animals can interact—e.g., they can manipulate objects and climb in a species-typical manner.[20] In these enrichment programs, zoos have different species-specific guidelines. The most pertinent for the story of Winky and Wanda is "Standards for Elephant Management and Care," the AZA's book of detailed rules for keeping African and Asian elephants.

Rapid Changes at the Detroit Zoo

In the late 1990s, the director of the Detroit Zoo and his staff began an extensive overhaul of Winky and Wanda's area in an attempt to bring them into line with the latest conceptions of an enrichment program and proper training. The first major change was a transition from "free contact" to "protected contact" training. Free contact training allows handlers to enter the elephants' enclosure and interact with them directly. In protected contact, keepers interact with the elephants through a barrier. In free contact, the elephants are usually free to leave if they choose, although sometimes they may be placed in an elephant restraint device if medical treatment is necessary.[21] The AZA requires that accredited zoos train their elephants to facilitate normal veterinary testing and care. Shortly after changing its training methods, the zoo also modified the barn and increased the size of the outdoor area to a full acre.[22]

Even with these improvements, zoo administrators determined that the habitat was not adequate and needed updating. In 2000, as part of a strategy to reorganize all programs of enrichment and training at the zoo, they considered building an elephant habitat at least four times the size of the expanded one. Over the next few years, a series of discussions with experts on elephant care and management led Kagan and his staff to conclude that an acceptable elephant enclosure should be between 10 and 20 acres, with a climate-controlled dome covering a significant portion of that area. While this would remain far smaller than an elephant's natural home range, it would allow more space for walking around, even in the winter. Altogether, "[the] price tag for such a facility in Michigan is likely to be 30–50 million dollars."[23] That much money was more than the Detroit Zoo could afford to spend remodeling a single exhibit, and it was never considered as a realistic financial possibility.

Nothing seemed seriously wrong with either Winky or Wanda. Wanda had arthritis, and Winky had some foot problems, but these are common ailments for captive elephants, and both were receiving treatment. There were no reports of abuse by the keepers, no elephant attacks against humans, no rampaging escapes from the enclosure. The Detroit Zoo could afford to maintain the existing elephant facilities, which already exceeded the AZA's minimum requirements, as well as a moderate upgrade, such as the one proposed in 2000.

The problem, according to Director Kagan, is that we now know that elephants have much more extensive and expensive needs than most other creatures. He argues that "we see elephants constantly damaged—physically and psychologically—from captive environments."[24] He states that the Detroit Zoo cannot satisfy three basic elephant needs: (a) a comfortable climate, (b) a wide area for roaming, and (c) a large social group. In each of these areas, there was a significant disparity between the conditions in the elephants' natural habitat and those at the zoo, and Kagan believes that this gap caused a failure to thrive in the elephants.[25] Winky and Wanda had avoidable foot and joint ailments, he had come to think, and they lacked any form of opportunity to form complex relationships with a herd.

ELEPHANT WELFARE

Captive Settings vs. Natural Environments

In the ideal, though to varying degrees, zoos attempt to recreate a species' natural environment. One of their goals is educational. They seek to teach visitors more about animals' natural habitats. Naturalistic exhibits enhance animal welfare in some cases. Providing animals with appropriate surroundings allows them to perform species-typical behaviors, such as roaming, foraging, and hiding. Being able to act naturally reduces the incidence of undesirable actions, such as stereotypies[26] (repetitive, purposeless movements) and acts of aggression. Some scientists also maintain that animals in naturalistic settings are less prone to stress, which can hinder immune system functioning. The important problem is how to distinguish among the optimal, the merely acceptable, and the suboptimal in recreating a natural environment. This is the key issue at the Detroit Zoo and beyond, raising questions about whether elephants belong in zoos at all.

For elephants, there is no denying that captive environments can only approximate nature to a limited degree. Currently, Asian elephants are found in scattered pockets in India, Southeast Asia, and some parts of Island Asia.[27] The climate is much warmer than in most parts of North America. Because it is so cold in Detroit, "the elephants can't even be outside for a number of months every year."[28] Kagan believes that this is not an acceptable state for animals that are used to living their entire lives outside. The Alaska Zoo—which has never applied for AZA accreditation—has also faced this problem with its African elephant, Maggie. Louis "Tex" Edwards, the director of the Alaska Zoo, says that he and his staff are concerned because their elephant is confined indoors for six months every year.[29] However, Maggie is allowed outside for brief periods even in moderate cold, and she seems to enjoy playing in the snow.[30] The deputy director of the Milwaukee Zoo in Wisconsin believes that elephants are well equipped to handle colder temperatures, with proper management. Milwaukee allows the elephants out of the barn a few times per day, even at 20° F (−6.7° C), and they leave all the doors inside the barn open so that the elephants can wander from room to room.[31]

Another concern is space to roam. The median home range for wild Asian elephants is 43.63 sq mi (113.0 sq km).[32] In more tangible terms, elephants typically range over an area roughly three-quarters the size of Washington, DC, or about 18,600 times the size of the Detroit Zoo's elephant enclosure, including the barn. However, the problem for zoos is more nuanced than the problem of how to approximate an animal's typical natural range of roaming space. Some elephant experts do not believe that elephants need that much space to live happily. The largest elephant sanctuary in the United States, the Elephant Sanctuary in Tennessee, has only 2,700 acres (about 11 sq km), and that space is divided in half so that the Asian and the African elephants can live separately.[33] Wild Asian elephants cover their territory at a rate of only about two miles per day unless there is a famine or drought, so the elephants do not seem to need as much space if they have a steady supply of food and water.[34] If the elephants travel only as far as necessary to find nourishment, then, arguably, a relatively small area with a constantly replenishing food source might suffice.

Steve McCuster of the San Antonio Zoo, which loaned Wanda to the Detroit Zoo in 1994, believes that the issue is primarily one of *exercise,* not *space.* He is concerned that sending the elephants to a sanctuary could have the result that they would simply stand still on a larger piece of land.[35] Similarly, John Lehnhardt, the animal operations director for Disney's Animal Kingdom® in Florida, stresses the importance of properly managing the available resources. For example, each day keepers spread 800 pounds of freshly cut grass across Disney's seven-acre elephant enclosure—the largest in any AZA accredited institution—so that the herd must walk across the entire area to eat all of the grass. The result is that the elephants receive as much exercise as they would in the wild. Lehnhardt also notes that zoo elephants receive benefits that are not always available in the wild, such as freedom from poaching and a steady food supply.[36] However, reliable feedings may not be such a boon. Wild elephants wander around grazing as many as 18 hours per day. Since Disney's feeding practice is the exception rather than the rule, most captive elephants in America lose their most common practice in exchange for large servings at isolated feeding times. This lack of routine makes the elephants prone to foot and joint impairments that would be less likely to occur if the elephants exercised more.

Kagan has also cited sociability as a concern about elephant welfare. Although male elephants usually live alone or in small groups, wild females live in matriarchal family herds throughout their lives, and they often communicate through vocalization and touching. Asian herds usually include six to eight elephants, consisting of a matriarch, her adult daughters, and juveniles of both sexes.[37] Since Winky and Wanda are both older females and have no other companionship, the Detroit Zoo staff was concerned that they were lacking an important component of social and psychological health.

While it is generally agreed that female elephants should be allowed to live within a social group, the minimum number of group members is debated among elephant keepers. There is wide disparity among recommendations found in different elephant care manuals. The Elephant Managers Association standards state only that "[elephants] should have access to other elephants, females should not be housed alone."[38] AZA rules specify that zoos should try to keep at least three females, but the AZA allows some leniency owing to the dearth of captive elephants.[39] The Elephant Sanctuary standards insist that "[any] herd of less than five individuals is not considered a viable social group. Every effort should be made to house elephants in groups no smaller than five."[40]

There is a parallel debate concerning the appropriate and acceptable ages of herd members. The Elephant Sanctuary mentioned above does not breed elephants, and there are no calves in its herd. Lehnhardt, of Disney's Animal Kingdom, argues that raising calves is the main job of wild elephant herds. He notes that the birth of a young calf to the Disney herd has stimulated maternal behaviors in all of the cows, not just the mother. The baby has also tied the herd together as a more cohesive group. He maintains that "the introduction of the calf has been critical to the social fabric of the herd."[41]

Free Contact and Protected Contact as Training Techniques

In addition to climate, space, and social concerns, the Detroit Zoo argued vigorously that Winky and Wanda should go to an institution that employs protected contact training, in which there is a barrier between the elephants and keepers at all times. Captive elephants must be trained to follow commands because they are too strong to be overpowered by almost any human device. This fact has practical importance. For example, it is effectively impossible for zookeepers to administer necessary medical testing and treatment to untrained elephants.

The traditional method of training is free contact, where the keepers interact with elephants without a barrier separating them. This method was derived historically from the mahouts (elephant drivers) of Southeast Asia; for millennia they had captured and trained elephants for a variety of tasks. Wild elephants are extremely dangerous, so the mahouts focus on dominating the elephants.[42] Similarly, free contact trainers in America say that dominance is absolutely essential to ensure safety.[43] Despite the danger, the ability to move freely in the elephants' space has important advantages. Proponents of free contact emphasize how routine bathing and medical tests are facilitated. Training with free contact also makes emergency medical care and scientific research easier.

However, free contact training has increasingly come under fire since the early 1990s. One concern is that free contact lends itself to excessive methods of control. Richard Farinato, a former elephant trainer who used free contact, says that a trainer must employ "attitude adjustment sessions" whenever an elephant misbehaves.[44] Joyce Poole, a very experienced elephant researcher at Amboseli National Park in Kenya, thinks that such language is not strong enough to capture the realities of free contact methods:

> Smaller individuals attempt to rank above larger individuals not by gaining the elephant's respect but through the use of discipline and fear. I have often heard it commented that elephants "discipline" their young and that discipline being natural in elephant society is therefore something that an elephant can understand. I have no idea how this myth was started, but I have never seen calves "disciplined." Protected, comforted, cooed over, reassured, and rescued, yes, but punished, no. Elephants are raised in an incredibly positive and loving environment.[45]

Poole's point is that dominance and punishment are not natural parts of elephant social structure and that training elephants in this fashion could be disastrous. This concern is echoed in a study conducted by the Royal Society for the Prevention of Cruelty to Animals (RSPCA) in the United Kingdom. This study notes that there appears to be a connection between elephant aggression against humans and the dominance training employed in free contact, an especially likely outcome if the trainer employs physical pain or deprivation as punishment. Statistical data from 1991 show that handling elephants was, at that time, the most dangerous job in the United States, outstripping police officers, firefighters, and fishermen in percentage of work-related deaths.[46]

Because of these problems with free contact, many zoos have switched to protected contact. Protected contact separates the elephants and keepers by a barrier at all times. The elephants are free to walk away from the barrier if they choose, so they can escape punishment. This forces the handlers to rely on positive reinforcement. Proponents of protected contact claim that positive reinforcement can be as effective as dominance training, but this claim is controversial.

Some elephant keepers have suggested that protected contact may have a fatal flaw— literally. If handlers cannot enter the elephant yard, then they may be unable to render assistance if elephants become sick or begin to attack each other. Another worry about protected contact is concerned with human, and perhaps elephant, emotion; elephant keepers develop close relationships with the elephants, and the keepers say that such relationships are mutually felt and mutually beneficial. There is fear that critical features of the relationship are lost when keepers and elephants are separated by bars.

ETHICAL ISSUES

Is Elephant Captivity Morally Justifiable?

The most basic ethical issue about zoos and elephants is whether it is justifiable to keep these animals in captivity. The question is whether these animals can justifiably be kept under the conditions they are now generally kept by zoos—not whether it would be justifiable to maintain them under ideal conditions, such as thousands of acres to roam, perfect vegetation, perfect climate, and the like.

Keeping elephants in zoos seems justifiable, and even commendable, from the perspective that zoos provide room for them when none is left in their dwindling habitats. To generalize, if zoos improve the conditions animals experience over what they would experience in their native habitat, then zoos are bettering rather than worsening their lives. An example is arguably found in countries in which elephant herds must be culled to keep the elephants from eating themselves out of house and home.[47]

However, to critics of current zoo policies it is not justifiable even for animals from overpopulated areas to go to zoos. In 2003, protestors tried to prevent the San Diego and Lowry Park Zoos from importing a herd of African elephants that were scheduled to be culled. The protestors maintained that death would be better for the elephants than captivity in zoos.[48] Presumably the judgment here is that, on balance, immediate death is preferable to some circumstances of lingering harms. If this view seems too extreme or implausible, there is a weaker version: Zoos uniformly worsen the conditions of elephants over what they would experience in their natural habitat, and therefore they ought not to be confined in zoos. This view may not be sustainable, but it does open up an important moral problem—one that needs to be addressed much in the way Kagan has raised this issue at the Detroit Zoo. It seems reasonable that zoos be held responsible for ensuring that the benefits of captivity outweigh the harms caused to elephants by captivity.

In many zoos elephants suffer stress, loss of freedom, and a foreign habitat when they are placed in captivity. They are also more likely to develop joint and foot problems in captivity than in the wild. On the other hand, captive elephants in decently managed zoos receive food and medical care daily, are freed from predators, and have congenial, if not the most natural, environments. There are, then, some clear benefits to captivity in these institutions. It is possible, of course, that no set of benefits could outweigh the harms, but this needs to be established by a careful collection of facts and by moral argument about how to array and assess those facts.

Do Elephants Have Rights?

Independent of these questions of balancing utilities (good and bad conditions), other reasons to not keep elephants captive deserve consideration. Perhaps elephants possess rights that we must respect before any considerations of utility are in order. Rights (as discussed in chapter 1) flow from having properties such as intelligence, sentience, and emotion. Elephants are clearly intelligent, sentient, and passionate creatures. They can learn to recognize and follow a large number of commands, both verbal and nonverbal, and they are capable of forming complex herd relationships such as those seen in human families. These facts lend credence to the thesis that elephants have a moral status that affords them some limited range of rights. Even a weak duty to respect an elephant's right not to be harmed could be enough to support the claim that keeping elephants captive is morally impermissible.

Historically, it seems safe to say that elephants have not been regarded as having moral rights. But historically slaves in many, and almost certainly most, societies were regarded as not having rights. Just as there has been a revolution in the way we now view the practice of slavery, so it might be time to recognize a broader set of rights—even if a diminished set of rights—for animals held captive in zoos, such as elephants.

It might be thought that the benefits for humans from elephant captivity are more important than and override any animals' interests and rights. One major benefit to people is entertainment value; another is educational value. No one doubts that these benefits exist, but what exactly do these benefits justify? One question is whether it is morally fair that benefits for humans be balanced against harms caused to animals; this kind of balancing of harms and benefits looks more like a moral prejudice than a fair weighing of utilities for all affected parties. The argument that benefit for people justifies captivity for animals is especially hard to make if elephants have rights. It is a generally accepted principle in rights theory that *some* rights are so basic that ordinary justifications for interference by a community or state, such as lessening inconvenience or promoting utility, are not sufficient to override the right(s). The right not to be harmed is almost universally accepted as such a right. The stakes must be very significant indeed to justify causing harm to individuals, because rights are valid claims held by an individual against the projects and utilities of others. Rights function to guarantee that individuals cannot be sacrificed to government or communal interests. Rights are, so to speak, above utilitarian goals.

Obviously the deepest question here is whether animals have rights of this strength.

Is the Choice One of Zoos or Sanctuaries?

Even if keeping some elephants captive is justifiable, questions remain about the most appropriate type of captivity. Specifically, should elephants be housed in zoos or in sanctuaries (as we know them today)? Is either an appropriate environment?

Consider Wanda and Winky and the Detroit Zoo, in particular. Both of the sanctuaries recommended by the Detroit Zoo as preferable are warmer and reasonably appropriate in climate (although the Elephant Sanctuary in Tennessee does receive snow during most winters). The Performing Animal Welfare Society (PAWS) sanctuary in California is semi-tropical. This smaller sanctuary has over 100 acres of land dedicated to Asian elephants, and both have herds of several elephants.

Many important differences exist between zoos and sanctuaries. Zoos allow more scientific research than sanctuaries. Sanctuaries do not allow scientific research on the grounds that it interferes with the elephants' activities (although observational studies are permitted). Zoo veterinarians can provide full medical treatment at any time, whereas sanctuary veterinarians have to locate elephants and their problems when they are wandering. These animals also may have to be transported to a barn—a considerable undertaking under the conditions of sanctuaries. Sanctuaries refuse to breed their animals because there is no chance that the calves will be reintroduced into the wild. This is in contrast to zoos, which sometimes include calves in their elephant social groups. As a result, elephants in sanctuaries have no chance to interact with young elephants.

Another difference—though it is not so clearly a morally relevant difference—centers on opportunities to view the animals and the implications of those opportunities. The public is allowed to view zoo animals. Only keepers, some scientists, and a few generous donors see sanctuary elephants. This fact, however, does not seem to decide the major moral issues about elephants. The AZA argues that people will donate more time and money for conservation if they can view the elephants personally, but this seems more a financial than a moral consideration.

Are Animals Ambassadors of Conservation and Education?

Michael Hutchins, the director of conservation and science for the AZA, writes that "zoo elephants can be seen as true 'ambassadors,' helping to educate the public and direct critical resources—human and financial—toward the conservation of their cousins."[49] He believes that elephants like Winky and Wanda are ambassadors in the sense that they bring conservation issues before the public, which in turn results in contributions of money made by the public to benefit elephants in the wild.

"Ambassadors" is a questionable metaphor in this setting. Unlike human ambassadors, these elephants are removed from their habitats, confined, and used as subjects of scientific research. The metaphor of "sacrifice" might be a questionable metaphor in the opposite direction, but the conception of ambassador in this argument does seem to suggest that one group of animals is making a sacrifice of its interests for the interests of another group. Moreover, coming as it does from an AZA official, this argument seems a bit self-serving and could even put the AZA in a position of conflict of interest.

Setting aside these questions of appropriate metaphors and their source, there are important ethical questions about conservation that need to be addressed. The simplest conservation method seems to be "reintroduction." Endangered animals are bred in captivity and then released into the wild. This plan seems an ideal conception for the revitalization of the failing Asian elephant population. However, reintroduction is risky and difficult in practice. "The probability of successful reintroduction, even for animals that are prepared for release from birth, is low (mortality can exceed 80 percent in some species). This risk to individual welfare is precisely why reintroductions should only be attempted when the benefit to conservation is very high, as for example, in desperate attempts to save endangered species from extinction."[50] There is no point in attempting to reintroduce animals to natural habitats that are rapidly being destroyed or in areas where herds are being culled. Also, since zoos do not yet have a self-sustaining captive population of elephants, they have made a judgment that they cannot risk their calves on such attempts at reintroduction.

The AZA itself has no plans for a reintroduction program.[51] Even with a stable captive population, the AZA would have to import some wild elephants to prevent the loss of genetic diversity through inbreeding. Importing can undercut conservation, so this policy would be at once expensive and self-defeating.

There are also problems with the feasibility of reintroduction. Animals bred in captivity are subject to different evolutionary stresses, and they can develop traits that would be maladaptive in the wild. As several authorities have argued, "Captive breeding should be viewed as a last resort in species recovery and not a prophylactic or long-term solution because of the inexorable genetic and phenotypic changes that occur in captive environments."[52] Although the AZA carefully selects breeding partners among the elephants, some genetic drift is inevitable.

It is likely that elephants born in captivity would have a difficult time surviving in the wild. Reintroducing captive-born elephants would also increase the risk of exposing wild elephants to foreign diseases. At the same time, breeding does allow researchers to learn about elephant reproduction, contraception, and physical development, and this knowledge is potentially of practical assistance in regulating and preserving wild herds. Calves also help cement the relationships within captive populations, as well as allow the adult elephants to exercise their parental instincts.

If *wild* elephants should become extinct, it is possible that stable *captive* populations might be useful in reestablishing the species. But since there are no significant practical plans for reintroduction, the *conservation* value in keeping elephants is doubtful. Nonetheless, there is some conservation value in zoos, which contribute to conservation through research. Some zoo scientists perform field research, and some do research on the animals in the zoos. For example, veterinary scientists have learned much about elephant reproduction and contraception by working with zoo elephants. This reproduction research promises to increase the success of zoo breeding programs, and elephant contraception can be used to help control wild elephant populations.[53] Without captive elephants trained to submit to medical procedures, much of what we know about elephants would not be available.

POSTSCRIPT

So what became of Winky and Wanda? In December 2004, the AZA announced its final decision concerning Detroit's elephants.[54] After tests indicated that Wanda might be infected with elephant endotheliotropic herpes virus (EEHV), the Columbus Zoo refused to take either Winky or Wanda. Realizing that exposure to EEHV could be fatal to calves, zoo officials considered Wanda and Winky to be surplus to the managed breeding population. The San Antonio Zoo (which had historically only loaned Wanda to the Detroit Zoo) then decided to officially donate Wanda to the Detroit Zoo in the interest of keeping the two elephants together. Finally freed of all external considerations, the Detroit Zoo made arrangements for both of the elephants to be transferred to the PAWS sanctuary in California.

While the situation for Winky and Wanda was resolved to the satisfaction of virtually every human directly involved, the ethical questions about elephants in captivity were not resolved either in the community of zookeepers or beyond.

NOTES

1. American Zoo and Aquarium Association (AZA), *Standards for Elephant Management and Care,* May 5, 2003, www.aza.org/AboutAZA/ElephantsZoos/Documents/ElephantStandards.pdf, p. 2 (accessed July 29, 2004). AZA standards are more comprehensive and difficult to meet than the government requirements for an animal exhibitor license; this will be discussed in further detail later.

2. Detroit Zoological Institute, "Detroit Zoo Intends to Send Elephants to Elephant Sanctuary," *Detroit Zoological Institute Press Releases and News,* May 20, 2004, www.detroitzoo.com/media/release_pages.asp?ID=330 (accessed July 27, 2004).

3. Ben Lefebvre, "Zoo to Free Elephants," *New York Times,* National Report/Midwest: Michigan, May 21, 2004; Richard Farinato, "Detroit Zoo Sends Its Elephants Packing; Should Others Follow Suit?" *Humane Society of the United States,* May 27, 2004, www.hsus.org/ace/21142 (accessed May 27, 2004).

4. Ron Kagan, interview by Paul Jude Naquin, telephone interview notes, June 3, 2004.

5. Peter Jennings, *ABC World News Tonight,* July 18, 2004; "Detroit Zoo to Give Up Elephants," *Discovery Channel News,* May 21, 2004, dsc.discovery.com/news/afp/20040517/detroitzoo.html (accessed August 21, 2004).

6. "Detroit Zoo Receives Long Awaited AZA Recommendation on Fate of Elephants," *Detroit Zoological Institute Press Releases and News,* September 7, 2004, www.detroitzoo.com/critters2.html (accessed October 16, 2004).

7. Karl Gröning and Martin Saller, *Elephants: A Cultural and Natural History* (Cologne, Germany: Könemann, 1999), p. 424.

8. Ron Kagan and Sue Marx, *From Animal Showboat to Animal Lifeboat,* directed by Sue Marx (26 mins.), Sue Marx Films, Inc., 2004 (videocassette).

9. Kay Houston, "How the Detroit Zoo's First Day Was Almost Its Last," *Detroit News,* 1938, info.detnews.com/history/story/index.cfm?id=204&category=locations (accessed July 27, 2004).

10. Michael Hutchins, e-mail correspondence with author, February 28, 2005.

11. In the traditional story, Noah saved the world's animals from death by taking two of each species of animal aboard his ship.

12. Eugene Hargrove, "The Role of Zoos in the Twenty-first Century," in *Ethics on the Ark: Zoos, Animal Welfare, and Wildlife Conservation,* ed. Bryan G. Norton, Michael Hutchins, Elizabeth F. Stevens, and Terry L. Maple (Washington, DC: Smithsonian Institution Press, 1995), pp. 13–19.

13. *Merriam-Webster Online Dictionary,* www.m-w.com/cgi-bin/dictionary?book=Dictionary&va=zoo (accessed July 27, 2004).

14. Max Block and Bijal P. Trivedi, "Former Pet Tigers Find Home in Tennessee Shelter," *National Geographic on Assignment,* November 17, 2003, news.nationalgeographic.com/news/2003/11/1117_031117_tvbigcats.html#main (accessed July 27, 2004).

15. "2005 Guide to Accreditation of Zoological Parks and Aquariums (and Accreditation Standards)," *AZA Accreditation,* www.aza.org/Accreditation/Documents/AccredGuide.pdf (accessed November 9, 2004).

16. "Current Number of Accredited Members," *AZA Statistics at a Glance,* www.aza.org/Newsroom/NewsroomStatistics/ (accessed August 23, 2004).

17. "FY 2002 Annual Report," *Animal Care Publications and Policy,* www.aphis.usda.gov/ac/2002ar/ar2002.pdf (accessed August 21, 2004).

18. Dale Jamieson, "Zoos Revisited," in *Ethics on the Ark,* ed. Bryan G. Norton, Michael Hutchins, Elizabeth F. Stevens, and Terry L. Maple, p. 62.

19. Michael Hutchins, "Characteristics of a World-Class Zoo or Aquarium in the 21st Century," in *International Zoo Yearbook* 38, ed. P. J. S. Olney and Fiona A. Fisken (London: Zoological Society of London, 2003), p. 136.

20. Food Security Act of 1985, Public Law No. 99–198, 7 USC § 2143. This law included amendments to the Animal Welfare Act of 1966 that animal exhibitors must provide for the psychological health of primates. AZA zoos attempt to extend this prescription to other species as well.

21. AZA, *Standards for Elephant Management and Care,* p. 8.

22. Detroit Zoological Institute, "Detroit Zoo Intends to Send Elephants to Elephant Sanctuary."

23. Detroit Zoological Institute, "Questions and Answers about Decisions to Move Elephants from the Detroit Zoo," *Detroit Zoological Institute,* May 19, 2004, www.detroitzoo.com/home_pg_article/index.html (accessed May 27, 2004).

24. Hugh McDiarmid Jr., "Detroit Zoo Elephant Decision: Director Answers Critics, Explains Why He Put Animals' Needs First," *Detroit Free Press,* June 17, 2004, www.freep.com/news/metro/kagan17_20040617.htm (accessed June 22, 2004).

25. Detroit Zoological Institute, "Questions and Answers about Decisions to Move Elephants from the Detroit Zoo."

26. For more on stereotypies, see chapter 7, in the case about large cats in circuses.

27. Michael Keele and Norie Dimeo-Ediger, *Asian Elephant (Elephas Maximus) North American Regional Studbook, Current as of December 31, 2000* (Portland, OR: Metro Regional Services, 2001), p. 5.

28. Ron Kagan, interview, June 3, 2004.

29. Louis "Tex" Edwards, interview by Paul Jude Naquin, telephone interview notes, June 18, 2004.

30. "Maggie's Corner," *The Alaska Zoo*, September 30, 2002, www.alaskazoo.org/maggie.htm (accessed July 29, 2004).

31. Bruce Beehler, interview by Paul Jude Naquin, telephone interview notes, June 1, 2004.

32. R. Clubb and Georgia Mason, *A Review of the Welfare of Zoo Elephants in Europe: A Report Commissioned by the RSPCA* [Royal Society for the Prevention of Cruelty to Animals] (Oxford: University of Oxford, 2002), p. 16.

33. "Frequently Asked Questions," *The Elephant Sanctuary*, www.elephants.com/questions.htm, question 6 (accessed July 30, 2004).

34. Clubb and Mason, *A Review of the Welfare of Zoo Elephants in Europe*, p. 16.

35. Steve McCuster, interview by Paul Jude Naquin, telephone interview notes, June 23, 2004.

36. John Lehnhardt, interview by Paul Jude Naquin, telephone interview notes, June 29, 2004.

37. Clubb and Mason, *A Review of the Welfare of Zoo Elephants in Europe*, p. 59.

38. Elephant Managers Association, "Standard Guidelines for Elephant Management," *Journal of the Elephant Managers Association* 10, no. 3 (1999): 203.

39. AZA, *Standards for Elephant Management and Care*, pp. 4–5.

40. Elephant Sanctuary, *Guidelines for Captive Elephants*, October 13, 2001, www.elephants.com/TESGuidelines.doc (accessed July 30, 2004).

41. Lehnhardt, interview, June 29, 2004.

42. Gröning and Saller, *Elephants: A Cultural and Natural History*, pp. 292–304.

43. Richard Farinato, interview by Paul Jude Naquin, telephone interview notes, June 1, 2004.

44. Ibid.

45. Joyce Poole, "Elephant Managers Association," *Circus Watch WA*, www.circuswatchwa.org/managers_assoc.htm (accessed February 10, 2005).

46. Clubb and Mason, *A Review of the Welfare of Zoo Elephants in Europe*, p. 232.

47. Gröning and Saller, *Elephants: A Cultural and Natural History*, p. 450.

48. Michael Hutchins, "Better Off Dead than Captive Bred?" *Communiqué* (June 2004): 47.

49. Ibid., p. 53.

50. Michael Hutchins, "Keiko Dies: Killer Whale of *Free Willy* Fame," *Communiqué* (February 2004): 55.

51. Michael Hutchins, telephone interview by Paul Jude Naquin, June 16, 2004.

52. Noel F. R. Snyder, Scott R. Derrickson, Steven R. Beissinger, James W. Wiley, Thomas B. Smith, William D. Toone, and Brian Miller, "Limitations of Captive Breeding in Endangered Species Recovery," *Conservation Biology* 10 (April 1996): 338.

53. Brandie Smith and Michael Hutchins, "The Value of Captive Breeding Programmes to Field Conservation: Elephants as an Example," *Pachyderm* 28 (January–June 2000): 103–5.

54. "American Zoo and Aquarium Association Announces Elephant Resolution," *Detroit Zoological Institute Press Releases and News*, December 3, 2004, www.detroitzoo.com/critters2.html (accessed January 7, 2005).

7

Ringling Brothers' Big Cats

On July 11, 2004, the crowds in Phoenix, Arizona, cheered for Clyde the lion. Only two years old, he was one of the youngest lions performing with Ringling Bros. and Barnum & Bailey Circus.[1] Clyde had been acquired from a lion troop in Spain and since January had been traveling with the circus. He was still a few years short of mating age and had probably not reached his full adult size.[2] Clyde was still rather new to performances, but he bore the charismatic majesty native to his kind, and the crowds cheered.

The next day, Clyde died. Feld Entertainment, Inc., which owns Ringling Bros., issued a press release saying that he had died on the circus train of unknown causes. The press statement also said that the remaining cats would be transported by truck until an internal review of conditions of transportation by train was conducted.[3] People for the Ethical Treatment of Animals (PETA) alleged that the young lion succumbed to heatstroke as the circus train crossed the Mojave Desert.[4] Frank Hagan, a former Ringling employee, issued an affidavit to the U.S. Department of Agriculture (USDA) supporting PETA's claims. He said that a circus supervisor had ignored repeated requests to stop the train so that the cats could receive water and that he was instructed not to speak to USDA investigators after Clyde's death. Hagan also stated that Ringling had installed mist sprinklers in the train before USDA agents arrived to investigate the incident.[5] Jim Andacht, vice president of circus operations for Ringling Bros., disputed the accuracy of Hagan's story, claiming that Hagan was not even an animal handler[6] and that he "was dismissed on July 21, 2004 for endangering his life, as well as the lives of other Ringling Bros. employees, arena personnel, and four of our lions."[7]

Exactly how and why Clyde perished is still unclear. Hagan has insisted that the lion's death resulted from reckless negligence on the part of Ringling employees. Ringling's representatives have claimed that the event was a tragic accident, blown out of proportion by a disgruntled, and possibly unbalanced, former employee.[8] Investigators for the USDA have offered no comments, and they are not allowed to discuss ongoing investigations. Animal advocacy groups across the country have asserted that Clyde's death marked the latest in a long history of animal abuses by Ringling and circuses in general.

THE HISTORY AND LEGACY OF ANIMAL SHOWS

Background History

Big cats have long been prized display items. In ancient Rome, lions and tigers were used for battles in the amphitheaters. The animals had to be starved for several days prior to battle to make them aggressive, because otherwise they would simply lie down in the arenas. Motivated by hunger, the large cats would then be pitted against humans or other animals, inflicting and sustaining deep and often fatal wounds. Well beyond Rome, and for many centuries, animals were kept as status symbols in private menageries, often living in small cages with nothing to do as years passed. Some of these animals were trained through brutal techniques of domination to perform tricks for the amusement of the wealthy.[9]

Near the beginning of the nineteenth century, traveling troupes of performers—the forerunners of modern circuses—began touring Europe, bringing exotic animals to attract spectators. Crowds came to ride some of the animals and watch them perform tricks, and circuses as we know them began to emerge.[10] In 1870, P.T. Barnum's Grand Traveling Museum, Menagerie, Caravan, and Circus began showcasing human and animal exhibitions.[11] It eventually became Ringling Bros. and Barnum & Bailey "The Greatest Show on Earth." Altogether, Ringling Bros. has now been displaying animal shows in America for over 135 years.

Defenses of Big Animals in Big Shows

Today's Ringling Bros. circus purports to break the mold of historical animal treatment. Ringling boasts of excellent animal care, both on the circus train and at the winter quarters in Florida. Ringling takes pride in its retirement facilities as well. Ringling sponsors a Center for Elephant Conservation and Big Cat Rescue, which is a separately owned nonprofit facility. Many circuses claim to encourage animal education and conservation by fostering strong emotional bonds between humans and animals.

Going to the circus is a tradition in many countries, and animal acts are at the heart of this tradition. For many attendees, the animals draw more interest than the human performers. Crowds flock to the circus to see lions, tigers, and elephants perform incredible feats of strength and agility. Circus advocates claim that there are often unnoticed human benefits to animal performances in circuses. At a time when sex, violence, and offensive humor are pervasive throughout most forms of entertainment, the circus seems to many to be one of the last wholesome family outings available. Many people also believe that seeing animals firsthand provides a connection to nature that cannot be supplied by television, and that this connection is especially important for children living in our increasingly urbanized society.

Circus advocates also believe that the animals can be more relaxed and happy because they need not fear starvation or thirst. Satisfying the appetites of lions, tigers, and elephants is costly and requires expertise. The big circus has an advantage over most zoos in that prohibitively expensive animal care is offset by paying customers. Circus enthusiasts also note that since many circus animals are members of endangered species, circuses can promote endangered species conservation both by caring for individual animals and by fostering public concern for endangered species.

Criticisms of Big Animals in the Circus

Whatever their benefits, for several years, Ringling Bros. and many other circuses have been the object of protests by animal advocacy organizations alleging inhumane treatment. Charges of inhumane treatment derive from two basic types of worry about animal participation in circuses. First, critics claim that the animals are improperly trained or cared for. Either the handlers are not conforming to the legal requirements of the Animal Welfare Act (AWA), or the law itself is insufficient to guarantee the animals' well-being. Second, critics contend that circuses, by their nature, are *inherently* unsuitable for animals. Both are strong condemnations requiring adequate supporting evidence. We will be looking only at the evidence in the case of Ringling Brothers and its treatment of big cats.

THE RECORD AT RINGLING BROTHERS

Some circuses have been accused of violating the AWA, which provides minimum guidelines for animal care. Ringling Bros. has been the biggest target of such accusations, perhaps because it is the largest circus. Ringling rejects these charges entirely, stating that "in the over 30 years of current ownership, Ringling Bros. has never been found in violation of the AWA for abuse, neglect or mistreatment of its animals."[12]

Ringling's official statement is correct in that the organization has never been *convicted* of an AWA violation. However, records from the USDA's Animal and Plant Health Inspection Service, Animal Care division, which is charged with enforcing the AWA, suggest problems in recent years.[13] In 1998 Ringling Bros. was issued an official warning for "[failure] to use an appropriate method of euthanasia."[14] More specifically, a handler fired five shotgun shells into a tiger that had bitten his brother.[15] Not long after this incident, Ringling was charged with forcing a sick elephant named Kenny to perform. Kenny had been bleeding from the rectum before the show, and he died later that evening. The case was settled out of court for $20,000, though Ringling was not required to admit fault in the incident.[16]

Has Ringling Brothers learned from the mistakes made in these cases? Consider a clause of the AWA regulations: "[Live] animals shall not be subjected to surrounding air temperatures which exceed 29.5° C. (85° F.) . . . for a period of more than 45 minutes."[17]

Ringling has two traveling groups, the Red Unit and the Blue Unit. According to a research study conducted through Texas A&M University and partially funded by the USDA, on June 21, 2000, the temperature in the Red Unit's tiger train car rose above 30° C (86° F) for more than 10 consecutive hours.[18] The same report shows that just a few weeks later, the temperature again stayed above 30° C for more than six hours. During that same summer, the Blue Unit was cited once in a USDA inspection report because two tigers injured themselves trying to escape the heat in their transport trailer; one broke off a tooth and tore the cage door off its track.[19] The USDA cited the Blue Unit again, one week later, for providing only a temporary solution to the problem.[20] After the second inspection report, Ringling decided to transport the tigers in the Blue Unit by truck instead of by train, giving Ringling time to address the cooling and ventilation issues on the circus train.

Four years later, Clyde died. PETA reported that a whistleblower told them that Clyde died in a poorly ventilated boxcar while traveling in high heat through the Mojave Desert.[21] Frank Hagan, the recently dismissed Ringling employee, supported this claim. In response, Ringling stated: "Hagan continues to completely misrepresent the facts surrounding his termination from Ringling Bros. circus during its run in Los Angeles, California."[22] Ringling also claimed that the results of Clyde's necropsy[23] by an independent pathologist were inconclusive as to the cause of death and that the other twelve lions on the train were found healthy in an examination. Nevertheless, Ringling once again decided to transport the big cats by truck, as a temporary measure.[24] It added a short clarification of animal care during transportation to its website: "The enclosures provide room for ample freedom of movement and appropriate social interaction with other animals, proper ventilation, and protection from the elements."[25]

An examination of records from 1990 to 2002 shows that Ringling was cited every year during this period by the USDA's Animal Care division.[26] Despite these citations, the Feld Entertainment website continued to advertise that "in all aspects of animal care and safety, Ringling Bros. meets or exceeds all federal animal welfare standards set by the United States Department of Agriculture (USDA) under the Animal Welfare Act."[27] (This statement was later revised to say, "In all aspects of animal care and safety, Ringling Bros. meets all federal animal welfare standards."[28])

BARRIERS TO IMPOSING ANIMAL CARE LAWS ON CIRCUSES

The AWA sets out the *minimum* legally permissible standards of animal care. These standards are not presented as optimal standards. Questions about applicable laws have centered less on the inadequacy of these standards than on their proper enforcement. There are several barriers to imposing animal care laws on circuses. Circuses rarely remain in one place long enough for state and local authorities to inspect the facilities, and even federal inspectors may have difficulty keeping up with the shows, which often travel to a different state every few days.

The USDA's procedure for handling AWA violations presents another problem of enforcement. When a circus is inspected, the inspector records any AWA violations in a formal report. The inspector's remarks include a date by which the problem must be addressed, usually between 7 and 30 days after the initial inspection. A copy of the report goes to a circus official, but no sanctions are imposed at that time. Unless the offense is particularly serious, the USDA will only issue an official warning. No fines or other punishments are imposed unless the same violation is evident at the next inspection. After such a report or warning is imposed, the circus might not be inspected again for several months.

As noted above, despite having received a number of citations, Ringling has almost never been brought up on formal charges. Ringling was not charged with violations related to the high heat during tiger transports, even though the July 2000 inspection report stated that the tigers were in immediate danger.[29] Questions have been raised about Ringling's other animals as well. For example, USDA undersecretary Mike Dunn has stated that Ringling Brothers had violated the Animal Welfare Act in allowing physical harm and behavioral stress to occur to baby elephants.[30] Even in the case of Kenny, the young elephant who died after performing when he needed medical care, Ringling Bros. avoided any legal conviction through a settlement.

Circus critics also challenge claims that Ringling and other circuses exhibit excellence in animal handling. The website Circuses.com lists violation records for 28 different circuses, including Ringling Bros. and Barnum & Bailey, Universoul Circus, and Carson and Barnes Circus. These violations run the gamut from having unsanitary facilities to allowing public interaction with animals that have communicable diseases (such as tuberculosis) or that have attacked humans in the past.[31]

ETHICAL ISSUES

Not meeting the basic physical needs of captive animals for food, water, and shelter has long been, and remains, the main ethical issue about circuses. However, other aspects of the circumstances and well-being of the animals also raise issues. What, then, are the major ethical issues?

Environments Suitable to Animal Well-Being

The maintenance of an appropriate ambient temperature in animal enclosures and the provision of environments that allow expression of the animals' normal range of bodily movement and behavior are of critical importance. Large cats, and indeed all circus animals, must maintain certain body temperatures in order to survive. Excesses of hot or cold can kill just as easily as starvation or dehydration, and in far less time. Even extreme temperatures that do not kill can have serious health effects on an animal. Also, in a performing environment with large animals, every structure and prop must be adapted to accommodate constant travel. Otherwise, there is risk of injury to both humans and animals.

The aforementioned research study from Texas A&M University indicates that the tiger transport temperatures were outside of the AWA limits on almost half of the relocation trips studied. Only one of the six circuses participating in the study had no incidences of extreme temperatures lasting longer than 45 minutes during transport.[32] Temperature maintenance is not usually a problem in milder seasons or more temperate areas; however, circuses continue to travel many thousands of miles throughout the winter and summer. Temperature control is not only difficult to provide but can be very expensive. This fact raises questions about when, if ever, it is permissible to cut costs at the expense of animal welfare.

Stereotypic Behavior

Another major concern for large cats—and for other captive animals—is stereotypical behavior. "The term *stereotypy* refers to behavior that is characteristically repetitive, is invariant in form, and has no obvious goal or function."[33] The most common stereotypy is pacing, in which the animal walks over the same path repeatedly. Rainer Maria Rilke captures the nature of stereotypic pacing in his poem *The Panther,* about a close cousin of both lions (*panthera Leo*) and tigers (*panthera Tigris*). The poem begins, "His weary glance, from passing by the bars, / Has grown into a dazed and vacant stare."[34]

Stereotypies are generally considered an indication of boredom or distress, and animal behaviorists have invested a great deal of time in learning how to reduce them.[35] Most experts believe that an animal develops stereotypic behaviors when it cannot express enough of its natural behaviors. Many keepers try to reduce stereotypies, therefore, by providing their charges with toys, exercise areas, or pools of water.

Recently, a different explanation of stereotypic behavior has surfaced. Ted Friend, a professor in Texas A&M University's animal science department, thinks that stereotypies may signify excitement and anticipation rather than unhappiness. He has conducted research on elephants that indicates that stereotypic behaviors increase just prior to feeding, watering, and performing. Friend claims that this is an indication that the elephants, and other animals such as large felines, are acting like small children bouncing in excitement.[36] For example, tigers often pace excitedly when they see small children (who look like easy prey).[37] Friend's unique viewpoint is as yet unsubstantiated, and a significant body of scientific research suggests that most stereotypic behaviors are an indication of distress.[38] They clearly result from maintaining captive animals in confining, barren enclosures that frustrate the expression of normal behaviors.

Exercise and Freedom of Normal Bodily Movement

Some critics of circuses argue that the requirements of the AWA do not prevent various forms of inhumane treatment. In particular, they claim that the AWA has extremely limited provisions for exercise, which are critical to animal welfare. The AWA requires animal exhibitors to provide "sufficient space to allow each animal to make normal postural and social adjustments with adequate freedom of movement."[39] Included in this clause is the freedom to exhibit normal bodily movement. But mobile circuses do not, and probably cannot under most circumstances, transport lions, tigers, and elephants in cages that allow them to walk around freely, let alone climb or jump. For this reason, the USDA has developed a policy that allows animals to be kept in travel cages that permit only "postural and social adjustments"; however, the animals must be allowed to exercise outside of the cages at least once per day (the period of time for exercise is not specified). It is not required that these travel cages permit movements such as rearing up on hind legs, which large cats periodically do.[40]

Animal welfarists have argued that these animals are being denied a basic necessity: the ability to exercise and move naturally at regular intervals. Circus supporters reply by arguing that animals do not walk for exercise in the wild, but, rather, they walk to find food. Since food is provided for them in the circus, the animals do not need to walk or exercise as much. In addition, they argue, large cats sleep for about 18 hours per day, so they do not need to spend much time in the exercise pen.[41]

Clearly there is an important empirical question as well as a moral question in this controversy: How much exercise does an animal need to remain healthy in mind and body? Many large cats in circuses exercise during performances for only about eight to ten minutes per day.[42] Might this be enough to stay fit? If trainers keep their animals fit at this level, have they discharged their moral obligations to the animal?

Training Methods

Animal performances in circuses have sparked controversy over the methods used to teach the animals the tricks that the crowds so enjoy. Which means of training are acceptable and which are unacceptable? Critics of circus methods claim that the animals are routinely subjected to pain and deprivation by being coerced to obedience. Critics have produced several videotapes documenting inappropriate treatment of circus animals.[43] Tom Rider, a former Ringling Bros. worker, has sharply criticized practices of training. He claims that the lions and tigers are only docile because "the cats are beat into submission as babies."[44]

Ringling's website presents a strikingly different view of corporate practices of animal training. "Our expert handlers watch closely as their animals socialize, then create routines based on natural behavior. We use voice recognition and rewards to encourage the animals to learn a set routine."[45] The website does not mention whether forms of punishment are used to train animals. Since there is no impartial observation of animal training techniques, it is difficult to know what happens under the big top. Is positive reinforcement the most basic tool used in the training of lions and tigers? Do standard training and care practices conform to AWA standards? Answers to these questions are largely unknown.

A Systemic Problem?

Another moral worry is whether circus performances should be allowed at all, even if the animals' environment and care are up to the latest standards and recommendations. There are concerns that both humans and animals are being placed at unnecessary risk in these performances. These worries are set forth in a report from the American Zoo and Aquarium Association's Tiger Species Survival Plan (SSP):

> During the 2002 Tiger SSP master plan meeting in Portland, there was a discussion of the appropriateness of handling tigers in public places. . . . There was complete consensus of all members in attendance that such actions place the viewing public at risk of injury or death, that there is no educational message of value being delivered, that such actions promote private ownership and a false sense of safe handling of exotic big cats, and that the animal itself loses its dignity as an ambassador from the wild. As a result, the committee resolved [that tiger shows are] inappropriate.[46]

The SSP's report focuses first on human safety. Wild animals, such as lions, tigers, and elephants, are extremely dangerous. Tigers killed nine people in the United States between 1999 and 2004.[47] There are many other cases of nonfatal attacks. Effectively, every one of these attacks was the result of some owner's inattention to the animal.[48]

(There are no wild lions or tigers in the United States, only captive ones.) In some cases, the public is not in danger, but tiger handlers are. For example, consider a much discussed (in the media) tragedy that befell Roy Horn of *Siegfried and Roy*, the entertainers who performed regularly at the Mirage Casino in Las Vegas. On October 3, 2003, Horn was performing with a tiger he had raised from birth, but the tiger still bit him on the neck, nearly killing him.[49] Large cats are extraordinarily adept natural predators. Placing them within close proximity of people is always dangerous.

But of what moral importance is this fact? Does it mean that no one should train lions and tigers or place them in circumstances of human contact? Why is danger to humans in these circumstances alarming? People voluntarily accept these jobs, just as they eagerly perform various dangerous jobs in other entertainment industries. Movie stunt actors and racecar drivers are examples. The dangers they undertake may indicate only that inexperienced people should not be allowed to do what they do. Perhaps the same is true with animal trainers?

The Role of Circuses in Education and Conservation

Setting aside questions of animal and human well-being and safety, there are moral questions about whether animals should be kept in circuses at all. Many circuses acknowledge that entertainment alone does not justify animal captivity, but they argue that circuses provide more than entertainment; they promote both education and conservation of endangered species.[50] For some people, especially those living far from a significant zoo, circuses provide a rare opportunity to see exotic animals. Circus proponents maintain that such experiences provide incentives for individuals to learn about endangered species and to contribute to their survival in the wild. Some circuses also participate in conservation efforts directly. For example, Ringling Bros. owns and operates the Center for Elephant Conservation, which is used for retirement, breeding, and research.[51] (For a discussion of problems with animal breeding and research, see chapter 6 on elephants in zoos.)

Circus critics counter that people should be wary of the message that is being taught. Watching deadly predators act like tame pussycats is deceptive; it gives the impression that wild animals have humane instincts and can be domesticated. One concern here is that lions' and tigers' natural beauty is diminished and that they seem like mere toys for human use. Instead of educating people about animal welfare and conservation, using animals for entertainment in this way might make them out to be mere objects for our amusement.

Animal advocacy groups also fear that watching tigers perform tricks may fuel the exotic pet trade. Under current market conditions, a person can buy an unusual kitten— that is, lion or tiger cub—for around $2,500. (The cub itself accounts for only a fraction of an adequate initial investment. The full price, including such items as a proper enclosure, transport vehicle, veterinary care, and insurance costs may rise to $100,000.) In a matter of months, the gorgeous kitten becomes a several-hundred-pound carnivore that costs at least $8,000 per year in food and nonemergency veterinary care.

Because these cats are so expensive to maintain, owners often cut corners on animal care, usually with disastrous results. According to one estimate, 98% of all exotic pets in the United States die within the first two years.[52] Every year, large cat sanctuaries turn away hundreds of people who are trying to rid themselves of their too-demanding pets.

These owners may love these pets and wish them well, but they cannot take care of them and often are not qualified to care for them.

The Dignity of Lions and Tigers

Thus far we have considered the effects that circus practices have on the health of lions, tigers, and human beings. Also important is whether such performances detract from the animals' dignity or otherwise disrespect the animals. This may be the most abstract and the most difficult consideration, because there is no way to measure these aspects, and the ideas of indignity and disrespect are difficult to define and to address in concrete ways.

Critics of circuses claim that training lions and tigers to perform tricks in front of an audience amounts to treating the animals like pets and playthings, rather than as powerful and majestic animals worthy of respect. A contrast can be made here between the way many producers of films about animals present the animals they film and the way circuses present animals. The concern is that big-cat shows encourage people to view the felines as objects that are human-controlled like other parts of nature, and in sharp contrast to humans. If people develop the view of animals as mere objects and playthings, then they will be unlikely to either understand or respect animals in the wild.

Circus proponents claim that the opposite is true. Ringling Bros. summarizes the conservation goals of animal performances on its website.

> Independent studies have shown that the public display of animals heightens public awareness of the animals and of our responsibility for their well being and protection. This is especially true for children, who not only become more aware of the animals and their special needs and abilities, but also experience firsthand the importance of caring for and respecting all animals.[53]

Ringling claims that people who see lions and tigers at the circus, especially people who rarely see animals elsewhere, gain a respect for the cats' incredible power and grace. This respect then spurs individuals to become aware of the need to protect endangered species.

It has never been carefully studied whether circus performances enhance or diminish human respect for large cats. In the absence of research studies, claims cannot be properly evaluated. However, this research would be very difficult to conduct, because it would be practically impossible to track appropriate beliefs about and actions toward exotic cats and other animals based on peoples' experience with circuses.

Crowds cheered for Clyde the lion the day before he died. Was his death a random, inexplicable occurrence? Did he have an undiagnosed disease? Did he die of heat exhaustion? Was his death the result of some form of neglect by Ringling employees? These factual questions about Clyde may have beneath them pressing ethical concerns. For example, does the Animal Welfare Act provide for adequate care of exotic cats, and even if it does, was Clyde adequately cared for? Does Ringling Brothers have appropriate moral standards for the treatment of animals? Do the needs of large felines and other circus animals make them unsuited to how they will be treated in circus life?

There are many strategies to address these ethical concerns, but all would involve a substantial change of direction in the way circuses operate and in the way the law is formulated and applied. Is it worth it?

NOTES

1. Several attempts were made during the writing of this case study to contact Ringling Bros. and Barnum & Bailey Circus, as well as its parent company, Feld Entertainment, Inc., for interviews and comments on this case. No responses were received.

2. "Life Cycle/Social Structure," *Africa: African Lion* (Oakland, CA: Oakland Zoo, 2003), www.oaklandzoo.org/atoz/azlion.html (accessed July 22, 2004).

3. "July 21 Updated Lion Statement," *Feld Entertainment—Press Room*, www.feldentertainment. com/LAVA/PRELE/00012039.HTM (accessed July 22, 2004).

4. "Ringling Lion Suffers Horrifying Death in Circus Boxcar," *PETA—Action Alerts*, www. peta.org/alert/automation/AlertItem.asp?id=1072 (accessed July 22, 2004).

5. Marc Kaufman, "USDA Investigates Death of Circus Lion," *Washington Post*, August 8, 2004.

6. Jim Andacht, "Taking Care of the Animals," *Washington Post*, August 14, 2004.

7. "Ringling Bros. and Barnum & Bailey Statement on Frank Hagan's Accusations of Wrongful Termination," *Feld Entertainment—Press Room*, October 11, 2004, www.feldinc.com/telescope//Public%20Relations/pr_ingest/00012738.HTM (accessed February 17, 2005).

8. "Court Grants Feld Entertainment's Motion to Dismiss Emotional Distress Claim in Employee Termination Case," *Feld Entertainment—Press Room*, April 21, 2005, www.feldinc. com/telescope/Public%20Relations/ehawksworth/HaganDistressClaim-Court%20Hearing.htm (accessed July 20, 2005).

9. Karl Gröning and Martin Saller, *Elephants: A Cultural and Natural History* (Cologne, Germany: Könemann, 1999), pp. 254–59.

10. Ibid., pp. 258–59.

11. "Bailey and the Ringlings," *Ringling Bros. and Barnum & Bailey: History and Tradition*, www.ringling.com/explore/history/bailey_2.aspx (accessed July 22, 2004).

12. "Ringling Bros. and Barnum & Bailey Animal Care Fact Sheet," *Feld Entertainment—Press Room*, www.feldentertainment.com/pr/mog/AnimalCareFactSheet.htm (accessed July 20, 2004).

13. People for the Ethical Treatment of Animals (PETA), *Ringling Bros. and Barnum & Bailey Circus: History of Animal Welfare Violations* (Norfolk, VA: PETA, 2004).

14. USDA, APHIS, Animal Care, "Official Warning: Violation of Federal Regulations, March 24, 1998," in PETA, *Ringling Bros. and Barnum & Bailey Circus*, p. 48.

15. "Second Tragedy Hits Circus Family," *BBC News*, February 25, 1998, news.bbc.co.uk/1/hi/uk/60162.stm (accessed July 22, 2004).

16. *USDA v. Feld Entertainment, Inc., dba Ringling Bros. and Barnum & Bailey Circus*, AWA Docket No. 98-0020, April 16, 1998, in PETA, *Ringling Bros. and Barnum & Bailey Circus*, pp. 39–41.

17. 9 CFR § 3.142(a)(1) (May 13, 2002). A review of the *Federal Register* revealed no changes to § 3.142 of the Animal Welfare Regulations between 1998 and 2004. Gregg Goodman of the USDA's Animal Welfare Information Center was helpful in clarifying the appropriate time limit during ground transport. (Since Ringling is generally considered to be an animal exhibitor rather than a transporter and the circus animals live on the train, it is possible to argue that Ringling should only be held accountable for meeting the temperature requirements outlined in § 2.131 of the AWA, which requires that handlers take action only if the ambient temperature is outside of the acceptable range for more than four hours. This possibility will not change the legal status of the actions reported later in the text. Denise Sofranko has my thanks for the clarification.)

18. Christian Heath Nevill, "The Effects of Exercise on Stereotypic Pacing in Circus Tigers and the Effects of Transport Environments on Body Temperature of Circus Tigers," Master's thesis, Texas A&M University, May 2002, pp. 44–48.

19. USDA, APHIS, Animal Care, "Inspection Report: Ringling Bros. Barnum & Bailey Circus Blue Unit, July 5, 2000," in PETA, *Ringling Bros. and Barnum & Bailey Circus*, p. 11.

20. Ibid., pp. 9–10.

21. Associated Press, "Ringling Bros. Lion Dies," 07/14/04: "A lion with Ringling Bros. was found dead after crossing the Mojave Desert in the circus train, en route from Arizona to Fresno, CA. The lion is believed to have died from heatstroke and dehydration. The circus is awaiting the results of a necropsy." Available at Animal Protection Institute, www.api4animals. org/facts?p=430&more=1 (accessed August 29, 2007).

22. "Ringling Bros. and Barnum & Bailey Statement on Frank Hagan's Accusations of Wrongful Termination."

23. A necropsy is an autopsy performed on an animal rather than a human.

24. "July 21 Updated Lion Statement."

25. "Transportation and Housing," *Ringling Bros. and Barnum & Bailey The Greatest Show on Earth*, www.ringling.com/animals/transportation/transportation.aspx (accessed February 19, 2005).

26. USDA, APHIS, Animal Care, "Inspection Report: Ringling Bros. Barnum & Bailey Circus Blue Unit, July 12, 2000."

27. "Frequently Asked Questions about Animals and Ringling Bros. and Barnum & Bailey," *Feld Entertainment—Press Room*, www.feldentertainment.com/pr/aca/FAQ1.htm (accessed August 20, 2004).

28. Ibid. (accessed February 17, 2005).

29. USDA, APHIS, Animal Care, "Inspection Report: Ringling Bros. Barnum & Bailey Circus Blue Unit, July 12, 2000," p. 10.

30. U.S. House Committee on the Judiciary, *Testimony of Pat Derby, President of the Performing Animal Welfare Society (PAWS)*, June 13, 2000, www.house.gov/judiciary/derb0613.htm (accessed July 22, 2004).

31. "Factsheets," Circuses.com, www.circuses.com/facts.html (accessed July 23, 2004).

32. Nevill, "Effects of Exercise on Stereotypic Pacing," pp. 41–105.

33. Kathy Carlstead, "Determining the Causes of Stereotypic Behaviors in Zoo Carnivores," in *Second Nature: Environmental Enrichment for Captive Animals*, ed. David J. Shepherdson, Jill D. Mellen, and Michael Hutchins (Washington, DC: Smithsonian Institution Press, 1998), p. 172.

34. Rainer Maria Rilke, "The Panther," *Poems*, trans. Jessie Lemont (New York: Columbia University Press, 1943), p. 69.

35. Marthe Kiley-Worthington, *Animals in Circuses and Zoos: Chiron's World?* (Essex, UK: Little Eco-Farms Publishing, 1990), pp. 71–73, 179–98; Carlstead, "Determining the Causes of Stereotypic Behaviors," pp. 172–83; Ted Friend and Melissa L. Parker, "The Effects of Penning versus Picketing on Stereotypic Behavior of Circus Elephants," *Applied Animal Behaviour Science* 64 (1999): 213–25.

36. Ted Friend, "Behavior of Picketed Circus Elephants," *Applied Animal Behaviour Science* 62 (1999): 73–88.

37. Denise Sofranko, interview by Paul Jude Naquin, telephone interview notes, July 15, 2005.

38. Laurie Gage, interview by Paul Jude Naquin, telephone interview notes, July 23, 2004; Denise Sofranko, interview by Paul Jude Naquin, telephone interview notes, July 7, 2004; Carlstead, "Determining the Causes of Stereotypic Behaviors," pp. 172–83; Kiley-Worthington, *Animals in Circuses and Zoos*, pp. 71–72.

39. 9 CFR § 3.128 (May 13, 2002).

40. USDA, APHIS, Animal Care, "Policy #6: Space and Exercise Requirements for Traveling Exhibitors, October 13, 1998," www.aphis.usda.gov/ac/policy/policy6.pdf (accessed July 26, 2004).

41. Michael Kernan, "Trailing the Big Cats," *Smithsonian Magazine* (January 1999), www.smithsonianmag.si.edu/smithsonian/issues99/jan99/mall_jan99.html (accessed September 22, 2005).

42. Denise Sofranko, interview, July 15, 2005.

43. For an example, see PETA, *Circus Elephants: Training and Tragedy* (Norfolk, VA: PETA, 2004).

44. Tom Rider, interview by Paul Jude Naquin, notes from telephone interview, July 19, 2004.

45. "Get the Answers," *Ringling Bros. and Barnum & Bailey The Greatest Show on Earth*, www.ringling.com/animals/answer.aspx (accessed October 2, 2005).

46. Tiger Species Survival Plan, "2003 ARCS (Annual Report on Conservation and Science) Report," *AZA Species Survival Plan*, www.aza.org/ConScience/ConScienceSSPFact/ (accessed July 26, 2004). This report is contained in the members-only section of the AZA (Association of Zoos and Aquariums) website and is therefore not immediately available to the general public.

47. Richard Farinato, "The Whims and Dangers of the Exotic Pets Market," *Humane Society of the United States*, www.hsus.org/wildlife/issues_facing_wildlife/should_wild_animals_be_kept_as_pets/the_whims_and_dangers_of_the_exotic_pets_market.html (accessed February 17, 2005).

48. Ibid.

49. "Feld Entertainment Continues to Cooperate with USDA Review into October 3, 2003 Injury of Roy Horn of Siegfried and Roy," *Feld Entertainment—Press Room*, August 25, 2004, www.feldinc.com/telescope//Public%20Relations/pr_ingest/00012239.HTM (accessed February 17, 2005).

50. For more information about conservation, see chapter 6, about elephants in zoos, and chapter 10, about bonobos in the wild.

51. "Center for Elephant Conservation," *Ringling Bros. and Barnum & Bailey The Greatest Show on Earth*, www.ringling.com/cec/ (accessed February 19, 2005).

52. "How Much Is that 'Kitty' in the Window?" *Big Cat Rescue*, May 18, 2004, www.bigcatrescue.org/buy_a_big_cat.htm (accessed July 26, 2004).

53. "Conservation Commitment," *Ringling Bros. and Barnum & Bailey The Greatest Show on Earth*, www.ringling.com/animals/conservation/conservation.aspx (accessed October 2, 2005).

PART IV

COMPANION ANIMALS

8

Cosmetic Surgery for Dogs

"Robbed of Their Tails, Robbed of Their Lives": This headline was accompanied by a photograph of 11 transparent body bags (for puppies) in a row, each with its own label, RH 1–11. All had died after their tails had been surgically amputated without anesthetic or without long-term pain relief that would be normal for humans after a surgical amputation, say for a finger. The effects of a few seconds of intense pain and maybe a few days of moderate pain and aches at and around the site of surgery are seen as being acceptable by many breeders, and few questions are asked. Much less commonly (nobody knows exactly how often), docking can be followed by side effects that may even result in animals having to be euthanized months or years later. This chapter begins with an actual case that is quite common.

DOCKING WORKING DOGS

An amateur breeder of weimaraners in the United Kingdom, Ms. A. was uncertain whether to have the tails of the litter of her pregnant bitch docked shortly after their birth. She telephoned her vet to arrange an appointment, only to be told that the vet did not dock unless it was for therapeutic reasons, that is, only when the tail had been damaged in some way and surgery was required for it to heal properly. Ms. A explained that she was complying with the Kennel Club's breed standard and that she was worried she might not be able to sell the pups if they were not docked. The vet explained that she considered it unethical to mutilate an animal in this way simply for cosmetic or financial reasons and that her professional body (the Royal College of Veterinary Surgeons [RCVS]) backed her up, and that if caught doing it she could be struck from the RCVS Register to practice. Ms. A did not know what to do, as she had always been to this vet and respected her abilities and opinions. However, her vet also told her that there were vets who did dock despite the prohibition by the RCVS. Ms. A eventually found Dr. S, a "docking vet," and after the litter had been born she took the bitch and her pups to him for the operation.

Ms. A arrived at Dr. S's clinic at the end of a surgery and the receptionist took her, the bitch, and the basketful of pups into the operating room. Dr. S made no enquiry as to why she wanted the pups docked but asked that the bitch be taken back to the car. He then applied a tourniquet tightly around the base of each puppy's tail, one by one, and then returned it to the basket. Every puppy squealed and struggled during this procedure and still remained rather noisy in the basket. Each pup was again removed from the basket, a dab of disinfectant was applied to the tail, and a pair of scissors was used to cut off part of the tail. The U.K. standard for weimaraners states that enough tail should be left to cover the vulva of bitches or the scrotum of males. The U.S. standard,[1] on the other hand, is as follows:

> *Docked.* At maturity it should measure approximately 6 inches with a tendency to be light rather than heavy and should be carried in a manner expressing confidence and sound temperament. A non-docked tail shall be penalized.

According to the owner, Dr. S docked many of the pups' tails much too short.

At each amputation every puppy squealed "very loudly," and also when Dr. S stitched the stump to stop the bleeding from the cut surface. The pups were returned to their basket, whimpering. Dr. S advised Ms. A on aftercare and told her that if there were any problems she could bring the pups back. The vet then asked for his fee, but as Ms. A did not have the whole amount in cash (only $200 instead of $320), she agreed to settle the outstanding amount later. Ms. A returned home, rather unhappy about what had happened, but the puppies were all asleep snuggling up to the bitch after suckling. Two days later one puppy died for no apparent reason, although it had not been as strong as the rest. Then a second puppy died a week or so after the first. The other nine seemed fine.

Some weeks later, after weaning, all the pups went to their new homes except for one that Ms. A was keeping and another that had been placed in a home, but the new owners were away for a week. The tail of this latter pup started to ooze pus and blood, so Ms. A took it to her regular vet, having to confess that she had had the litter docked by another vet. The pup was given antibiotics and, after a few days, all seemed well. The pup duly went to its new owner, Ms. W, who was informed of the problem that now seemed to have cleared up. About a month later, Ms. W called to say that the problem had recurred and that her own vet was dealing with it. Ms. A responded by offering to buy back the puppy, but that offer was rejected, so she offered to pay their vet's bills and sent a check for $300 to Ms. W. Four months later a second bill arrived, this time for $800 for ongoing treatment, and both agreed that it should be the responsibility of Dr. S to pay these invoices. The tail still did not heal and the puppy was referred to a specialist vet, who carried out X-rays, an MRI scan, and therapeutic surgery (removal of damaged and dead bone and a remaining suture) and presented his bill for $3,000. At about the same time, Dr. S sent a reminder to Ms. A about the outstanding $120.

Ms. A was so outraged by what had occurred that she reported the vet to the RCVS for breaking its ethical rules as well as for negligent practice. She was also clearly remorseful about what she had done.

HISTORICAL BACKGROUND AND MAJOR ISSUES

Docking has been practiced for centuries.[2] Captain Jocelyn Lucas wrote in 1920 in his book *Hints on Dog Management* that "all running dogs such as Hounds, Greyhounds and Retrievers—animals used to catch as well as pursue game—have their tails left long so they can twist and turn, using their tails as 'rudders.' Dogs such as the Spaniel used for hunting out game but not for catching it, formerly had their tails cut to impede them. Thus the bobtailed Sheepdog was originally docked to prevent them [from] catching hares."[3]

Dogs that were used for hunting and shooting frequently damaged their tails in this work. It is thought that docking reduces the chance of injury in some breeds. Spaniels, for example, put up game by going into thorny hedgerows, and they are thereby more likely to damage their tails than are retriever-type dogs, which work in the open and bring back game after it has broken cover and been shot. Consequently, spaniels, but not retrievers, are normally docked. Today docking is carried out for a variety of other reasons, including not wishing to break with tradition, improving appearance, better hygiene, and providing for more harmonious cohabitation with humans in confined living conditions. At present, some 50 breeds are customarily docked.

On the surface, docking puppies seems a relatively trivial issue, a few seconds of significant pain shortly after birth, but all is soon forgotten. So what are the major issues?

1. Why are the tails removed, and why in some breeds and not others?
2. Does docking have any adverse effects on the animals?
3. Who should dock, how should it be done, and at what age?
4. Finally, ought docking to be carried out at all?

MEDICAL ASPECTS OF DOCKING

The tail is formed from a line of 15 to 20 vertebrae, with flexible joints, strengthened by ligaments and covered by muscles that move the tail in all directions. The tail serves as an organ of balance and for communication with other dogs and humans. Its position and actions, together with body stance, can signal pleasure, friendliness, dominance, playfulness, unhappiness, lack of well-being, defensiveness, inquisitiveness, aggression, nervousness, and submissiveness. The tail also carries a scent gland used to mark out a dog's territory. Although animals appear to adapt well to docking, the lack of a tail can adversely affect their balance, speed of movement, and communication.

Docking is the surgical process by which a varying length of tail (depending on the breed) is removed by means of scissors, scalpel, razor, knife, or rubber rings.[4] It is normally carried out without anesthetic in the first few days of life; the stump may be stitched or treated to stop the flow of blood and to reduce the chance of infection. Rarely is an anesthetic or analgesic (pain reliever) given before, at the time, or afterward.

Pain is a characteristic property of higher vertebrates, including mammals, birds, reptiles, amphibians, and fish, and pain sensors are located in skin and other tissues. Pain perception is biologically essential for survival to alert an animal to potential or actual physical injury, helping prevent further damage. After a painful stimulus, with impulses traveling to the brain at over 100 mph, an animal normally shows an immediate unconscious withdrawal reflex, followed a second or so later by responses that enable the animal to consciously locate the source of the pain and to take further evasive actions. An underlying question is whether a puppy in the first week or so of life is capable of feeling pain or whether its nervous system is too immature. That the pups could feel pain in the present case seems clearly indicated by their behavior during docking, because each pup squealed. Others argue that such squealing is a reflex response and does not necessarily indicate pain. However, as the pups whimpered for some time afterward and sought comforting behavior from the dam (female parent),[5] it seems unlikely to be a simple reflex, because that would occur within a fraction of a second and then cease. More recent scientific evidence from work in neonatal rats and humans suggests that puppies feel more, and not less, pain because of this immaturity.[6]

Docking by means of rubber rings rather than by surgical methods has been advocated as not being painful, but evidence for pain has been found in lambs, calves, and goat kids for at least two hours after ringing shortly after birth, lasting for two days or so, hence the need for longer term postoperative analgesia.[7]

LAWS AND POLICIES ON DOCKING

National laws in many European countries and recently in Australia, New Zealand, and Scotland totally ban tail docking in dogs, but elsewhere, including the United States and Canada, there are no specific laws. In some countries it is legal for dog breeders to dock their own litters, but the conditions under which the procedure is carried out are often far from ideal.[8] Veterinarians are often given the responsibility to carry out docking because it is an act of veterinary surgery. Some veterinarians carry out docking because, they argue, it would be worse for the animals if they, as trained surgeons, left it to the owners to perform the procedure. Despite there being a financial inducement to carry out docking, the profession as a whole is against the procedure on the grounds that it causes unnecessary suffering.[9] A 1989 survey by the Australian Veterinary Association found that 86% of respondents opposed nontherapeutic docking and described it as "archaic, barbaric and pointless." A similar survey conducted in 1992 by the British Small Animal Veterinary Association showed that 92% of U.K. veterinarians agreed with a ban and 56% stated that they refused to dock at the present time.[10]

In June 2005 the American Veterinary Medical Association (AVMA) posted the following on its website:

> Ear cropping and tail docking in dogs for cosmetic reasons are not medically indicated nor of benefit to the patient. These procedures cause pain and distress, and, as with all surgical procedures, are accompanied by inherent risks of anesthesia, blood loss, and infection. Therefore, veterinarians should counsel dog owners about these matters before agreeing to perform these surgeries.[11]

The Canadian VMA state as follows on their website:

> The Canadian Veterinary Medical Association (CVMA) opposes surgical alteration of any animal, for purely cosmetic purposes . . . and believes that cosmetic surgery is unnecessary,

e.g., tail docking in the canine species. The CVMA recommends that breed associations change their breed standards so that cosmetic procedures are not required.[12]

Animal welfare organizations have occasionally made policy statements. For instance, in the United States, the Association of Veterinarians for Animal Rights has labeled docking and cropping as "cruel and needless rituals."[13] Other animal welfare organizations have written position statements but do not appear to have mounted significant campaigns. Notable exceptions are the U.K. RSPCA and the British Veterinary Association, which had several joint anti-docking initiatives during the passage of the Animal Welfare Act in 2006. The RSPCA also has a list of breeders willing to supply undocked puppies.

INTERESTED PARTIES AND THE POLITICAL LANDSCAPE

Several reasons for and against docking are found in the literature on the subject. These reasons are not always *moral* reasons, but they generally do have ethical implications.

Proponents of Tail Docking

What seems not to be in contention on both sides of this debate is that if the tail has been damaged in any way, and it is in the dog's best interest for it to be docked, then "therapeutic" docking should be carried out as part of normal veterinary practice.[14] However, even when there is no therapeutic reason, national kennel clubs and breeders favor the retention of dog tail docking. The kennel clubs regulate the registration and showing of pedigree dogs through their breed standard councils (made up of "leading" breeders). Docking is not required to conform to any breed standard, according to the U.K. Kennel Club (KC). It is left as optional, and breed societies have started to give guidance on what sort of tail a judge should favor. The American KC, on the other hand, seems determined to protect the status quo.[15] It rejects any legislation that proposes a ban.[16] Its official position is as follows: "The American Kennel Club recognizes that ear cropping, tail docking, and dewclaw removal, as described in certain breed standards, are acceptable practices integral to defining and preserving breed character and/or enhancing good health. Appropriate veterinary care should be provided."

Improved appearance is probably the most common reason that breeders give (and are now learning not to give) to justify removing or shortening the tail, believing that it makes an animal look more attractive, hence the language of "cosmetic" docking. Traditionally, breeders have determined the breed standard, in conjunction with their national kennel club, and so when breed standards are revised, they tend to perpetuate the traditional view of what an animal of that breed should look like. With changes in national legislation and other pressures, the word "optional" has crept into the standard in some countries, but it is what wins at shows that matters. If docked animals continue to win, the message sent out is that it is important to dock dogs.

Prevention of injury is another major argument for docking puppies, particularly in breeds used in hunting and shooting, such as spaniels and pointers. The injuries occur because when the dogs go into dense cover, briars can become tangled in the long fur (feather) and damage the tail. This can also occur in field trials, where courses are set out by the organizers. Because docking has been prohibited in some countries for more than 15 years, relevant evidence is now available for comparing older, docked dogs with younger, undocked dogs. For example, in Sweden, where docking has been banned since 1989, a 1991 survey in veterinary clinics showed that 73% of tail injuries were in undocked animals.[17] However, these figures were not related to the proportion of undocked versus docked dogs attending the clinic. Until we can establish accurate figures for tail injuries in docked and undocked dogs, together with the circumstances surrounding the injury (i.e., whether the injury occurred at home or during field work, the extent of tail damage, etc.), we are unlikely to have the sort of data that would substantiate further commentary. As of this writing, there are still no peer-reviewed papers on the incidence of tail injuries.

Improving hygiene is the third reason advanced to support docking in the Old English sheepdog, Yorkshire terrier, and Australian silky terriers. Fouling and retention of feces in perineal (area in front of the anus) hairs may lead to maggot infestation, as well as an unwelcome smell. It can be argued that owners of breeds with this potential problem can, by thorough and regular grooming, prevent this problem from occurring, but owners have not proved to be reliable in attending to their animals in these ways. The hygiene argument, like the prevention argument, has attracted suspicion because there are various breeds with the same potential hygiene problem that are not docked (for example, Pekingese, bearded collies, and border collies).

Reasons for Not Docking

The pain inflicted at the time of docking is likely to be significant for the animal as far as we can ascertain. It may persist as discomfort for a day or more, particularly if rubber rings are used, so that animals may suckle or sleep less. Breeders lack adequate training in surgical technique, and they are not always aware of the potential adverse consequences of docking and how to recognize, assess, or avoid them. Tails docked improperly can become infected, but in most cases infection is not a common problem. In extreme cases infection can ascend the spinal cord or spread to other places, and the animal may have to be humanely killed. This is more likely to happen in those breeds where the tail is cut very short, e.g., the Old English sheepdog and the rottweiler.

Fatal hemorrhaging has been recorded in genetic lines that carry a blood-clotting defect, and chronic pain and self-mutilation have also been reported.[18] Some dog psychologists believe that a dog with no tail, such as an Old English sheepdog or a rottweiler, can miscue other dogs. These severely docked animals may appear to other dogs to show unwarranted aggression by not being seen to wag their tails, and so may become the victim of attack.[19]

Docking also appears to be ineffective if the goal is preventing injury. A study of one clinic's records, extracted between 1965 and 1985, showed that 0.41% of undocked dogs and 0.31% of docked dogs sustained injuries of the tail or stump; the authors concluded that docking could not be recommended as a prophylactic measure.[20] If docking is truly a preventive measure, then complete removal of the tail should be even more successful because it would eliminate all risk of injury, and this would hold true for all breeds. However, both breeders and international breed standards vary considerably (even within a breed) as to how much tail to remove. Normally, this is between one-third and three-quarters of the tail, depending on the breed.[21] Furthermore, many of the breeds that commonly injure their tails are not traditionally docked (e.g., Great Danes, Greyhounds, Labradors), and even with this risk of tail injury, breeders will not entertain the idea of docking these breeds.

The logic of removing part of the body to prevent injury has obviously got to have some limits, but where are they? Would it be acceptable to remove other limbs or organs to prevent commonly occurring injuries to them, e.g., to ear flaps, or paws, or teeth?

ETHICAL ISSUES

The arguments for and against docking have now been discussed, but we have yet to consider applicable ethical norms and the moral problems involved in docking dogs.

Acceptable Criteria for Nontherapeutic Surgery

Many kinds of surgical procedures are carried out on animals. Those defending the docking of puppies often compare it with the docking of other species, such as lambs, piglets, horses, and cattle. In addition, the docking of puppies is compared with neutering, as well as with trimming the beaks of caged laying hens. Is the justification for the surgical intervention the same in each of these cases? If not, what are the key differences?

The following ten criteria have been suggested as appropriate ways of addressing the moral justifiability of docking (and other surgeries sometimes said to be "mutilations").[22] The criteria look at justification for the proposed interference and can be seen as tests of necessity to ensure that the proposed benefit is real, effective, valuable, and attainable. The assumption is that if all of the criteria are satisfied in a particular case by answering "yes" to questions 1–6 and "no" to questions 7–10, then docking would likely be justified.

1. Is there compelling evidence that leaving the animal intact (i.e., leaving the tail on) predisposes those individuals to harmful consequences, e.g., to some form of damage to its tail?
2. Is there compelling evidence that leaving the animal intact (i.e., leaving the tail on) predisposes other animals, e.g., in a flock or herd, to harmful consequences (e.g., it might attract flies or be the focus of attention for other animals in the herd to harm such as tail biting in pigs)?
3. Is there evidence that the proposed intervention (docking the tail) is in the best interest of that animal (i.e., it would confer a benefit such as not having a tail to be bitten, or being able to escape faster from a threat) and that the benefits outweigh the predicted harms, as in (1) and (2) above?
4. Does the proposed intervention cause a greater harm than repairing the damage one is trying to prevent (e.g., when docking as an adult)?
5. Would the less harmful consequences or the benefits occur in a significant proportion of the population at risk (e.g., a litter of pups), or should a particular subset of dogs be considered (e.g., breeds that are more likely to damage their tails because they will go hunting, or those animals in a litter that are going to work in the field)?
6. Is the increase in "value" as a result of carrying out the proposed interference (an economic value being an increase in monetary value and a social value being a better appearance) sufficient to offset the harm done to the animal?

7. Is the reason for docking due to the way in which animals are kept and used? If so, can the environment be altered rather than the animal?

A second set of criteria (beyond 1–7 above) relates to the method of docking. Can any suffering be avoided by using a less painful way of achieving the desired end (e.g., by preventing tail damage)?

8. Is there an alternative means with no adverse effects (e.g., clipping tail fur, breeding, or genetic manipulation for bob-tailed dogs) that would achieve the same objective?

9. Is there a less harmful alternative way of carrying out the proposed interference (docking) that would achieve the same end (e.g., by giving a local anaesthetic or sedative), or even changing the way in which we use the dogs?

10. Is the method used to achieve the end one that should *never* be used, on grounds that it is either inherently objectionable (e.g., debases the person doing it) or causes so much pain and suffering that it should simply not be done?

The Principle of Protecting Structural and Functional Integrity

One principle that seems to have little or nothing to do with balancing harms and benefits is the following: It is important not to destroy or unnecessarily disturb the structural and functional integrity of an animal. This is a notably strong principle. Is it acceptable? What are its implications?

Many reasons might be offered in support of this principle. A major reason might be derived from the reasoning outlined in the introduction to this volume (pp. 24–25) pertaining to the inherent value of animals: Removing parts of animals would not seem respectful of the inherent value of animals (or, perhaps, of their *telos,* as some prefer to say).[23] A practice of significant structural or functional alteration suggests that the animal was imperfect in some way beforehand and that it is necessary to alter it to make it perfect (at least in light of certain human purposes). There are also limits to what would be morally permissible in light of the standards of preventive medicine: Removal of limbs to avoid damaging them or removing teeth to avoid the possibility of decay are not considered acceptable veterinary practices—that is, they deviate from standards of practice, which are usually regarded as determining morally appropriate actions, not merely medically recommended ones.

What are the implications of this reasoning? Can the hair of poodles not be trimmed to an owner's taste—or even hair cut away to unblock the eyes of Old English sheepdogs or bearded collies? Perhaps these particular examples are not matters of structural integrity. If not, then what about cropping dogs' ears to "improve" their appearance? What are we to say about the removal of claws from indoor cats, or the removal of poisonous mechanisms from pet snakes? What is the scope of the principle of not disturbing the structural and functional integrity of an animal?

On the other side of these questions is this question: Ought breeders be able to alter or even mutilate a dog merely because it is their property under law? Does the principle of property rights and ownership have no standing or defense whatever in the way of supplying a moral constraint on the conduct of breeders? Of veterinarians? If no pain and suffering are involved in making functional or structural changes, would that make it morally acceptable?

It is likely that some surgical mutilations will require more justification than others. Those who hold stringent positions on animal rights will maintain that it is always wrong to intervene and likely will defend some version of the principle requiring that the structure and functional integrity of animals not be altered. The grounds likely would be that animals have an inherent right not to be caused to suffer or to be surgically altered unless the surgical intervention is ultimately in their best interest (e.g., a therapeutic intervention). But would this be the only acceptable interpretation of the principle? Should the principle be specified in a different way, or should it be abandoned?

Alternative Possibilities and Slippery Slopes

There may be alternative ways to avoid the very harms that docking is thought to minimize. For example, sportsmen could be encouraged to trim the hair from the tail and to examine their dogs more frequently to remove briars, and so minimize tail damage. They could also avoid using their dogs in thorny cover or choose a more appropriate breed or strain with different coat characteristics. Pet owners could be taught to groom and trim their animals effectively so that fecal material did not become trapped. Breeders could breed (even genetically engineer) for sensible tail shape, tail feather, and tail length (for example, shorter tails, as in the Pembrokeshire corgi). If effective, would these alternatives be preferable to docking, and should they become standards of practice?

Another question about alternatives arises from the thesis that some forms of surgical intervention are *necessary*. A strong thesis is that a surgical harm can be judged necessary only if it is in balance with any gain *for the animal*. A weaker principle is that a surgical harm can be judged necessary only if it is in balance with any gain for the *animal and/or human*. From either perspective, the claimed benefit and the animal suffering have to be carefully evaluated and balanced, one against the other.

But there are additional problems, too. At what level of probability of injury would it be agreed that docking is a justifiable preventive measure: 10%, 20%, 50%, or 80%? Studies on sheep suggest a test case: Can the docking of lambs be justified if, as now appears to be the case, more than 40% of undocked lambs are affected with larvae (maggots) eating the animals' flesh, compared with less than 12% in docked controls?[24] Could preventive docking in dogs be justified if similar proportions were to apply to certain breeds or in certain circumstances?

One problem with this test case is that so few dogs will ever be used for hunting, probably less than 1%. Moreover, of the class of dogs that hunt, only a small proportion will damage their tails or require a therapeutic intervention at a later date. However, the results of two surveys (neither was peer reviewed or published in a scientific journal) carried out by the Swedish KC and the Veterinary School at Uppsala between 1990 and 1994 have been submitted to the Swedish Department of Agriculture for their consideration to lift the docking ban for German Pointers.[25] They found in a total of 368 hunting dogs that some 28.3% of animals sustained tail damage (although the extent and nature of that damage were not specified) and up to 70% had actual tail injuries. In such cases, if the activities in these ways of using dogs are themselves justified, the test case of necessity for lamb docking might apply to some subset of dogs in a population that would be affected. However, there would still seem to be no point in docking dogs that will never be used in hunting.

On a utilitarian basis, this conclusion might seem to receive additional support: The total amount of suffering (pain and discomfort) caused by docking every puppy in a "susceptible" breed is likely to be greater than the suffering of the few adults needing this operation therapeutically. The pain caused by therapeutic docking also could be justified, because it was in that individual animal's best interest, and also the pain could be mitigated through the use of anesthetics and postoperative analgesics to a point where it should be relatively insignificant. Using a similar utilitarian logic, it could be argued that the benefit gained from having a tail by the majority of intact dogs would outweigh the disadvantage to the small number of dogs that would have to be docked therapeutically.

A larger utilitarian picture incorporates human interests. Docking for cosmetic purposes involves balancing human aesthetic sensibilities against animal suffering in a "cost-benefit analysis." Such preferences could be regarded as trivial or important, depending on the view taken. But accepting any human pleasure or aesthetic preference at the expense of an animal would also seem to open the door to a justification for many uses of animals that are now widely considered unacceptable and often legally prohibited, such as dog fighting. How does one draw a line on the limits of human benefits when balancing a wide variety of interests? Pursuit of this question will likely lead to questions of whether the consequences of accepting docking as an ethical procedure would lead down a slippery slope that would involve accepting other surgical interventions such as ear cropping or trimming and carrying out similar procedures in other breeds of dogs, or animal species, such as horses, cattle, and cats.

A final question about possible alternatives is whether decreasing the harms associated with docking would make docking any more justifiable. If we could refine the operation by relieving the pain associated with docking and by training those carrying out the procedure, thereby reducing the incidence of faulty technique and painful side effects, would this make docking any more justifiable?

Do Veterinarians Have a Special Moral Responsibility?

Many veterinarians take an oath stating that they will do their best to protect the welfare of animals in their care. "Welfare" can be interpreted in several ways, but it almost always includes not inflicting unnecessary or avoidable suffering on animals. Does society look to the veterinary profession for informed opinion on whether animals suffer during a particular procedure and whether it is really necessary? In the event of uncertainty, is it the professional responsibility of the veterinarian to give the benefit of that doubt to the animal or the owner? Does the veterinarian have an obligation to be either the animal's advocate or the owner's servant? For example, are veterinarians entrusted with the care and protection of animals in the same way that guardians are entrusted to protect vulnerable and incompetent persons? If not, what role do veterinarians have, and does anyone have special responsibilities assigned by society for the protection of animals?

Answers to these questions may depend on more general moral questions such as those about the *rights* of animals. If human rights trump animal rights, and if human rights are broad enough so that docking is a right, then it could be that a breeder has a right to insist that a veterinary surgeon do what the breeder wants—or, less drastically, the breeder's right must be balanced by the right of the veterinary surgeon to do what he or she judges to be right. Surely, though, an animal is some kind of stakeholder, and this way of casting the issue seems to suggest that the animal has no rights at all.

The docking veterinarian with whom we started this case knew that docking the puppies would cause them pain, and he did it solely for monetary gain. Should Dr. S be found guilty of bringing his profession into disrepute? Whose rights were trampled in this case?

NOTES

1. American Kennel Club, "Weimaraner Breed Standard," www.akc.org/breeds/weimaraner/index.cfm (accessed August 24, 2007).

2. *Dalziel's British Dogs*, 2nd ed. (original 1889), pp. 44–45, as in Drury's version of 1905; W. Youatt, *The Obligation and Extent of Humanity to Brutes*, written for the Society for the Prevention of Cruelty to Animals in 1839.

3. John Bower Evidence given to the Scottish Parliament, www.scottish.parliament.uk/business/committees/environment/inquiries/ahw/Bower__John.pdf (accessed August 24, 2007). Later Old English Sheepdogs were docked to indicate that they were working dogs and so exempt from tax. See George Jones, "History of the Old English Sheepdog," www.barkbytes.com/history/oldeng.htm (accessed August 24, 2007).

4. "Editorial: Guidelines for Tail-Docking," *Journal of the American Veterinary Medical Association* 152, no. 1 (1968): 60–61; "Standards for Docking Tails of Pups," *Australian Veterinary Journal* 46 (August 1970): 403.

5. Jean Irwin, John Irwin, and Ceri Irwin, "Puppy Behaviour at Docking Time," *Dog World* (May 22, 1987).

6. M. Fitzgerald, "Neurobiology of Fetal and Neonatal Pain," in *Wall and Melzack's Textbook of Pain*, 5th ed., ed. Stephen McMahon and Martin Koltzenburg (Amsterdam: Elsevier, 2007).

7. J. E. Kent, V. Molony, and I. S. Robertson, "Changes in Plasma Cortisol Concentration in Lambs of Three Ages after Three Methods of Castration and Tail Docking," *Research in Veterinary Science* 55 (1993): 246–51.

8. The Council of Europe's (46 member states) *Convention for the Protection of Pet Animals* (Strasbourg, 1988), Article 10.1.a specifically prohibits the docking of dogs' tails, and other sections ban ear cropping, devocalization, defanging (removal of canine teeth), and declawing (exceptions are made for all these operations if it is for therapeutic purposes). Derogation is permitted for docking under the convention (i.e., countries can sign the convention but need not implement the ban on docking). Furthermore, the convention prohibits surgical interventions that are primarily carried out for aesthetic reasons or for the personal convenience of the owner or the breeder, and it states that operations that involve severe pain shall be done under anesthesia by a veterinarian or under veterinary supervision.

9. F. B. Edwards, "The Practice of Docking," *Veterinary Record* 57, no. 17 (1945): 208.

10. Reported on the website of the Council for Docked Breeds, www.cdb.org/bsava.htm (accessed September 24, 2007). P. C. Bennett and E. Perini, "Tail Docking in Dogs: A Review of the Issues," *Australian Veterinary Journal* 81, no. 4 (2003): 208–18.

11. American Veterinary Medical Association, "Ear Cropping and Tail Docking," www.avma.org/issues/policy/animal_welfare/tail_docking.asp (accessed June 2005).

12. Canadian Veterinary Medical Association, "Cosmetic Surgery," November 2000, canadianveterinarians.net/ShowText.aspx?ResourceID=46 (accessed August 24, 2007).

13. Association of Veterinarians for Animal Rights, "AVAR Launches Campaign to Stop Docks and Crops on Dogs," *AVAR Directions* 32 (Spring 1993): 1–3.

14. Council for Docked Breeds, www.cdb.org (accessed August 24, 2007).

15. American Kennel Club Update, www.akc.org/canine_legislation/NY_action_center.cfm (accessed August 24, 2007).

16. American Kennel Club, News Article, June 28, 2006, "NY Crop/Dock Bill Dead for 2006," www.akc.org/news/index.cfm?article_id=2928 (accessed August 24, 2007).

17. Swedish Docking Survey, "Swedish Tail Injuries in Undocked German Pointers," *Dog World* (November 8, 1991): 4, 61.

18. T. L. Gross and S. H. Carr, "Amputation Neuroma of Docked Tails in Dogs," *Veterinary Pathology* 27 (1990): 61–62.

19. R. A. Mugford, personal communication to Mr. J. Bower, February 21, 1989; W. J. Netto, J. A. M. van der Bourg, and D. J. U. Planta, "The Establishment of Dominance Relationships in a Dog Pack and Its Relevance for the Man-Dog Relationship," *Proceedings of the Royal Netherlands Veterinary Association and the Netherlands Association for Companion Animal Medicine* 117 (1992): 51S-52S.

20. P. G. G. Darke, M. V. Thrusfield, and C. G. G. Aitken, "Association between Tail Injuries and Docking in Dogs," *Veterinary Record* 116 (1985): 409.

21. The English pointer, unlike the German pointer, is not docked. The show springer spaniel has a tail docked by two-thirds, whereas the working springer is docked by only one-third. Great Danes, greyhounds, wolfhounds, and Labradors are not infrequently docked as adults for thera-peutic reasons, but never as puppies.

22. D. B. Morton, "Docking of Dogs: Practical and Ethical Aspects," *Veterinary Record* 131 (1992): 301–6.

23. B. E. Rollin, *The Frankenstein Syndrome: Ethical and Social Issues in the Genetic Engineering of Animals* (Cambridge: Cambridge University Press, 1995).

24. See Al Vizard, "Tail Docking of Lambs in the Control of Flystrike," *Veterinary Record*, May 28, 1994, p. 583. Also see N. P. French, R. Wall, and K. L. Morgan, "Tail Docking of Lambs in the Control of Flystrike," *Veterinary Record*, July 9, 1994, p. 47.

25. Swedish Kennel Club Pointer Docking Survey, *Dog World*, November 8, 1991, pp. 4, 61. See also Nick Mays, "Sweden Is Set to Lift Docking Ban," *Our Dogs*, August 4, 1995.

PART V

RELIGIOUS USES OF ANIMALS

9

Animal Sacrifice as Religious Ritual

The Santeria Case

In the spring of 1987, a controversy arose in the city of Hialeah, Florida. It began when Ernesto Pichardo, the president and priest of the Church of the Lukumi Babalu Aye, issued a public statement describing the church's plan to build a worship and education center on city land that the church previously had leased. The announcement triggered discussion and debate among residents of Hialeah, some of whom were opposed to the church's plan.[1] Before the controversy subsided, the U.S. Supreme Court had become involved. The case raises issues about balancing the interests of nonhuman animals against the interests of humans—in particular, the human interests incorporated in the First Amendment protection of the free exercise of religion.

The original opposition was based on moral concerns about the sacrifice of animals, a practice associated with the Church of the Lukumi Babalu Aye. Members of the church practice a religion called Santeria. This religion began in the sixteenth century among Cuban slaves who had been removed from their East African homes. The slaves belonged to the Yoruba people, who practiced a traditional religion in Africa. In Cuba, the Yoruba were not permitted to practice their religion openly. They were often baptized without their consent as Christians before being forced onto the Spanish ships that took them to Cuba. In response, many Yoruba practitioners incorporated their traditional faith into the Roman Catholic religion. In this merging of the two religions, traditional spirits and symbols among the Yoruba became identified with various Christian saints and symbols. The assimilated references to Christian doctrine enabled Santeria believers to practice their religion more openly, reducing the possibility of persecution and stigma.[2]

The exact number of Santeria believers in the United States is unknown. According to one estimate, by the 1980s there were about 50,000 to 100,000 practitioners in the southern part of Florida. Other areas with a concentration of Santeria believers are New York City, northern New Jersey, northern Virginia, and California.[3] Santeria also has adherents in Cuba, Puerto Rico, and Venezuela.[4]

THE RITUAL SACRIFICE IN SANTERIA

The ritual sacrifice of animals is a traditional activity that remains important to the practice of Santeria. According to Santeria, God has a destiny for each person. To fulfill their destinies, people rely on the help of certain spirits, called orishas. Animal sacrifice is viewed as an important way to express one's devotion to the orishas. Indeed, because the orishas are seen as living beings, their very survival is dependent on receiving food from their devotees.[5] Ceremonies involving animal sacrifice are conducted when new members enter the church; to mark births, deaths, and marriages among members; to heal the sick; and as part of a yearly holiday observance. Based on figures provided by Pichardo, an estimated 12,000–15,000 animals are sacrificed each year as part of church initiation ceremonies conducted in the Hialeah area.[6]

Partially due to the stigma and persecution experienced by Santeria practitioners, the church does not have a central authority, a training system for its priests, or written documents setting forth its principles, rituals, and ceremonies. At the present time, much Santeria worship is conducted in private, in groups whose members and priests often have little contact with other Santeria practitioners. As a result, there is variation among different groups in how animal sacrifice is performed.

According to the statements of Pichardo, as well as other documents admitted as evidence in legal proceedings on the church's building proposal, chickens, pigeons, goats, doves, guinea pigs, ducks, sheep, and turtles are sacrificed in Santeria rituals. Priests are taught the method of sacrifice as apprentices, through observing and assisting more experienced priests. In the most common sacrifice, the animal is held on its side, while the priest raises the animal's head with one hand and with the other hand inserts a knife about four inches long into the right side of the animal's neck and then pushes the knife through the entire neck. The knife is not inserted into the animals' throat, but into an area behind the throat and in front of the vertebra. The goal is to puncture the animal's two main neck arteries with one movement, producing death rapidly.

A veterinarian and scientist from the Humane Society of the United States participating in the legal proceedings testified that "this method of killing is not humane because there is no guarantee that a person performing a sacrifice in the manner described can cut through both carotid arteries at the same time."[7] In addition, certain physiological events may occur in the animal, particularly in young goats and sheep, to prolong the experience of pain and distress prior to death. Moreover, chickens have four carotid arteries, which makes it more difficult to achieve success with one cut.

Because numerous animals may be sacrificed at a single ceremony, various species of animals are at times gathered in one room prior to sacrifice and exposed to the noise and bodily secretions produced by the nearby animal being killed. As a result, they may detect that animal's pain and fear, and they may themselves experience fear and distress prior to their own sacrifice. Many animals killed in Santeria ceremonies are raised specifically for sacrifice, and they may receive inadequate food, water, and housing during the course of their lives.

RESPONSES IN THE HIALEAH COMMUNITY

Some Hialeah residents were disturbed by possible health consequences of animal sacrifice. They were also worried about the practice's impact on people in the community. In the usual Santeria procedure, the sacrificed animal's blood is collected in clay pots, which are then offered to the orishas. The animal's head is cut off, and the blood and body remain present for a longer period. In some ceremonies, flesh from the animal is cooked and eaten; in others it is discarded. According to court testimony, animals' remains are often found in public places in Hialeah, creating a possible health hazard. Concern was also expressed about the possible psychological effects the sacrifice procedures could have on children observing the ritual.

Concern that members of the Church of the Lukumi Babalu Aye would engage in animal sacrifice led members of the Hialeah City Council to take a series of formal actions designed to discourage the practice. Two resolutions and four ordinances were enacted by unanimous vote. The resolutions expressed the city's desire to prohibit and oppose "public ritualistic animal sacrifices" and "all acts of any and all religious groups which are inconsistent with public morals, peace or safety."[8]

The ordinances (1) incorporated Florida's anticruelty statute, which provides for criminal punishment of anyone who unnecessarily or cruelly kills animals;[9] (2) prohibited the possession of animals for the purpose of ritual slaughter, whether or not the animals were to be eaten as food, with an exemption for slaughtering of food animals carried out by licensed facilities; (3) made it illegal to sacrifice animals (defined as "to unnecessarily kill . . . an animal in a . . . ritual or ceremony not for the primary purpose of food consumption") within city limits, based on a finding that the activity conflicted with "the public health, safety, welfare and morals of the community;"[10] and (4) permitted animal slaughter solely in places zoned for that activity, with an exemption for commercial establishments processing "small numbers of hogs and/or cattle" each week, in accordance with state law.

In addition, the city obtained an opinion from the state attorney general asserting that "ritual sacrifice of animals for purposes other than food consumption" should be defined as "unnecessary" and a violation of the state's anticruelty law.[11] Persons found guilty of violating any of the four ordinances could be imprisoned for up to 60 days and fined up to $500.

Pichardo went to federal court to challenge the ordinances as impermissibly interfering with the constitutional right of Santeria believers to practice their religion. Although the trial judge found that the ordinances had the effect of burdening church members' religious conduct, he determined that the Hialeah City Council's actions were justified by four compelling governmental interests: (1) protecting the health of city residents, who might be exposed to disease from the decaying bodies of sacrificed animals, as well as the health of participants in the Santeria ceremonies, who could become ill from ingesting uninspected meat; (2) protecting the emotional health of children exposed to animal sacrifice; (3) protecting animals from inhumane killing methods and living conditions; and (4) restricting animal slaughter to areas zoned for that activity. Moreover, the judge determined that a total prohibition of animal sacrifice was constitutionally permissible because any less restrictive attempt to regulate the activity to protect the city's interests would be ineffective, due to the private nature of most Santeria ceremonies.[12]

This decision was appealed to the U.S. Court of Appeals for the Eleventh Circuit, which affirmed the decision without discussing it in detail.[13] Pichardo then petitioned the U.S. Supreme Court to hear the case, and it agreed.

THE SUPREME COURT DECISION

Six years after the church announced its building plans, the Supreme Court issued an opinion striking down Hialeah's ordinances on grounds that they unconstitutionally interfered with the Santeria religion. All nine Supreme Court justices agreed that the ordinances violated the Constitution. Justice Anthony Kennedy wrote the majority opinion. In it, he cited a number of problems with the ordinances, based on the Court's previous decisions construing the First Amendment's ban on any law that prohibits the free exercise of religion.

Three years before deciding the Santeria case, the Supreme Court had issued an important decision interpreting the Constitution's Free Exercise Clause. In *Employment Division v. Smith*,[14] the Court ruled that laws having the effect of restricting religious practices must be both neutral and generally applicable to be valid exercises of state authority. In *Smith,* the Court applied this requirement to uphold Oregon's refusal to exempt from its drug laws the use of peyote in Native American religious ceremonies.

In the Court's view, however, the Hialeah ordinances did not qualify as neutral and generally applicable. First, the Court found that the ordinances' text and their probable practical effect supported the contention that they were enacted to suppress religious conduct, instead of to address legitimate governmental interests. The city's failure to enact laws addressing the animal welfare concerns raised by other practices such as hunting, slaughter of animals for food, pest control, euthanasia of unwanted companion animals, fishing, and other accepted practices "devalues religious reasons for killing by judging them to be of lesser import than nonreligious reasons."[15] Thus the ordinances constituted an improper singling out of religious sacrifice for punishment, while permitting other activities to continue even though they posed equivalent harms to animals.

Second, the Court found the ordinances impermissibly overbroad, in that they restricted more religious conduct than was necessary to protect legitimate government interests. For example, if the city wanted to address animal welfare issues, it could create and enforce regulations governing how animals are cared for, treated, and killed within city limits, rather than impose a ban on ritual sacrifice. Similarly, it could implement rules on disposal of organic waste to advance any public health concerns. In response to Hialeah's claim that the secrecy of the Santeria ceremonies made such regulation impossible, the Court saw no reason why enforcing more narrowly drawn health regulations would be any harder to enforce than would a ban on animal sacrifice.

Third, the Court found that Hialeah's ordinances were too narrow in scope in their impact on the city's ostensible animal welfare and public health concerns. Again, if the city had a genuine interest in addressing these concerns, it could enact rules governing many secular activities as well, such as hunting. In addition, the Court found that records of the city council revealed that the object of the ordinances was to target ritual killing, based on city residents' hostility to the practices of the Santeria religion.

For the above reasons, the Court held that the Hialeah ordinances were not neutral and generally applicable. First Amendment doctrine holds that when laws burdening religious conduct fail the test of neutrality and general applicability, they may still be upheld as constitutional if they are necessary to advance a compelling state interest. But again, the Hialeah ordinances failed to meet the constitutional requirements. Laws needed to protect compelling state interests must be as narrowly drawn as possible to advance the relevant governmental interests. The Hialeah ordinances, however, were both overbroad in their effect on religious conduct and underinclusive in advancing the government's claimed interests.

The Court was also dubious about the city's claim that its ordinances were based on compelling interests in protecting human health and animal welfare. "Where government restricts only conduct protected by the First Amendment and fails to enact feasible measures to restrict other conduct producing substantial harm or alleged harm of the same sort, the interest given in justification of the restriction is not compelling."[16] In sum, before restrictions on ritual sacrifice could be upheld, Hialeah would have to enact comprehensive and consistent laws addressed to all activities, both secular and religious, that threatened its claimed interests in advancing animal welfare and public health.

In a concurring opinion joined by Justice O'Connor, Justice Blackmun expressed his disagreement with the *Smith* rule permitting neutral and generally applicable laws that burden religious practice. He stated his preference for the alternative standard, requiring the government to prove that any law burdening religious conduct is justified by a compelling state interest and is the least restrictive means available to advance that interest. Justice Blackmun agreed with Justice Kennedy's conclusions in the majority opinion that Hialeah's ordinances could not meet this standard, because they were "both overinclusive and underinclusive in relation to the state interests they purportedly serve."[17] But he noted that the case would present a more difficult question if members of the Church of the Babalu Aye were seeking to be exempted from the state's general anticruelty law. If government officials had prosecuted members of the church involved in animal sacrifice for violations of this law, and if the government could demonstrate that the anticruelty law "sincerely pursued the goal of protecting animals from cruel treatment,"[18] the Court might have reached a different result than it did in the actual case.

After the *Babalu Aye* opinion was released, news reports portrayed Hialeah's Santeria believers as "jubilant" and "plan[ning] to resume" animal sacrifices.[19] Although the Supreme Court's decision provoked concern among animal protection organizations,[20] lawyers affiliated with these groups emphasized the unusual characteristics of the *Babalu Aye* case, particularly the city's enactment of laws singling out ritual sacrifice for punishment. They echoed Justice Blackmun's assertion that the Court did not resolve the issue of whether religious motivation was sufficient to exempt from punishment those who engage in conduct harmful to animals that is otherwise punishable as a violation of general anticruelty laws. The Court's *Smith* decision, which upheld the constitutionality of applying state anti-drug laws to persons using peyote in religious ceremonies, suggests that the justices might be unwilling to exempt religiously motivated animal harm from anticruelty laws.[21]

Later developments, including the passage of a new federal law, have created new uncertainties about the precise legal status of animal sacrifice. In the Religious Freedom

Restoration Act of 1993,[22] Congress expressed its disagreement with *Smith*'s approach to evaluating the constitutionality of laws burdening religious conduct. The statute's explicit purposes are "(1) to restore the compelling interest test . . . in all cases where free exercise of religion is substantially burdened; and (2) to provide a claim or defense to persons whose religious exercise is substantially burdened by government."[23] This law could provide Santeria believers with a defense to *any* anticruelty prosecution they might face, as well as with a basis to challenge the constitutionality of any such government action. Courts are likely to reject such a defense or challenge from religious believers only if the government presents a convincing case that an anticruelty prosecution is the least restrictive means by which to advance the state's compelling interest in animal protection.[24]

ANIMAL USE AND THE FIRST AMENDMENT

In today's world, people use animals for a variety of reasons. In the United States, activities such as hunting; fishing; exterminating rats, mice, and other "pest" animals; euthanizing unwanted companion animals; and slaughtering animals for meat, leather, and fur are widely accepted as legitimate, based on the human recreational, sanitary, aesthetic, and related secular preferences that these activities satisfy.

In *Babalu Aye*, Santeria members claimed that a particular form of animal use was a crucial part of their religion. If the orishas are denied animal nourishment, they will be unable to help Santeria believers fulfill their individual, God-given destinies. As an analogy, imagine the impact if the government passed laws prohibiting Christians from participating in Holy Communion or baptism, or Jews from fasting on Yom Kippur. For Santeria adherents, the reasons for sacrifice are so vital that they, on balance, decisively find the infliction of harm on animals to be justified.

Yet Hialeah residents who opposed the church dismissed the distinctly religious justifications offered for animal sacrifice. At a Hialeah City Council meeting called to consider the church's building plans, speakers referred to Santeria as " 'foolishness,' 'an abomination to the Lord,' and the worship of 'demons.' "[25] In the eyes of the majority population, many of whom regarded Santeria as a strange and frightening cult, church members' religious beliefs were illegitimate and insufficient to justify how the animals were treated.

Similar disagreement surrounded the question of whether animal sacrifice qualified as a "necessary" use of animals. According to the attorney general of Florida, religious animal sacrifice performed for reasons unrelated to food consumption was an unnecessary killing within the meaning of this law. On the other hand, the Santeria religion defines animal sacrifice as "absolutely necessary."[26] According to Pichardo, animal sacrifice is "an integral part of our faith. It is like our holy meal."[27]

An explicit values preference is expressed in the First Amendment's refusal to allow laws that interfere with the free exercise of religion. Although judicial interpretations have permitted some absolute restrictions on religious practices, such as drug use and polygamy, the courts have set strict limits on government attempts to punish or otherwise constrain religious conduct. According to constitutional law, religious freedom is so important that the state may restrict it only when necessary to protect other extremely important values, and even then the state may apply only the most minimal restrictions on religious conduct necessary to protect the other values.

In light of this values framework, it is easy to see why the Supreme Court struck down the Hialeah ordinances. Hialeah's failure to enact laws interfering with animal harm in other commonly accepted activities revealed the hypocrisy of its claim that the ordinances were designed to protect animal welfare. As the Court noted, the Hialeah City Council's "careful drafting ensured that, although Santeria sacrifice is prohibited, killings that are no more necessary or humane in almost all other circumstances are unpunished."[28] It was clear to the Court that hostility to the Santeria religion, as opposed to the city's claimed interests in animal welfare and public health, motivated Hialeah's actions. In addition to its relatively small number of adherents, Santeria is "mostly a religion of poor people, mostly black Cubans."[29] Because the First Amendment was written to address religious beliefs in exactly such a situation, that is, to disallow a majority's use of its political power to target the religious freedom of an unpopular minority group, *Babalu Aye* turned out to be a simple case for the justices to resolve.[30]

ETHICAL ISSUES

Morally, however, the case is not so simple. The law does not determine moral right and wrong, and *Babalu Aye* raises a broad range of questions about how to evaluate the importance of various human interests in killing and otherwise burdening nonhuman animals.

Problems of Conflicting Rights

In essence, Hialeah officials claimed that animal sacrifice was unjustified and unnecessary because Santeria religious beliefs were not as important as many secular reasons for killing animals. Hialeah officials appear to have been thinking that the risks to the community and the harms caused to animals jointly outweighed benefits to members of the Santeria faith. Even if this balancing were accurate, however, it would not decide questions about the *rights* of the members of this faith—or, for that matter, questions about the rights of animals. The language of rights has long been used to assert claims that demand recognition, to secure moral and legal protections, and to carve out a zone within which individuals are protected against interventions that benefit the majority but present risks to minorities. (See the introduction, pp. 25–27, on rights theories.)

The Santeria case is notable for the way it raises questions of both rights of religious freedom and animal rights in circumstances in which a more powerful group seems to deny the importance of those rights. The government appears to deny that the adherents of Santeria have strong rights of religious freedom, and the adherents of Santeria seem to deny that animals have significant rights not to be harmed. Moreover, and perhaps paradoxically, Hialeah officials appear to have been appealing to the rights of animals (or at least obligations not to harm animals) as a basis for overriding rights of religious freedom.

Yet neither Hialeah officials nor other Florida officials have erected a significant framework of rights for animals. In Florida, state policy permits and even protects many types of animal use engaged in for secular reasons, but little in the Florida framework of policies protects animals against the forms of treatment involved in Santeria practices. For example, it is a criminal offense in Florida to assist an animal in escaping from a hunter,[31] and children are given the opportunity to learn hunting skills in state-sponsored camps.[32] In his opinion in *Babalu Aye,* Justice Kennedy referred to the determination of a Florida court that using live rabbits to train racing greyhounds was not a violation of the state anticruelty law's prohibition on "unnecessary" killing.[33] In oral argument on the case, Justice O'Connor challenged Hialeah's attorney to explain the city's rationale for banning religious sacrifice while permitting the boiling of live lobsters for consumption in area restaurants.[34] The Supreme Court ruled that the rights framework that underlies the First Amendment did not permit Hialeah officials to deem Santeria religious beliefs a less worthwhile basis for animal use than the preferences underlying practices such as hunting, greyhound training, and eating fresh lobster.

Human Interests and Animal Interests

Finding the proper approach to evaluating and balancing human benefits and obligations to animals becomes increasingly complex as the ethical perspective is broadened. In a brief on the Hialeah animal sacrifice case (filed with the Supreme Court), the Humane Society of the United States and other animal protection organizations asserted that "the 'necessity' of animal killing has generally been determined by reference to tangible human needs such as food, the prevention and treatment of disease, and safety."[35] The brief noted that human survival is the most compelling justification for killing or otherwise harming animals.

Human survival is not at stake in the Santeria case; and even when human survival is at issue, how probable must it be that a certain action toward animals, such as pest extermination or laboratory animal research on disease, will remove the threat to human survival? Does a 10% chance of success justify animal use? Do nonlethal health threats to humans furnish adequate justification for imposing pain, distress, or death on animals? For example, what level of importance should be assigned to the human desire to continue testing new cosmetics on animals to avoid the risk of eye damage? (See the cosmetics case, pp. 202–12.) What about interests other than human life and health? What significance ought to be assigned to recreation, pleasure, and aesthetic preferences?

Arguably, given a broad enough understanding of what constitutes a human *good,* almost any human need or desire can be viewed as being of *vital* importance to humans. Set against such broad understandings of human goods is the view that animals, like humans, have interests. If one admits that animals have interests, it seems necessary to find a way to balance human interests with the interests of nonhuman animals. This balancing might take a utilitarian or a nonutilitarian form (see the introduction, pp. 19–20, 23–25); but once one admits that both humans and animals have interests, it follows that one is committed to some scheme of balancing those interests.

The Standard of Harm to Animals

In assessing whether animal use is justified or necessary, virtually everyone agrees that consideration should be given to the level of harm imposed on the animal. Animals have interests in avoiding harm and enjoying benefits, interests that (theoretically) may be ranked in terms of importance. According to one commonly accepted ranking, the highest significance should be assigned to avoidance of extreme pain, deprivation, and distress, with interests in receiving species-appropriate living conditions, avoiding premature death, and other interests placed at lower points on the scale. Those who favor a *balancing* approach to the justification issue argue that a compelling justification is required for using animals in procedures and activities that pose a deep threat to animal interests.[36] Some who do not favor a balancing approach believe that a *threshold* or upper limit of pain, suffering, anxiety, fear, and distress (including the duration of each) should be a stable part of society's network of protections for animals. (See the introduction, pp. 29–31.)

In its *Babalu Aye* opinion, the Supreme Court relied on the belief that a variety of secular and religious practices subject animals to harm similar to the harm they experience from the Santeria sacrifice procedure. The Court noted that a similar method of killing adopted for Kosher slaughter, for example, is explicitly permitted by state and federal law.[37]

It is not clear whether the Court would have responded differently to a religious practice involving an extraordinary level of harm to animals, such as subjecting conscious animals to a lengthy period of extreme pain, thus amounting to a form of torture. Most state and federal laws are unclear on the matter, and very few ethical perspectives on animals (other than those that would prohibit such practices altogether) have presented a clear solution to such problems.

One probable response by the Court is suggested in its remark that "if the city has a real concern that [Santeria sacrifice] methods are less humane, . . . the subject of the regulation should be the method of slaughter itself, not a religious classification that is said to bear some general relation to it."[38] The Court implicitly acknowledges the legitimacy of official efforts to minimize pain and distress among animals used to advance various human interests, but it requires only that such efforts be consistently applied and narrowly targeted when they affect religious activities. The Court does not require that there be a limit or threshold and does not consider the underlying problems of how to handle extraordinary levels of harm to animals and whether human benefits can justify them.

Setting Policies on Animal Use

Traditionally, the rules governing animal care and use have reflected a social consensus regarding which human interests are important enough to justify imposing death and other harms on animals. Over the years, some governments have made some effort to forbid certain kinds of animal use, such as dog and cock fighting, presumably based on the judgment that the enjoyment of the human participants and observers is an insufficient reason to justify the harm such activities cause to animals. Overall, however, regulatory efforts in the United States have sought to minimize the pain, distress, and other burdens imposed as part of animal use, rather than to forbid certain forms of animal use or to set thresholds.[39]

As the Supreme Court pointed out in *Babalu Aye*, the current legal consensus seems to be that nearly any human interest can in principle qualify as an acceptable justification for animal use, although there may be legal requirements for humane treatment of the animals used to advance those interests. Whether there is a moral consensus in society to this effect is more doubtful. It also remains to be seen whether animal protection is of sufficient social importance for the citizenry to accept constraints on many now commonly accepted recreational and other pursuits so that the more consistent policies on animal use demanded by the Supreme Court could actually be devised.

NOTES

1. Except as otherwise noted, the facts in this case study are taken from the U.S. District Court and U.S. Supreme Court opinions in *Church of the Lukumi Babalu Aye, Inc. v. City of Hialeah,* 723 F. Supp. 1467 (S.D. Fla. 1989), *rev'd,* 113 S. Ct. 2217 (1993). For a historian's in-depth account of the legal case, see David M. O'Brien, *Animal Sacrifice and Religious Freedom: Church of the Lukumi Babalu Aye v. City of Hialeah* (Lawrence, KS: University Press of Kansas, 2004).

2. General descriptions of the Santeria religion and its history can be found in George Brandon, *Santeria from Africa to the New World* (Bloomington: Indiana University Press, 1993); Migene Gonzalez-Wippler, *Santeria: The Religion; A Legacy of Faith, Rites, and Magic* (New York: Harmony, 1989); and Miguel A. De La Torre, *Santeria: The Beliefs and Rituals of a Growing Religion in American* (Grand Rapids: Eerdmans, 2004). See also Joseph M. Murphy, "The Beliefs and Rituals of a Growing Religion in America," *Theological Studies* 67 (March 1, 2006): 211–13 (a book review of De La Torre); and Johnny Diaz, " 'This Is Mother Nature's Religion': Once-Secretive Santeria Faith Brings Its Healing Message into the Open," *Boston Globe,* November 4, 2004.

3. O'Brien, "Animal Sacrifice," pp. 19–21.

4. Joseph M. Murphy, "Santeria," in *The Encyclopedia of Religion,* ed. Mircea Eliade (New York: Macmillan, 1987), pp. 13, 67.

5. Murphy, "Santeria," p. 66.

6. 723 F. Supp. at 1473.

7. 723 F. Supp. at 1472.

8. 113 S. Ct. at 2234–35. The text of the Hialeah resolutions and ordinances can be found at 113 S. Ct. 2234–38.

9. Fla. Stat. Sec. 828.12 (West Supp. 2006).

10. 113 S. Ct. at 2237.

11. 113 S. Ct. at 2223. This opinion and the ordinances' definition of animal sacrifice were intended to exempt from punishment persons performing kosher slaughter, which officials claimed has food consumption as its primary purpose.

12. 723 F. Supp. at 1487 n.59.

13. 936 F.2d 586 (1991).

14. 494 U.S. 872 (1990).

15. 113 S. Ct. at 2229.

16. 113 S. Ct. at 2234.

17. 113 S. Ct. at 2251.

18. 113 S. Ct. at 2251.

19. Larry Rohter, "Santeria Faithful Hail Court Ruling," *New York Times,* June 13, 1993, p. A16.

20. Roger A. Kindler, "A Legal Defeat for Animals," *HSUS News* (Fall 1993): 10–11.

21. R. Ted Cruz, "Animal Sacrifice and Equal Protection Free Exercise," *Harvard Journal of Law and Public Policy* 17 (Winter 1994): 262–73.

22. Public Law No. 103–141, 107 Stat. 1488 (1993).

23. Religious Freedom Restoration Act, Sec. 2(b).

24. In 1987, a New York state court ruled against a Santeria group that brought a lawsuit challenging the constitutionality of an anticruelty prosecution against them for practices related to animal sacrifice. *First Church of Chango v. ASPCA, aff'd,* 521 N.Y.S.2d 536 (1987), *appeal denied,* 521 N.E.2d 443 (1988). The strength of this case as precedent is unclear, however, in light of the subsequent Supreme Court and congressional actions.

25. 113 S. Ct. at 2231.

26. Douglas Laycock, "Free Exercise and the Religious Freedom Restoration Act," *Fordham Law Review* 62 (February 1994): 890.

27. Linda H. Greenhouse, "Court, Citing Religious Freedom, Voids a Ban on Animal Sacrifice," *New York Times,* June 12, 1993, p. A9.

28. 113 S. Ct. at 2228.

29. Laycock, "Free Exercise," p. 890.

30. Stephen L. Carter, "The Resurrection of Religious Freedom?" *Harvard Law Review* 107 (November 1993): 127–28.

31. Fla. Stat. Ann. Sec. 372.705 (West 2000).

32. Laycock, "Free Exercise," p. 890.

33. 113 S. Ct. at 2229.

34. Henry M. Holzer, "The *Santeria* Case and the Cost of Contradiction," *International Society for Animal Rights Report* (Summer 1993): 2.

35. Brief for the Humane Society of the United States et al. at 51, *Church of the Lukumi Babalu Aye v. City of Hialeah,* 113 S. Ct. 2217 (1993) (No. 91–948).

36. Rebecca Dresser, "Standards for Animal Research: Justification and Assessment of Alternatives," *Journal of the American Veterinary Association* 200 (March 1, 1992): 668.

37. In enacting the federal Humane Slaughter Act, Congress permitted as a humane method "slaughtering in accordance with the ritual requirements of the Jewish faith or any other religious faith that prescribes a method of slaughter whereby the animal suffers loss of consciousness caused by the simultaneous and instantaneous severance of the carotid arteries with a sharp instrument": 7 U.S.C. sec. 1902(b) (2000). Florida has a similar statute: Fla. Stat. Ann. sec. 828.22, 828.23(6)(b)(1976).

38. 113 S. Ct. at 2230.

39. Jerrold Tannenbaum, *Veterinary Ethics* (Baltimore: Williams and Wilkins, 1989), pp. 92–94.

PART VI

ENDANGERED SPECIES

10

Bonobos

Humans' Closest Relatives
Face Extinction

In 2004, five trucks from a Western logging company pulled into Mompano, a town in Congo.[1] Mompano is in the center of the habitat of the bonobo—an extremely endangered species that, along with the chimpanzee, is the closest living relative of human beings. The trucks were laden with sacks of sugar, salt, and other supplies. The loggers offered the supplies to the villagers in return for an illegal permission to cut down all of the trees in the area.

The offer was tempting to the impoverished villagers. Congo has been torn apart by many years of a civil war that has left more than 3 million people dead. It has the highest infant mortality rate in Africa, and a per capita gross domestic product (GDP) that in the 1980s was only half of what it was in 1962; it continues to fall yearly. The vast majority of the population in Congo survives on less than two-thirds of the daily calories needed; 80% lack access to safe water, and 70% have little or no access to health care.[2]

Despite their poverty, the villagers told the loggers that this was part of an area controlled by a former ambassador to the United Nations, Nkema-Liloo, and that they would have to get his approval before any logging could take place. Nkema's family were chiefs of the Mongo people who lived in the region, and he purchased much of the surrounding land in order to prevent logging and habitat destruction while developing sustainable plantations and working to protect bonobos. Nkema told the villagers, "No!" The trucks drove away. However, the same company was able to convince other villagers nearby to allow the logging. This type of illegal logging is a major threat to endangered species such as the bonobo, but it is common in Congo, where companies often smuggle illegal logs.

Logging and mining companies, many of them Western, are one contributing cause of the near extinction of bonobos. Logging destroys their habitat, increases hunting of bonobos and other apes to feed work crews, and builds roads that enable hunters to penetrate into previously undisturbed habitat. Although these projects threaten the survival of bonobos and other endangered species, they offer a ray of hope for the impoverished people of the region. This situation in Congo raises profoundly difficult moral questions. How much should human beings sacrifice for the good of endangered species such as the bonobo? How can the needs of impoverished people be met without destroying the environment on which they depend? What responsibilities do people outside of Congo have toward both the bonobos and the people that live there?

WHO ARE THE BONOBOS?

Bonobos share over 98% of their genetic material with human beings, and we have a common ancestor 6 million years ago. Bonobos are very intelligent, social apes noted for their peaceful nature. Some researchers have proposed that bonobos may be the species that most resembles the common ancestor of bonobos, chimpanzees, and humans.[3] Bonobos have limb proportions more similar to those of human beings and very close to the human ancestor *Australopithecus*. They are often observed to walk bipedally. They also have a long gestation period like humans and a humanlike distribution of special neurons in the frontal cortex. Whether or not bonobos resemble our common ancestor more than chimpanzees and humans, they offer an alternative perspective to the theories of early human evolution based primarily on the study of chimpanzees.

Despite their demonstrably close relation to humans, bonobos remain relatively unknown. They live only in the rain forest of Congo, a nation torn by civil war and often inaccessible to the outside world. When bonobos were discovered by outsiders, they were often mistaken for chimpanzees. The ancestors of bonobos and chimpanzees split from each other only 2 million years ago, and they look similar enough that bonobos were not recognized as a separate species until the late 1920s.[4] Prior to that time they were simply thought of as small chimpanzees, as there is a great deal of overlap between the size distributions of the two species. Bonobo males average 95 pounds and females 82 pounds, both at the smaller end of the chimpanzee size distribution.[5] Because of the history of their discovery, small size, and similarity to the better-known chimpanzees with whom they were confused, bonobos were often referred to as *pygmy chimpanzees,* a term still occasionally used.

Ironically, Western scientists may have known bonobos for longer than any other ape. In 1641 Dutch anatomist Nicolaas Tulp became the first Westerner to dissect and describe an ape. Many scientists now believe that Tulp's ape was a bonobo. More recently, the American ape research pioneer Robert Yerkes raised a number of chimpanzees in the 1920s. One of them, whom he named "Prince Chim," was exceptionally bright and agreeable, and he is now recognized to have been a bonobo.

Despite their apparent similarities, bonobos and chimpanzees behave in markedly different ways. Chimpanzees are a violent and warlike patriarchal species; males often raid neighboring tribes and kill other males.[6] Even within their own group, chimpanzees often settle disputes through violence. Chimpanzees also hunt, sometimes even for monkeys.[7] Chimpanzee males form strong bonds, especially between brothers, and they often cooperate in fighting and hunting. For much of the past 100 years, chimpanzees have served as a model of human ancestors for evolutionary theorists, lending credence to the characterization of our ancestors as "man the hunter."

In contrast, bonobos are gentle and have been referred to as the "apes from Venus."[8] They have a more gregarious nature than chimpanzees, achieve a higher level of mutual tolerance, and excel at individual coexistence.[9] Instead of violence, bonobos often use sexual activity to resolve social tension. They display both heterosexual and homo-sexual activity, engaging in face-to-face copulation and tongue kissing not seen in chimpanzees and once thought to exist only among human beings. When two different groups of bonobos discover a food source in the forest, they often engage each other sexually instead of fighting; they then split the food (though displays of aggression do sometimes occur). Human beings are the only other primate species that have as diverse and frequent intergroup interactions as bonobos.

Bonobo society is peaceful and matriarchal, unlike the violent patriarchal alpha-male system found in chimpanzees.[10] Both chimpanzees and bonobos are male-philopatric, meaning that males stay in their native groups while females disperse to neighboring groups during adolescence. Female bonobos reach sexual maturity and first give birth at age 13 or 14, and they continue to give birth about once every five years thereafter. Infants nurse for four years and are carried around by their mothers even longer. They go everywhere that she goes. Bonobo society is characterized by very strong mother-son bonds and by friendships between adult females.

Bonobos live in groups of up to 40 individuals, and these groups exhibit a fission-fusion structure.[11] They travel together during the day in smaller groups of a few indi-viduals, regrouping with different individuals from the same larger group when these smaller groups break apart.[12] At night bonobos weave nests in trees to keep themselves safe from predators while they sleep. Whereas chimpanzees nest in small groups, bono-bos regroup in late afternoon and have been observed to sleep in as many as 26 different nests at one site. Some researchers think that they may be exchanging information for future foraging.

Bonobos eat a mainly vegetarian diet. The biggest single component in their diet is ripe fruit, which accounts for as much as 80% of their food intake. Most of the fruit is picked from trees, but some of it is massive—up to 60 pounds—and is consumed after it drops to the forest floor. Bonobos also eat large quantities of high-protein pith from plants known as terrestrial herbaceous vegetation (THV) in the form of leaf stalks and shoots. Humans living in the area also eat THV, and researchers say that these humans find an "incredibly delicious" taste in the vegetation.

While bonobos occasionally eat reptiles, shrews, squirrels, duikers, and maybe some fish, animal foods comprise only about 1% of their diet, and organized hunting is not a part of bonobo life. Bonobos have been observed playing with and grooming monkeys, but they have also been seen injuring and even killing them when the monkeys do not cooperate. Bonobos have also been observed digging for earthworms, which they appear to eat for enjoyment more than for food value. Because of their vegetarian diet, in addition to their large social clans, bonobos require a lush, large habitat.

Bonobos live in the tropical rain forest of the Congo River basin in Africa. Their entire range is contained within the Democratic Republic of Congo. The Congo and

Lualaba rivers form the boundaries of their distribution to the west, north, and east. To the south they are bounded by the Kasai River and also by a change in vegetation from tropical rain forest to grassland. Changes in vegetation may also play a role in their eastern boundary. Unlike chimpanzees, bonobos have not adapted to life in a wide range of habitats, perhaps because a lack of transition zones with intermediate vegetation along the borders of their range has prevented gradual adaptation. The distribution of bonobo populations may also have been influenced by pressures created by human hunting of bonobos ever since Bantu farming tribes migrated to the Congo forest 700 years ago. This appears likely in the southern parts of the bonobo range.

Climate and topography are almost invariable in the area inhabited by bonobos. One small group of bonobos (fewer than 100) lives in a tropical rain forest with temperatures between 68 and 86 degrees with hardly any monthly variation, and annual rainfall of over 60 inches, again with little variation. The altitude varies from 980 to 1,570 feet. There are two types of forest in the bonobo range, swamp forests and dry ground forests, though both are humid tropical rain forests. Swamp forests are found along rivers that frequently flood, permitting people to navigate their boats among the trees. Trees in swamp forests typically have roots like the arms of an octopus and are relatively low. The ground feels spongy to walk on when it is not flooded, and, because the canopy is low, there is more sunlight and undergrowth on the forest floor. Dry ground forests have solid ground, taller trees, and a more complicated array of plant species. Because of the taller canopy, dry ground forests are darker and have less underbrush. Both types of forests are currently being destroyed by loggers, reducing the land available for the bonobos to roam. The presence of the loggers has also made more common the hunting of these animals by humans.

HUMAN THREATS TO BONOBOS

For many years, bonobos have been protected by the fact that the indigenous people in the areas inhabited by bonobos have had strong taboos against eating them.[13] The local people have folk tales that emphasize the common ancestry of bonobos and people, and the good will between them. These stories relate that bonobos and humans used to live together in villages and that bonobos introduced people to many of the foods they eat.[14] These historical taboos have begun to crumble, however, in the face of economic desperation, war, and immigration of outsiders.

The major threats that human beings pose to bonobos are habitat destruction due to logging and mining and the hunting that often accompanies these operations as companies feed their workforce off the land. For example, Denzer, a German logging company, claims that its subsidiary SIFORCO feeds its employees millet, rice, and manioc (an edible root). However, the employees report that they receive no such supplies.[15] When Denzer refused to allow photographer Karl Ammann to visit its logging concession in the late 1990s, he entered the area on his own. He discovered that SIFORCO hired hunters to travel with its crews and encouraged its own workers to hunt for bush meat, including bonobos. The company also transported bonobo meat and live bonobos to market in the cities, and it provided the shotguns used to hunt them. Although bonobos are theoretically protected by law, "in reality all Congolese hunting laws [are] habitually and completely ignored."[16]

Mining also plays a role in threatening the bonobo. Colton is an ore containing the element tantalum, which is needed in electronics circuitry for such items as cell phones, video games, and laptop computers.[17] The release of the Sony PlayStation 2 videogame system was delayed by a supply bottleneck that sent the price of tantalum soaring. As a result, thousands of villagers abandoned farming and took up mining in the Kahuzi-Biega National Park, eating their way through virtually all of the large animals present, including apes.

A problem facing bonobos that is related to the destruction of their habitat is the fragmentation of their population into small, isolated pockets. When a species' range becomes broken up and discontinuous, as is currently happening to the bonobo, the species becomes much more at risk of extinction.[18] Small, isolated populations are more vulnerable to local catastrophes, and the lack of opportunity for gene flow between groups can lead to an increase of genetic diseases. For the bonobos, the lack of contact between groups can also reduce the birthrate by making it difficult for females to migrate to new groups. Small, isolated populations are also less capable of adapting to changing environmental conditions. Adaptive evolutionary change requires heritable genetic variation, of which there is much less in small populations. Small populations are also at risk of being wiped out by virulent pathogens, which are often introduced from other host species such as domesticated animals.[19]

STRATEGIES FOR PRESERVING THE BONOBOS

Actions can be taken to prevent this isolation from worsening and to slow the destruction of the bonobos' habitat. Conservationists see these actions as desperately needed, whereas others regard them as too costly and as harmful to humans.

Habitat Preservation

Habitat preservation is the fundamental problem. Because of the threats posed by population fragmentation, it is necessary not only that large amounts of habitat be preserved, but also that territories be contiguous so that groups of bonobos can exchange members. War and lack of access to the forest have made it difficult to determine the full extent and location of bonobo populations. In order to protect their habitat effectively, it is necessary first to gain a better understanding of where bonobos live as well as how the local human population utilizes the forest, including threats to bonobos such as hunting and snares.

Efforts to preserve bonobos are unlikely to be successful unless they are supported by the people who live in the area. Previous efforts to protect threatened species in Africa have often failed due to lack of local support. For example, during colonization, and after their independence, countries across Africa nationalized their game, not allowing them to be privately owned and controlled. Local people then had no incentive to conserve, and the results were alarming. Elephants, for example, represented a threat to farmers, who saw no benefit in preserving them. By contrast, in cases in which the elephants have been re-privatized, as in campfire programs in Zimbabwe in which sport hunters buy the right to hunt elephants from local villagers, local people have rapidly learned to manage and conserve the animals.[20]

The goal of developing local participation (though not through hunting) is one of the key strategies adopted by the Bonobo Conservation Initiative (BCI).[21] This group has been working for years with local populations to better understand indigenous needs and perspectives and to build local partners. As a result of these efforts, the people of Kokolopori recently signed an agreement with BCI to establish a reserve of over 1,000 square miles.[22] In return for their help with bonobo preservation, BCI and other groups are helping the people in the region by introducing a new variant of cassava, the staple crop in the region. Disease decimated the old variant and forced people to expand areas of cultivation into the forest in an attempt to compensate. The program will provide local people with food while also relieving pressure on the forest.

Preserving the habitat of bonobos would also have the effect of protecting many other species in its ecosystem, including a broad range of rare, endemic, or threatened species.[23] These include the forest elephant, water chevrotain, golden cat, giant ground pangolin, and Congo peacock. Within Africa, Congo ranks second in plant diversity and first in variety of species of mammals, primates, birds, amphibians, fish, and swallowtail butterflies. It ranks fourth in the number of mammal species worldwide. The presence of so much diversity within this single nation makes the bonobo what is termed an "umbrella species" whose protection would confer protection on many other threatened species and/or critical ecosystems. In the United States, umbrella species are often afforded special protection by law. For example, the protection of the northern spotted owl required limitations on forest harvest to protect the owl's ecosystem, thereby providing an umbrella benefit to other species that live there.[24]

Saving the habitat of umbrella species such as the bonobo often benefits humans, because a habitat rich in biodiversity has economic value. For example, 57% of the 150 most commonly prescribed drugs originated in wild species.[25] Scientists worry that, as biodiversity is lost, humanity may be destroying species that might provide remedies for many of the diseases that afflict us. Nonhuman plants and animals also provide critical benefits, termed ecosystem services, to humans. These services include the maintenance of fertile soil and water, climate control, the composition of the atmosphere, and pest control.[26] The U.S. Agency for International Development (USAID) estimates that ecosystem services are worth $33 trillion a year to the world, including $54 billion worth of pollination of just 30 of the world's major food crops every year and $250–500 billion worth of pest control.[27]

Of course, there is often no way of knowing what the effects of losing a species will be. Whereas a particular endangered species may seem to be of no consequence for human welfare, or may even seem to be a competitor, its extinction may lead to a domino effect of undesirable consequences. Consider the case of wolves in Yellowstone National Park.[28] As wolves have been reintroduced in recent years, a cascade of effects on the ecosystem has been documented. Wolf predation has eased overpopulation among elk while creating survival opportunities for smaller carnivores and scavengers such as coyotes and magpies. Riverside tree species such as aspen, cottonwood, and willow have also returned now that they are no longer subject to overgrazing by elk, and their return has led to a renewal of beaver populations.

No one knows what impact the decline of the bonobos is having or ultimately will have on the ecosystems in Congo. What is clear is that by preserving the bonobo habitat, people can also protect a myriad of other species whose interrelationships and potential benefit to human beings remain unknown.

Hunting

The bush meat crisis is as great a threat to bonobos as habitat destruction, and its halt is imperative for their immediate prospects of survival. Under international law, bonobos are protected by the Convention on International Trade in Endangered Species of Wild Flora and Fauna (CITES), effective in 1975.[29] CITES has three categories, or appendices, of endangered species. The bonobo is listed in Appendix I, which covers species threatened with extinction. International trade in species listed in Appendix I is permitted only in exceptional circumstances. Unfortunately, as the case of the bonobos illustrates, CITES has failed to save those species whose primary threat is from habitat destruction and/or direct predation. Its focus on stopping international trade does not address the market forces within countries that often prove more threatening. And, even when international economic pressures are a large part of the problem, banning trade in the specific species threatened often does little to help. Bonobos and many other endangered species are threatened by international demand for products that originate in their habitat, such as wood and Colton, not by international demand for the actual animals.

Bonobos are also protected by national laws in Congo; however, these laws often remain unenforced. Protecting bonobos from hunters is hindered by poverty, the lack of alternative sources of protein, and the need for education.[30] There is also a great need for training, salaries, equipment, and medicine for park guards, who sometimes go for months without pay and are confronted by well-armed poachers.[31] People who have worked in Congo emphasize that bonobos cannot be saved without both better enforcement of existing laws and the provision of education and alternatives for local people.

Captive Breeding Programs

Another possible strategy for preserving bonobos is through captive breeding programs.[32] Bonobos are not difficult to breed, and they can live long, healthy lives in captivity. However, there are only around 100 bonobos in the world's zoos. The average size of bonobo populations in zoos is now fewer than six. These small populations make it almost impossible to maintain genetic diversity, even with cooperative breeding exchange programs. Zoos are trying to build their populations up while maintaining social cohesion. They mainly exchange maturing females in order to preserve the mother-son bonds that are central to bonobo society. Furthermore, even if captive breeding programs were able to ensure the survival of the species, the different cultures of bonobos would be lost.

Assessing captive breeding requires careful consideration of its ultimate goal. Is the goal to maintain a captive population indefinitely, or is it to breed bonobos in relative safety in order to release them back into the wild to supplement remaining populations? Supplementation has sometimes been used as a method to increase the numbers of a threatened wild population by breeding them in captivity and then releasing them into the wild. Indeed, future supplementation is often cited as one of the justifications for keeping captive zoo populations of animals such as elephants (see pp. 109ff).

However, supplementation can cause significant problems that pose more of a threat than a benefit to the species.[33] Despite the best efforts of breeding programs, populations bred in captivity generally adapt themselves to the domestic environment created by human beings.[34] Animals raised in captivity often do not learn how to survive on their own in the wild. It may not be possible for humans to teach bonobos how to survive in the forests from which their ancestors were taken.

If a wild population is threatened because of loss of habitat, as the bonobos are, supplementation may, and probably will, only serve to increase population densities to unsustainable levels.[35] The end result will be competition for limited resources between the wild and captive populations, which may lead to a reduction in the wild population. Captive breeding and reintroduction work well only if there is plenty of unoccupied habitat available and threats to the species have been reduced or eliminated. This strategy was successfully used to reintroduce the peregrine falcon to much of North America. Supplementation is not an alternative to habitat preservation; it is a limited method of rebuilding natural populations where sufficient habitat exists.

ETHICAL ISSUES

The Moral Status of Bonobos

The intelligence and social capacity of bonobos raise questions regarding their moral status (see the introduction, chapter 1, pp. 15–19). Some philosophers maintain that sentience or conscious awareness make an animal a member of the moral community. Others believe that a higher level of intelligence or rationality is required. The considerable intellectual gifts of bonobos challenge the idea that a sharp line can be drawn between human beings and other animals on the basis of intelligence or any other trait. It may be that wherever one chooses to draw the line, either some humans will be left out of the moral community or some animals such as the bonobo will be included. There is a species difference between humans and bonobos, but does this difference mean there is a difference of moral status? If so, how big is the difference?

People who hold that sentience or conscious awareness is all that is necessary for membership in the moral community grant that an animal's advanced capabilities are relevant to how it can suffer and thus to how it ought to be treated. For example, while both slugs and pigs can feel pain, pigs have much more advanced cognitive capabilities that may also allow them to feel boredom and loneliness. Even if one holds that inflicting gratuitous pain on either species is morally unacceptable, it may also be morally obligatory to provide pigs with a stimulating environment and to increase contact with their fellows on pig farms. The same moral reasoning would apply to bonobos, which are known for their social interaction in large groups.

Bonobos have strikingly advanced intellectual and emotional abilities, and they appear to be more aware of and distressed by pain, suffering, and deprivation than even mammals such as pigs. To the extent that bonobos share characteristics with human beings, it may be "speciesist" to treat them in ways in which we would not treat similarly situated human beings. In addition to sentience and basic conscious awareness, another major criterion of moral status for humans and other animals has long been the possession of language. Bonobos are currently at the forefront of this discussion, because at least some bonobos manifest the cognitive ability to use simple signing, a form of language.

An example of bonobo intelligence is Kanzi, undoubtedly the most famous bonobo. Kanzi was raised at the Language Research Center at Georgia State University and is credited by many researchers with at least rudimentary knowledge of a language as well as many other cognitive abilities, such as imaginative play and toolmaking. Kanzi spontaneously learned to use a signboard by watching his adoptive mother work with researchers who were trying to teach her.[36] Kanzi can understand human commands, even when spoken through earphones to prevent unintentional clueing. He can also follow commands linking several objects. When commanded to "give the dog a shot," he picks up a syringe and injects his stuffed toy dog. On another occasion, Kanzi demonstrated that he can understand conditional sentences. Sue Savage-Rumbaugh, a scientist working with Kanzi, offered him a deal. "Kanzi, if you give Austin your monster mask, I'll let you have some of Austin's cereal." Kanzi immediately gave Austin the mask and then pointed at the cereal.[37]

To address skeptical concerns that bonobos are exhibiting a "clever Hans" phenomenon in which their human trainers are unwittingly clueing them in, Savage-Rumbaugh and her colleagues conducted a test in which she sat behind a one-way mirror while she read requests to Kanzi. The requests included commands such as "Get the balloon that's in the microwave" and "Go scare Matata with the snake." They were deliberately designed to be sentences he would not normally have encountered. The other experimenters in the room wore headsets so that they could not hear Savage-Rumbaugh's commands. Savage-Rumbaugh issued 660 requests, and Kanzi's responses were taped. He was able to carry out correctly 72% of the commands, while a two-and-a-half-year-old girl who was tested on the same sentences responded appropriately to 66% of them. Savage-Rumbaugh also points out that Kanzi has often made combinations of words that are unlike any to which he has been exposed. For example, he might request "milk hug" to indicate that he wants to be held and coddled with milk. She argues that this fact shows that he is not merely memorizing commands by rote, but rather that he actually understands what he is doing and has even invented his own simple rules of grammar. Language ability, it appears, is not all or nothing. Language involves a cluster of abilities of which an individual can have more or fewer. No one is claiming that Kanzi has the language skills of a normal five- or six-year-old human. But this does not imply that he has no language skills at all.

Kanzi has also exhibited the ability to make tools. Researchers presented Kanzi with a task requiring him to use either a knife or a sharp flake of rock. Kanzi figured out how to perform the task and then how to make flakes on his own by breaking rocks apart, either by throwing them against a wall or by striking them together.[38] Although bonobos have not yet been observed making stone tools in the wild, they apparently have the cognitive ability to do so.

The intellectual abilities of bonobos raise questions about how they ought to be kept in captivity. In order to have their abilities better studied, Kanzi and the other bonobos at Georgia have been moved to the newly established Great Ape Trust of Iowa, located outside of Des Moines.[39] Savage-Rumbaugh is the director of the bonobo research program. Scientists continue to study the bonobos' linguistic ability, and the bonobos are provided with musical instruments and art supplies to see if they can develop these talents often declared to be uniquely human. Savage-Rumbaugh contends that the experiment will show that language and art are not innate human abilities, but rather that our ancestors learned and developed them over time. The experiment is expected to last for several generations. The Great Ape Trust in Iowa strives to meet all of the bonobos' needs by providing an environment rich in intellectual stimulation while also encompassing acres of forest meant to mimic their native habitat. But despite these efforts, the bonobos are not free to roam as they would in the wild, and their opportunities for social interaction are constrained by the small population at the project.

Are Special Duties Owed to Captive Populations?

Arguably, human beings owe special duties to bonobos raised in captivity. Kanzi and his fellow captive bonobos are no longer fit to live in the wild. They have never lived in the forest apart from human beings, and they might do no better in the wild than a person from modern America would. The language experiments also may have created duties. It is possible that access to even rudimentary forms of language changes the subjective experience of animals. Now that Kanzi has been taught to use his signboard, would it be cruel to deny him the use of it or to place him in an environment without other signing apes or humans with whom to communicate? Furthermore, bonobos that have been taught to sign can indicate their desires, fears, and frustrations to human beings. To the extent that this makes it possible to understand how human treatment affects the bonobos, people may no longer be able to plead ignorance of an animal's subjective experience as an excuse for methods of treatment that may cause suffering.

Human interactions with bonobos in the wild may also create moral obligations. For example, Japanese researchers at Wamba in Congo supply provisions to the bonobos that live there in order to be able to study them more closely. The scientific benefit of this method is that it allows social groups to be studied over many years. Japanese investigators first uncovered many of the unique aspects of bonobo society. Provisioning may create dependency, however, and it may alter the bonobos' way of life, even though the researchers try to limit provisioning to several months a year. Once bonobos have come to structure their lives and expectations around provisioning, is there a duty to continue to provide it and to look out for their welfare? Is there a danger in creating a false sense of security among bonobos that may be hunted by other people?

Balancing the Interests of Bonobos and Humans

Preserving the bonobos in Congo potentially will yield vital human benefits. As one of our two closest living relatives, they provide us with a wealth of potential knowledge regarding our own origins, our nature, our diseases, and the like. As an economic concern, the biodiversity contained within their territory may yield valuable discoveries if it is preserved.

Nevertheless, preserving the bonobos in their native Congo will require sacrifice of many human needs such as land, fuel, and food. In any fair moral estimate of the situation, human needs in Congo will be recognized and taken into consideration. The people of Congo are poor and often malnourished, and few alternatives for food and livelihood remain after decades of civil war and tyranny. Morally, it is problematic to ask that they make sacrifices in order to safeguard an animal species, even one as important as the bonobo. How much should they be asked to do if it makes their situation worse? Many of the people who benefit from studying bonobos are not from Congo. Even if preserving bonobos protects economically valuable biodiversity, it is not clear that the benefits derived will flow to the people of Congo. People from the developing world also point out that the developed world has already reaped the benefits of despoiling nature within its borders, and they express concern that preserving nature will come at the expense of poor people.

Responsibility for Remote Regions of the World

Many people who learn of the bonobos' plight think it would be a shame to lose such an animal, but they feel no personal sense of responsibility because these matters are so far away. Despite the distance, however, the developed world bears a great deal of responsibility for the plight of the bonobo—perhaps almost all of it. Bonobos are threatened in part because of habitat destruction fueled by the demand for wood and Colton in the developed world. The demand for these products results from individual decisions that almost all of us, as consumers in the developed world, make every day.

Strategies for preserving bonobos in the wild will have to take account of facts about both the developed world and countries like Congo. Consumers in the developed world face a moral decision every time they choose to consume products whose production threatens endangered species. Investors face moral decisions when they buy stocks in companies that are involved in habitat destruction or that contribute to the conditions that force people to choose between their immediate self-interest and the protection of the environment. As citizens, our judgments concerning foreign aid, trade agreements, and geopolitical policy all have the potential to affect species such as the bonobo. One hundred years from now, will humanity's peaceful relatives still roam the forests of Congo, or will the few survivors be relegated to a living museum? Does it make any moral difference?

NOTES

1. Michael Hurley, Bonobo Conservation Initiative, personal communication, June 16, 2004, and May 31, 2005.

2. World Bank Country Brief on Congo, available under specific countries at web.worldbank.org/wbsite/external/countries/0,pagePK:180619~theSitePK:136917,00.html (accessed June 29, 2005).

3. Frans de Waal, *Bonobo: The Forgotten Ape* (Berkeley: University of California Press, 1997), pp. 24–25.

4. Sue Savage-Rumbaugh and Roger Lewin, *Kanzi: The Ape on the Brink of the Human Mind* (New York: John Wiley and Sons, 1994), pp. 93–97.

5. De Waal, *Bonobo*, p. 24.

6. Christopher Boehm, "Segmentary 'Warfare' and the Management of Conflict: Comparison of East-African Chimpanzees and Patrilineal-Patrilocal Humans," in *Coalitions and Alliances in Humans and Other Animals,* ed. Alexander H. Harcourt and Frans de Waal (Oxford: Oxford University Press, 1992); Frans de Waal, *Chimpanzee Politics: Power and Sex among Apes* (Baltimore: Johns Hopkins University Press, 2000); Christophe Boesch, "Behavioral Diversity in *Pan,*" in *Behavioral Diversity in Chimpanzees and Bonobos,* ed. Christophe Boesch, Gottfried Hohmann, and Linda F. Marchant (New York: Cambridge University Press, 2002).

7. De Waal, *Bonobo,* p. 65.

8. Ibid., pp. 99–123.

9. Takayoshi Kano, *The Last Ape: Pygmy Chimpanzee Behavior and Ecology,* trans. Evelyn Ono Vineberg (Stanford, CA: Stanford University Press, 1992), p. 89.

10. De Waal, *Bonobo.*

11. Kano, *The Last Ape,* p. 71.

12. De Waal, *Bonobo.*

13. Ibid., pp. 173–75.

14. Some of these stories are related on the Bonobo Initiative's website; see "Stories and Songs," www.bonobo.org/storiesandsongs.html (accessed June 29, 2005).

15. Dale Peterson, *Eating Apes* (Berkeley: University of California Press, 2003), pp. 118–20.

16. Ibid., p. 127.

17. Ibid., p. 121.

18. Committee on Scientific Issues in the Endangered Species Act, Board on Environmental Studies and Toxicology, Commission on Life Sciences, Natural Research Council, *Science and the Endangered Species Act* (Washington, DC: National Academy Press, 1995), chapter 7.

19. Rosie Woodroffe, "Managing Disease Threats to Wild Animals," *Animal Conservation* 2 (1999): 185–93.

20. Matt Ridley, *The Origins of Virtue: Human Instincts and the Evolution of Cooperation* (New York: Penguin Books, 1996), p. 236.

21. Interview with Sally Coxe and Michael Hurley, July 30, 2004.

22. A description of programs is available on the Bonobo Initiative's website; see "Principles and Concepts," www.bonobo.org/howwework.htm (accessed June 19, 2005).

23. N. Thompson-Handler and R. K. Malenky, *Action Plan for Pan Paniscus: Report on Free Ranging Populations and Proposal for Their Preservation* (Milwaukee, WI: Zoological Society of Milwaukee County in cooperation with the Primate Specialist Group, SSC, IUCN, 1995).

24. Committee on Scientific Issues in the Endangered Species Act, *Science and the Endangered Species Act*, p. 199.

25. U.S. Agency for International Development, "Biodiversity Conservation: A Guide for USAID Staff and Partners" (Washington, DC: USAID, 2003), p. 2, www.usaid.gov/our_work/environment/biodiversity/pubs/biodiversity_guide_2003.pdf (accessed June 29, 2005).

26. Committee on Scientific Issues in the Endangered Species Act, *Science and the Endangered Species Act*, pp. 188–89.

27. USAID, "Biodiversity Conservation," p. 2.

28. John Pickrell, "Wolves' Leftovers Are Yellowstone's Gain, Study Says," *National Geographic News* 4 (December 2003). See also Robert L. Beschta, "Cottonwoods, Elk, and Wolves in the Lamar Valley of Yellowstone National Park," *Ecological Applications* 13 (2003): 1295–1309.

29. Richard Littell, *Endangered and Other Protected Species: Federal Law and Regulation* (Washington, DC: Bureau of National Affairs, 1992), pp. 101–6.

30. For information on the bush meat crisis, see The Bonobo Conservation Initiative (Washington, DC), "Bushmeat," *Bonobo Initiative*, www.bonobo.org/bushmeat.htm (accessed August 30, 2007).

31. See "Salonga National Park Support," Zoological Society of Milwaukee, www.zoosociety.org/Conservation/Bonobo/BCBI/Salonga.php (accessed June 29, 2005).

32. De Waal, *Bonobo*, pp. 175–76.

33. Committee on Scientific Issues in the Endangered Species Act, *Science and the Endangered Species Act*, p. 137.

34. Noel F. R. Snyder et al., "Limitations of Captive Breeding in Endangered Species Recovery," *Conservation Biology* 10 (April 1996): 340–41.

35. Committee on Scientific Issues in the Endangered Species Act, *Science and the Endangered Species Act*, p. 139.

36. Sue Savage-Rumbaugh, Stuart G. Shanker, and Talbot J. Taylor, *Apes, Language, and the Human Mind* (Oxford: Oxford University Press, 1998).

37. Savage-Rumbaugh and Lewin, *Kanzi: The Ape at the Brink*, p. 170.

38. De Waal, *Bonobo*, p. 37.

39. See Great Ape Trust of Iowa, www.iowagreatapes.org/index.php (accessed June 1, 2005).

PART VII

BIOMEDICAL RESEARCH AND COSMETIC TESTING

11

Head Injury Experiments on Primates at the University of Pennsylvania

Rapid social change is often stimulated by commanding events. The case presented below, involving baboons, marks a critical turning point in the history of twentieth-century animal experimentation. The stakeholders include a respected scientist, an Ivy League university, the federal government, and the newly formed (at the time) activist group People for the Ethical Treatment of Animals (PETA). PETA's actions, as it turned out, triggered major changes in public attitudes toward animal welfare issues and regulation by public policy and law.

THE USE OF BABOONS IN RESEARCH

Baboons (along with chimpanzees and monkeys) are among the closest relatives to human beings. They are native to Africa and are bred in the United States for research. They are among the most expensive research species, costing between $3,500 and $5,000 each, in 2007 dollar values.[1] Their protection in the context of biomedical research has been a major objective for animal activists.[2] Despite pressures from these activists, the numbers have remained fairly constant at around 55,000 per year in the United States for the last 20 years.

The baboons discussed below were involved in head injury experiments. Head injuries to humans are widespread and serious. Commonly they result from car accidents, cheerleaders' accidents, and contact sports. Since the brain has limited potential for self-repair, trauma can leave survivors with permanent brain damage and persistent motor and cognitive dysfunction. According to NIH assessments, approximately 1.4 million people in the United States experience traumatic head injury, and approximately 50,000 people die each year.[3]

At the same time, neuroscience is one of the leading biomedical areas in which amazing discoveries have been made in recent years. Modern noninvasive research methods such as magnetic resonance imaging are much less invasive in comparison with the seemingly crude method of forcefully hurling and striking an animal's head as featured in this case. However, the place of primates in such research is still under active discussion today.

THE LABORATORY RAID

During the early morning hours of the 1984 Memorial Day weekend, five men and women crept across the deserted University of Pennsylvania campus in Philadelphia. They entered the university's Head Trauma Research Center, where head injury studies on baboons were conducted under the direction of Thomas A. Gennarelli, associate professor of neurosurgery. They stole approximately 30 videotapes that had been made by the researchers to record the day-to-day experiments. The videotapes showed baboons in states of paralysis and incapacity and researchers who seemed indifferent to the distress of the animals. Before they left, the intruders also vandalized equipment used in the experiments and wrote their initials on the lab wall: ALF, short for Animal Liberation Front.

The ALF is a radical organization whose members conduct laboratory raids. Because it is a clandestine group, another national animal rights group, PETA, handled the ALF's publicity and negotiations. PETA claimed that the videotapes received from the ALF provided documentation of repeated, significant violations of federal policies governing the humane use of laboratory animals, including inadequate anesthesia and disregard of legally required surgical asepsis. Mandates come from two federal government agencies, the National Institutes of Health (NIH),[4] which has rules for researchers receiving its grants, and the U.S. Department of Agriculture (USDA), which administers the Animal Welfare Act (see chapter 1, pp. 36–37).[5] Gennarelli's baboon studies were part of a larger program headed by Thomas W. Langfitt, chair of neurosurgery, that covered both human and animal studies. In 1984, the total NIH annual grant award to Langfitt was approximately $1 million, of which Gennarelli's portion was approximately $330,000 per year.

The investigators had developed a special device that produced sudden jerking movements to the animal's head, which had been cemented into a helmet. This impact inflicted acceleration injury as in whiplash. The device could generate the equivalent of up to 2,000 times the force of gravity. The neurological damage to the brain resulted in paralysis and coma, which meant that the baboons could not feed themselves. The animals were maintained in their helpless states for up to two months, when they were killed and their brains analyzed. The investigators maintained that the purpose of the research was to develop an animal model to study the functional and anatomical effects of the head injuries that can occur in automobile accidents, football, and boxing. The research was intended to provide basic information about pathological events in an important area of human disability.

Television networks showed shocking excerpts from the videotapes stolen during the raid. One excerpt showed a baboon repeatedly writhing on a table as a hydraulic piston hit the animal's head. Just before the head injury, the animals were seen with their eyes open, twisting on the table in an attempt to turn their bodies over. Some animals received repeated head blows. PETA made a 20-minute film from footage of tapes titled *Unnecessary Fuss*.[6] Gennarelli had stated that he was "not willing to go on record to discuss the laboratory studies because it had the potential to stir up all sorts of unnecessary fuss among those who are sensitive to those kinds of things."[7]

Disclosure of the facts in this case stunned the biomedical community. Worldwide media attention was intense. It became a *cause célèbre* that brought public sympathy for PETA and other animal experimentation critics. But within days of the raid, a University of Pennsylvania spokesperson said that the ALF had leveled false, misleading attacks on both the quality and integrity of the research and asserted that the treatment of the animals conformed to the NIH guidelines for the humane care of experimental animals. Langfitt himself went on record claiming that the experiments had provided extremely valuable information on the nature of severe and often irreversible brain damage.

The most influential and oft-quoted defense of the research came from the director of the NIH, James B. Wyngaarden, who said that the University of Pennsylvania's head-injury clinic is considered to be "one of the best labs in the world."[8] Wyngaarden's comments were denounced by spokespersons for the animal rights movement, primarily on grounds of conflict of interest: Before he took the position of NIH director, he had been the chair of the Department of Medicine at the University of Pennsylvania Medical School.

Congressional Hearings

Congress held hearings on the research only a few months after the raid. Representatives from both NIH and USDA presented testimony. In the past, NIH external review teams had repeatedly found scientific merit in the baboon experiments, and none had raised issues about animal welfare. A few days before the raid, USDA inspectors had uncovered only four violations of USDA regulations. However, spurred by the publicity surrounding the raid, the same veterinary inspector found 74 violations a few days later.[9]

PETA wanted to show the film *Unnecessary Fuss* at the congressional hearings, but NIH and USDA would not attend if this showing was permitted. PETA then arranged public showings at a nearby church during the hearings' lunch breaks. PETA's press release for this event stated: "The graphic footage shows violations of federal regulations and federal and state laws. Researchers perform painful surgery on animals without proper pain relief."[10] In one sequence in the film, a researcher can be heard to say, "The animal is off anesthesia," just before infliction of the brain injury. The film records the laboratory personnel ridiculing the injured animals for their inability to use their limbs. It was hard going for many to watch the film. Newspaper columnist Henry Mitchell reported that he could not watch it all.[11] A reporter for *Science* described the tapes as ranging from "embarrassing to disastrous."[12]

Even without the videotape at the congressional hearings, the evidence presented about the treatment of these baboons and of other primates captured in an earlier ALF raid led directly to important new amendments to the Animal Welfare Act (see chapter 1). Enacted in 1985, the amendments mandate stronger institutional oversight committees, better pain control, consideration of alternatives to animal use, and housing for nonhuman primates that promotes their psychological well-being.

Ongoing Conflicts

Throughout the time that Congress was preparing new legislation, PETA was engaged in conflicts with NIH, the university, and USDA. A month after the congressional hearings, NIH's Office for Protection from Research Risks wrote to PETA stating that they had been unable to confirm the alleged misconduct. NIH demanded that PETA unconditionally hand over the 60-hour version of the tape. NIH refused to view the edited 20-minute version on grounds of biased and unfair editing. PETA requested that NIH include a person in their investigation who was acceptable to both NIH and PETA "to assure that the investigation is verifiably fair and impartial."[13] NIH refused this request.

The next month, under pressure from the University of Pennsylvania's Law School, the university's vice provost for research, Barry Cooperman, formed a panel of faculty members to examine the controversial head injury experiments. However, Cooperman refused to allow *Unnecessary Fuss* to be shown at the meeting. Thirteen law school professors, including animal activist Gary Francione, accused the university of stifling debate and suppressing evidence. Law professor Arnold Morris said, "It seems pretty peculiar that the tape that generated the discussion not be shown."[14] The meeting was angry and inconclusive.

Defenders of this type of research were heavily invested in this case. The Society of Neuroscience, a professional association that included Gennarelli and Langfitt as members, established a three-person investigative committee. Their report stated that Gennarelli had made "a convincing case that the procedures represent an ethical and humane way to produce an animal model of human head trauma."[15] Shortly after the raid, Gennarelli was awarded the National Head Injury Foundation's 1984 Caveness Award for outstanding contribution to head injury. Other awards followed.

PROTESTS BY ANIMAL PROTECTION SYMPATHIZERS AND NIH POLICY DECISIONS

A full year after the raid, there was no progress toward a resolution. No investigations were completed by NIH, USDA, or the university. Animal protection sympathizers were frustrated by the nature and slowness of the scientific establishment's response. By comparison, in response to the 1981 ALF raid on an animal facility, known as the "Silver Spring Monkey" case, NIH halted government funding after only four weeks. However, there were now different NIH officials, and more cautious attitudes prevailed.

Animal activists and others were disgruntled when they discovered that NIH was set to renew Gennarelli's grant for another five years, starting August 1, 1985. More baboons were to be used in head injury studies. At this point members of the animal rights movement urged Congress to act. Some 60 members of Congress then petitioned Health and Human Services secretary Margaret M. Heckler to stop the funding.

NIH Sit-In

When no government action was forthcoming, activists undertook a campaign of civil disobedience to press their case. Some 14 months after the initial raid, "it became obvious to PETA leaders that they were getting nowhere with letter writing, lobbying and the usual means of protest."[16] About 100 animal activists from around the country decided to occupy several NIH offices. As the hours passed, fellow activists brought food baskets that were hauled up on ropes through the NIH office window. Their signs were readily seen from the heavily trafficked main road. Drivers passing by expressed their support, and media coverage was intense. After four days of this sit-in and media attention, Secretary Heckler instructed NIH to suspend federal support for the University of Pennsylvania project.[17]

Secretary Heckler's actions created new levels of controversy. Among the critics, the American Association of Medical Colleges protested that this capitulation to the demands of an "irresponsible advocacy group" increased the vulnerability of academic institutions to further property destruction. The organization also claimed that Heckler's decision meant a loss of research of incalculable value.[18] Other groups made similar claims.

Penalties Imposed

About a year after the original raid, PETA gave the tapes to USDA and NIH officials. In May 1985, NIH conducted a site visit to investigate compliance with NIH policy and report its findings. Inspectors found a "material failure" of the University of Pennsylvania to comply with NIH animal welfare policy.[19] Among the areas of noncompliance were deficiencies in anesthesia management during both the pre- and post-injury periods; failure to achieve a sterile environment; inadequacies in the laboratory environment and laboratory personnel training; failure to consistently ensure that experiments were conducted under the immediate supervision of qualified scientists; and unreliable nursing care.

In September 1985, the president and provost of the university issued a joint public reprimand of Gennarelli and Langfitt for "less than satisfactory discharge of the responsibility expected of research faculty at the university."[20] USDA fined the University of Pennsylvania $4,000 for violations of the Animal Welfare Act in the baboon head injury lab.[21] The university had received $70 million in grant support that year from NIH. The fine, though small, was symbolically important as a signal of wrongdoing and culpability.

Within nine months of the funding suspension, the university made corrections to its laboratory animal program. In turn, NIH removed its funding restrictions.[22] The baboon studies were not resumed because the university had decided to suspend all head injury research using nonhuman primates.

ETHICAL ISSUES

The Weatherall Report, a 2006 report from the U.K. Medical Research Council, examined the general justification for use of nonhuman primates in medical research. It found that "there is a strong scientific case" for maintaining the use of nonhuman primates in "carefully selected" neuroscience problems "at least for the immediate future."[23] How strong is this case, and what kind of case is it? Is it strong enough for moral justification? However strong the case, what limits, if any, should be placed on the use of primates in research? And what should we take away, morally, from developments at the University of Pennsylvania?

Standards of Behavior of Laboratory Personnel

The videotape from Professor Gennarelli's laboratory showed workers mocking and laughing at the brain-damaged animals. Such lack of respect for injured animals is widely believed to be inappropriate. But some observers excused the researchers on the grounds that it was the same sort of "gallows humor" that is found among surgeons in the operating room and among people taking care of comatose patients. This humor is a way of coping with difficult and unsettling tasks. The ethical problem is that "humor" of this sort may foster a general disrespect for vulnerable subjects, human and nonhuman. Does it therefore deserve a rebuke wherever it is found? Do persons encountering disrespectful circumstances have a responsibility to speak up about observed infractions of standards by co-workers and to see that they are corrected?

The American Association for Laboratory Animal Science, a membership organization for laboratory veterinarians and technicians, has a code of ethics.[24] The code requires the "highest standards of personal conduct" and a responsibility to encourage the "highest levels of ethics within the profession of laboratory animal science." Specific directives to see that observed infractions either be corrected or reported to higher officials are unstated, but they could be implied. Infractions could be anything such as breaking the law, misrepresentation, fraud, or unethical behavior.

The Problem of Severely Harmful Experimental Procedures

Antivivisectionists hold that *all* harm-inflicting animal experiments are unacceptable. But even among non-antivivisectionists, there are those who believe that *some* experiments that cause particularly severe pain or distress are unacceptable. An analogy is often made to human experimentation, where certain procedures can never be justified, regardless of the level of potentially useful scientific findings.

According to one view, as long as certain conditions are satisfied—the scientific merit is high, the researchers are competent, and the potential for major human benefits in the form of vital knowledge or therapeutic treatment exists—there should be no restrictions on upper limits of permissible animal pain or suffering. On this view, no research procedures are absolutely unacceptable. Since humans enjoy a dignity not enjoyed by other animals, it is permissible to use these animals freely for human benefit. (See chapter 1, pp. 14, 16, 24.)

In the head injury case at the University of Pennsylvania, many people thought that these experiments so *severely* harmed the primates that they should not have been done. In their eyes, the ethical costs were too great. When assessing ethical harms of severe experimental procedures, the general harms of captivity, loss of freedom, loss of control over an environment, lack of social interaction, and loss of life should all count. As is often the case with animal experiments, all costs are *certain* for each and every animal used; they are not merely *potential,* as is generally the case with the human benefits that research might produce.

The laws of several countries outlaw certain research procedures either because they are too severe or because the purpose of the research is too trivial.[25] Some animal advocates seek to place on such a list severe brain or spinal cord injury, prolonged deprivation resulting in disabling, abnormal mental states, and lethal radiation doses. But this proposal is highly controversial. How should society resolve this disagreement about acceptable procedures? Who should decide whether to approve proposed projects? Should it be up to some combination of animal researchers, scholars, the public, and representatives from the animal welfare community?

The Promise of Basic Research

Professor Gennarelli's work was basic research, and there was controversy over the level of benefit the study produced. Basic research provides an understanding of physiological and pathological processes that may lead to future ideas for prevention or treatment. Scientists are more likely than the general public to recognize that basic research can contribute to original knowledge. Gennarelli told the university and the public that the information gained from the baboon model was a major contribution toward understanding the basic mechanisms responsible for brain damage in head injury patients. The researchers and some NIH funding committees held that it was reasonable to project that there was social benefit from this work. In particular, they maintained that this original work would lead to treatment that would help head injury patients, but no evidence was forthcoming to show that study results had specific human applications. If this work had presented a more direct contribution to applied therapies for human head injury, it might have been viewed by the public more sympathetically.

The ethical question is not whether basic research is of great benefit for purposes of the accumulation of knowledge. It is. The ethical question is whether the procedures essential to such research are warranted when they produce significant harms to animals.

The Three Rs: Replacement, Reduction, and Refinement

The adequacy of NIH and institutional prior review and approval of Gennarelli's baboon experiments raised questions about whether the Three Rs conception has ever been discussed or used.

Replacement

Since these experimental procedures involved severe pain, would it have been more ethical, and within the scope of truly scientific work, to restrict study of such head injury to clinical interventions in naturally occurring human injuries? Studying human survivors of naturally occurring trauma is productive, but it has serious limitations. The primary concern of physicians taking care of such patients is to help their patients, not to conduct research on them. Many ethical and legal restrictions apply to human subjects that do not apply to animal subjects. In particular, human subjects are protected from the levels of harm that are imposed in animal research. This limits the information that researchers can derive from human studies. But if these concerns apply to human subjects, why do they not also apply to baboons, given their evolutionary proximity to human beings? Is it truly necessary to use primates? Could another species be substituted?

Substitution of another species was accepted by Gennarelli in another round of NIH review. Between 1991 and 1996, after the NIH restored his funding, he adapted his head injury accelerator device so that he could study minipigs, a breed developed for laboratory use. He believed that minipigs were a reasonable substitute for baboons, and NIH reviewers agreed. Physiologically and anatomically, pigs have been found to be reasonably good human substitutes. But this substitution may have been more for public relations than grounded in good ethics. Experiments on pigs do not receive the same level of public criticism as work on primates, because pigs arouse less moral concern. Pigs also may suffer somewhat less than baboons because pigs have less well-developed cognitive abilities. But just how far apart pigs and baboons are in cognitive capabilities and capacity to suffer is difficult to judge. Pigs and baboons share 99% of their genes. Pigs are very sensitive animals (see chapter 2), and if they were subjected to the head injuries in the baboon experiments, they clearly would suffer, much as the baboons did.

Another replacement option is to study nonanimal models. Gennarelli stated that he used some replacement alternatives, including mathematical and computer models and gelatin simulations of brain material. Such studies can decrease the number of sentient animals used, but they are insufficient to replace animal studies on all topics.

Some have suggested that more use could be made of human autopsy studies. There are serious limitations, however, in studying nonliving subjects. Nerve responses cannot be studied and blood does not flow, both of which are important indicators of normal and abnormal function. Also, many families would probably refuse to allow their loved ones' bodies to be used in such research.

In short, replacement is a difficult goal to achieve in head trauma studies.

Reduction

Could fewer animals have been used in the head injury experiments? Gennarelli used 200 baboons over the four years preceding the raid, approximately one animal per week. Whether fewer would have sufficed has never been determined. The number of experimental subjects used in procedures carrying high ethical costs is significant. In these cases, several strategies are available to an institutional ethics committee to help keep the numbers of animals to a minimum. The committee could establish special restrictions, such as requiring pilot studies to demonstrate that animal welfare is satisfactory. It could allow only highly competent laboratory personnel to do the work (Gennarelli's technician training was inadequate, according to the NIH review). It could use a professional statistician to address the minimum number of animals needed to establish statistical validity. Or it could provide careful oversight and re-review at frequent intervals.

There is no indication that the university's oversight committee used any of these strategies. The number of baboons used may have been determined by the convenience of the investigators, rather than by an attempt to reduce the numbers.

Refinement

If, before approving the project, the review committees of NIH or the university had addressed the issue of refinement, there would have been fewer grounds for criticism. A basic principle of refinement is that adequate anesthesia be provided. If anesthesia and other standards had not been violated, as was eventually established by a postraid NIH review, there would have been less harm to the baboons. Perhaps other refinements could have been devised, such as using less force of impact of the accelerator device, fewer head blows, a shorter period of survival time for the baboons, and an earlier endpoint.

Institutional Issues

The University of Pennsylvania responded to allegations of animal mistreatment in several ways. The day after the raid, university officials strongly defended the work; 16 months later, when official government investigations had established infractions of the Animal Welfare Act, the university issued a reprimand of the two primary researchers. In between, the university resisted inquiries, backed away from an outside investigative team, refused entreaties from the university's law school to open up the case with evidence for discussion, and conceded only minor infractions of the Animal Welfare Act. The university never conceded the inadequacy of the anesthetic regimen found by the NIH investigation.

Civil Disobedience

In the years following the head injury raid, activists raided several other biomedical facilities, including the University of Oregon, the University of California at Davis, and the University of Arizona. They also raided the University of Pennsylvania again, to protest controversial sleep research on cats. In 1989, a PETA spokesperson argued that civil disobedience such as raids and other illegal activities belongs to a long tradition of permissible responses to social injustices.[26] These strategies are last resorts used only when repeated legal approaches have failed to yield results. There is no evidence that PETA tried legal strategies before the raid to resolve the problems in Gennarelli's laboratory. The objective was to stop the experiments, not to improve them.

NIH director Wyngaarden said that the raid on the head injury laboratory "carried civil disobedience to a level this society cannot tolerate."[27] To those who believed there was no wrongdoing by the researchers, all these illegal activities were wrong. But the justification for illegal activities depends, at least in part, on the wrong that is being protested and the level of injustice involved. Still debated today is whether the clearly illegal activity at the University of Pennsylvania was warranted.

In the twenty-first century, a few ALF activities have proposed arson and personal harassment of researchers. Researchers have not only suffered the loss of months or years of experimental results but have been publicly maligned in their neighborhoods and publicly threatened. In a raid on November 14, 2004, at the University of Iowa, a widely circulated ALF communiqué included the names and addresses of seven of the university's faculty members and ten of their laboratory assistants.[28] These tactics were intimidating for those named. The ALF has claimed that such exposure is a public safety measure, on the grounds that there is an established link between violence toward animals and that toward humans. Although in the United States it is believed that no person has yet suffered physical harm from animal rights activists, the anguish and mental suffering of these laboratory personnel and their families is itself a moral consideration.

Conclusion: Enforcement of the Law

By law, USDA conducts regular on-site inspections of research facilities where some infractions, usually small violations, are found and then corrected. But historically, vigorous USDA monitoring of research laboratories is usually undertaken only after an animal protection group has provided evidence of legal violations. The federal inspector general's office conducted an audit of USDA's animal care program and regular on-site inspections. The 2005 report[29] criticized the inspection and enforcement efforts during fiscal years from 2002 to 2004. For instance, the report states that an unnamed university in Illinois, with assets of $6.2 billion in 2002, was fined $9,400 to cover 12 "serious" violations related to veterinary care and deaths of a monkey and a pig. The average fines levied for animal welfare violations were about $2,300 in the eastern region of the United States and $1,300 in the west. The report states that many animal facilities viewed the fines as "a normal cost of conducting business rather than a deterrent for violating the law."

At NIH, enforcement of the animal welfare regulations is the responsibility of the Office for Laboratory Animal Welfare. According to a 2005 *Washington Post* report,[30] PETA, using undercover agents, produced video footage of federal law violations in two successive years at the same research facility. After receiving the first year's evidence, this NIH office sent what was called a "damning report" to the university. No sanctions were made, and the NIH office determined that the problems had been corrected. In the second year, PETA sent in another undercover agent who produced evidence of continued violations. Although NIH has the authority to stop the research, a spokesperson from NIH stated that his office "doesn't work in a punitive fashion," preferring instead to "work with the institution" to bring it into compliance.

NOTES

1. National Academy of Sciences, "Demands for Rhesus Monkeys in Biomedical Research: A Workshop Report" (workshop held April 19–20, 2002), p. 16, dels.nas.edu/ilar_n/ilarjournal/44_3/v44n03workshop.pdf (accessed August 30, 2007).

2. See, for instance, Stop Animal Exploitation Now! "Primate Experimentation in the U.S.—The National Picture (2005 Edition)," www.all-creatures.org/saen/fact-primate-05.html (accessed February 18, 2007).

3. National Institutes of Health, "Traumatic Brain Injury: Hope through Research," www.ninds.nih.gov/disorders/tbi/detail_tbi.htm (accessed February 15, 2007).

4. The NIH Guide for the Care and Use of Laboratory Animals (1979) was in effect at the time. Among the requirements were that each facility maintain an oversight committee and that pain-relieving agents be used where indicated.

5. The Animal Welfare Act (7 U.S.C. 2131–2156) was in effect at the time, as amended December 24, 1970. Among the legal provisions were use of pain-relieving agents and use of aseptic surgery for nonhuman primates.

6. People for the Ethical Treatment of Animals, *Unnecessary Fuss*, video, www.peta.org/mc/videoDisplay.aspx?type=testing (accessed February 14, 2007).

7. Paul Palango, "Brunt of Research Borne by Monkeys," *Toronto Globe and Mail*, March 5, 1983, p. 1.

8. Jeffrey L. Fox, "Lab Break-In Stirs Animal Welfare Debate," *Science* 224 (June 22, 1984): 1319–20.

9. Jeffrey Goldberg, "Report Shows Violations in Animal Care: USDA Cites Lab with 74 Infractions," *Daily Pennsylvanian*, April 8, 1985, p. 1.

10. People for the Ethical Treatment of Animals, "Violations of Federal Law Shown in Footage to be Released Wednesday, Capitol Hill," News Release, September 17, 1994.

11. Henry Mitchell, "Any Day," *Washington Post*, September 21, 1984, pp. C1, C4.

12. Jeffrey L. Fox, "Lab Break-In Stirs Animal Welfare Debate," p. 1319.

13. Alex Pacheco, Chairperson, PETA, letter dated November 13, 1984, p. 1, to Honorable Margaret Heckler, Secretary, U.S. Department of Health and Human Services, Washington, DC.

14. Jeffrey Goldberg, "Profs Blast Constraints on Animal Panel," *Daily Pennsylvanian*, December 6, 1984, pp. 1, 10.

15. Robert E. Burke, "The Philadelphia Raid—The 'Next Taub Case'?" *Neuroscience Newsletter* (September/October 1984): 9. The Taub case refers to a 1981 ALF raid, the evidence from which, as with this 1984 case, was critical to the passage of the 1985 amendments to the Animal Welfare Act.

16. Jim Mason, "Baboons Win Reprieve: Civil Disobedience, Protests Pay Off," *The Animals' Agenda* (September 1985): 9–10.

17. "Statement by HHS Secretary Margaret M. Heckler on the University of Pennsylvania Head Injury Clinical Research Center Grant," *HHS News*, July 18, 1995, p. 1.

18. Quoted in "An Update on the Head Injury Laboratory," *Almanac Supplement*, September 3, 1985, p. 2. Published by the University of Pennsylvania.

19. "Evaluation of Experimental Procedures Conducted at the University of Pennsylvania Experimental Head Injury Laboratory 1981–1984," Report Submitted to the Office of the Director, National Institutes of Health, July 17, 1985, p. 5.

20. Sheldon Hackney and Thomas Ehrlich, "On the Head Injury Laboratory: To the University Community," *Almanac*, September 24, 1985, p. 1. Published by the University of Pennsylvania.

21. U.S. Department of Agriculture, Office of Information, "University of Pennsylvania Settles USDA Animal Welfare Act Charges," *News*, November 18, 1985.

22. "Lab Animal Research Funding at University of Penn Re-instated," *NABR Update*, March 24, 1986, p. 1. Published by the National Association for Biomedical Research, Washington, DC.

23. U.K. Medical Research Council, "The Use of Non-Human Primates in Research—The Weatherall Report," December 12, 2006, www.mrc.ac.uk/Utilities/Documentrecord/index.htm?d=MRC003440 (accessed March 15, 2007).

24. American Association for Laboratory Animal Science, "AALAS Code of Ethics," *Contemporary Topics* (January 1995): 20, www.aalas.org/association/about.asp#AALAS%20Membership%20Code%200f%20Ethics (accessed February 16, 2007).

25. Outlawed procedures include painful procedures on anesthetized animals paralyzed with curariform drugs; killing an animal using strychnine, potassium chloride, or some other injectable agents (1985 law of the United States); use of animals for testing weapons, cosmetics, washing powders, and tobacco products (1986 law of Germany); experiments leading to intense suffering, anxiety, or severe pain (1993 law of Denmark); many uses of animals to gain manual skills (1985 law of the United Kingdom); and use of animals to produce monoclonal antibodies (1995 law of Switzerland).

26. Christine M. Jackson, "The Fiery Fight for Animal Rights," *Hastings Center Report* 19, no. 6 (1989): 37–39.

27. John K. Ingelhart, "Health Policy Report: The Use of Animals in Research," *New England Journal of Medicine* (August 8, 1985): 398.

28. Americans for Medical Progress News Service, "University of Iowa Vandalism—Situation Report," November 19, 2004, Alexandria, VA.

29. U.S. Department of Agriculture, "Audit Report: APHIS Animal Care Program Inspection and Enforcement Activities," Report No. 330002–3-SF, September 2005. See also Jeffrey Brainard, "Report Knocks Agriculture Department's Protection of Research Animals," *Chronicle of Higher Education*, November 11, 2005, p. A27.

30. Rick Weiss, "Lab Violations Decried: Activists Urge NIH to Sanction University for Repeat Offense," *Washington Post*, December 2, 2005, p. A21.

12

What Does the Public Have a Right to Know?

The Progressive Animal Welfare Society (PAWS), a nonprofit organization in the state of Washington, and the University of Washington (UW) in Seattle have generated controversy over several issues regarding the organization's access to information about the university's procedures and positions. Major questions are: Does an activist animal welfare organization have a legal or moral right to information about newly proposed or renewed animal experiments conducted at the university? Should such organizations be present at oversight committee meetings where animal experiments are either approved or disapproved?

PAWS presents itself as representative of a segment of the community that is concerned about the welfare and protection of laboratory animals. It maintains that it should have a voice in what is done to animals at the university. The university is partially funded by revenues from state taxes and therefore is publicly accountable. But the university does not agree that PAWS has anything to do with questions of accountability. University officials view PAWS as an antivivisection group prone to distort information about animal experiments. John A. Coulter, executive director of health sciences administration for the university, says that the university is not opposed to divulging information, but it is opposed to giving certain types of information to PAWS and to having PAWS participate in university affairs. PAWS might raise public opposition to already approved animal experiments, which might result in unwanted confrontation and even stoppage of animal experiments and embarrassment to the university.

This conflict is representative of battles in several states in the United States (and other countries) between animal research facilities and animal protection organizations. PAWS, like other animal protection groups, believes that animal research should not be conducted behind closed doors. The Physicians Committee for Responsible Medicine distributes a fact sheet titled, "Your Right to Know: Understanding Animal Experiments in Your Community,"[1] which instructs the public on how to obtain information about animal experiments. "Your taxes and contributions to foundations support the overwhelming majority of these experiments, and you have a right to information about them." In Washington State, these issues have been pressed perhaps further than anywhere else in the United States, attracting national attention.[2]

PAWS concentrated on the university's institutional oversight committee—the Animal Care Committee (ACC), as it was called at this institution when these controversies began in the 1980s. (The term now universally used is Institutional Animal Care and Use Committee (IACUC), and this is the term used below except for references to the PAWS versus UW activities.) These committees have a central role in the oversight of animal experiments. They are legally required to see that anesthetics are administered where more than momentary pain exists (unless the anesthetic compromises justified research goals), that animals are killed humanely by prescribed methods, and that certain standards of animal husbandry are maintained. Their legal role is to approve or disapprove animal experiments conducted at that facility. PAWS pursued several goals: to obtain the committee records, to attend its meetings, and to have a vote in the decision making.

ISSUES ABOUT ACCESS TO MEETINGS

PAWS first attempted to obtain committee membership and therefore a vote, citing the legal requirement that the committee must have at least three members—a scientist, a veterinarian, and a noninstitutional member (variously called noninstitutional, public, or community member). PAWS applied to UW for the noninstitutional slot but was turned down. By law, committee membership is controlled by institutional officials, without rights of appeal granted to others.

PAWS then lowered its sights and applied for observer status on the ACC, which at least would give it access to information. This petition was initially denied. At that point, PAWS sued the university under Washington State's Open Meeting Act, which permits public observers to attend certain decision-making meetings. In the first of a succession of legal battles spanning seven years, PAWS in 1987 won the legal right to observer status.[3] The major protagonist, Mitchell Fox, and other representatives of PAWS then started attending every meeting as observers.

UW officials deplored the 1987 court ruling.[4] A prevalent view within the university was that the ACC would be hindered if outside observers were present. John Lein, vice president for health sciences, feared harassment of the university's researchers and their families. His fears were well founded. For several weeks preceding the court ruling, some people picketed the homes of the chair of the ACC and an anesthesiologist whose work on dental pain had been particularly disturbing to some activists. The scientists had received phone calls from people who harassed them and even threatened them with death. The local press reported that the Northwest Animal Rights Network was responsible. PAWS itself was not involved.

For the eight months following the first open ACC meeting, *PAWS News* reported that only "a handful" of projects were discussed and that "the remaining [projects involving animal experimentation] have been summarily approved without even a mention. To the observer they are nonexistent: no title, no investigator, no purpose, no method. But in this void exist thousands of animals, unprotected by even the most cursory public scrutiny."[5] PAWS' opinion was that the ACC's most meaningful deliberations were actually taking place behind closed doors.

Rights of Access to the Full Text of Protocol Review Forms

In a second suit, PAWS sought access to the ACC records under Washington State's Public Disclosure Law.[6] After a contentious battle, PAWS successfully established a legal right to disclosure of the protocol forms used by the ACC in which investigators describe their proposed animal experiments, the number and species of animal to be used, whether alternatives to animal use are available, the reason for using animals, and the care and treatment the animals will receive.

According to court documents, UW officials contested this ruling, arguing that the forms constituted a preliminary draft (and are therefore exempt from the law) and that the forms contain valuable research designs that are proprietary. Attorneys warned that release of the forms would result in the loss of research funds to UW, harm to its researchers' livelihood and careers, and a decline in the university's ability to ensure the humane treatment of animals.

Sunshine Laws Requiring Open Meetings in Washington State

The laws that PAWS used to achieve its goals of access to meetings are the so-called sunshine laws of Washington State. These laws require that meetings of certain public agencies be open to the public, and also that certain records be made public—commonly called Open Meeting and Public Disclosure Laws. These laws include state statutes (all states have sunshine laws) and the federal Freedom of Information Act, often used by watchdog organizations.

The underlying philosophy of these disclosure laws is that the public has a right to know what its government is doing and how its tax dollars are being spent. These laws are intended to preserve the central tenets of representative government. In her 1994 ruling on the PAWS v. UW case, Judge Barbara Durham wrote that without tools such as disclosure laws, "government of the people, by the people, for the people, risks becoming government of the people, by the bureaucrats, for the special interests."[7]

The federal Freedom of Information Act has been widely used by activists to obtain information about the use of federal tax dollars by the National Institutes of Health (NIH) in support of animal experiments. On request, NIH is required to provide copies of funded grant applications, including the project title, the grantee institution, the identity of the principal investigator, and the amount of the award.

The Federal Advisory Committee Act, another statute promoting public access, has also been used to challenge the procedures of the committees that establish national policy. Over the years several court cases had, without success, challenged the lack of public access to the meetings or representation on the committees that prepare the *Guide for the Care and Use of Laboratory Animals,* the manual that sets national policy for handling and monitoring the treatment of laboratory animals by NIH grantees. The first edition was issued in 1963, and revisions have been issued approximately every five years up through the seventh edition in 1996. All seven editions have been prepared by committees composed overwhelmingly of members who were animal researchers, and they lacked formal representation from the animal protection movement.

On January 10, 1997, the U.S. Court of Appeals for the District of Columbia ruled in favor of the Animal Legal Defense Fund and others who together had sought broader representation on the *Guide* committee.[8] For a brief period, it seemed that the committee preparing the eighth edition would be required by law to include formal animal welfare representation. However, that was not to be. On December 17, 1997, Congress passed a bill to amend the Federal Advisory Committee Act to exclude any such committee requirement.[9] This bill effectively voids the victory in the case of the Animal Legal Defense Fund case.

The U.S. Department of Agriculture (USDA) is also required under the Freedom of Information Act to disclose publicly reports of its federally mandated inspections of animal research facilities. These reports include information about facilities' noncompliance with the Animal Welfare Act. Armed with this information, watchdog organizations can exert pressure to help ensure that federal agencies perform their mandated responsibilities.

At the state level, sunshine laws vary in their impact, depending on the provisions of the law.[10] Few universities have opened up their meetings unless they were under a court order to do so. The University of Florida in Gainesville is an exception. This university recognized that the Florida sunshine laws (which are notably open) would cover the IACUC. When a group of activists composed heavily of faculty and students at the university petitioned to attend the meetings, the university permitted them to do so, believing that it would have no hope of winning a legal challenge. Since 1985, the meetings have been open, and the times and places of future meetings are publicly announced. Although there have been some additional faculty protests, the policy has caused no ill effects to the university.

THE LEGACY OF PAWS' LEGAL CHALLENGES

The legacy of PAWS' legal challenges has changed over time. At the last ACC meeting attended by Mitchell Fox before leaving PAWS in 1994, he said that the committee is "our only window" into the UW research laboratory and that protocol review had moved from being "a mockery" to being more professional.[11] The "unrelenting sunshine the UW committee had to endure" had benefited both the animals and the university; ACC discussion was "more serious, spirited and substantive."[12] Some barriers had been crossed. At the ACC meetings, scientists and animal advocates met on a regular basis and, to some extent, got to know each other, which they had not done before. This interaction increased mutual understanding and respect.

After Fox's departure, the organization changed its course and ceased to focus on animal experimentation. However, members of the Northwest Animal Rights Network continued. Psychologist Wayne Johnson was the founding board member of this broad-based animal rights organization. Their perspectives and strategies are different from PAWS, and the two groups sharply disagree over tactics: a protest method used by

Johnson's organization is to conduct what he claims to be peaceable but nevertheless intimidating demonstrations outside UW researchers' homes.

The University of Washington's Perspective

In 2005, UW spokesperson for the IACUC (previously ACC), Nona Phillips, the director of the Office of Animal Welfare and executive secretary of the IACUC, related some history and current practices. She reported that in compliance with state law, committee meeting dates are publicly announced. As of May 1, 2005, the 15-member IACUC is comprised of a chair, a nurse not involved in animal research, two non-UW affiliated members (both retired teachers, of whom one is a former high school biology teacher), two veterinarians, six animal researchers, one budget officer, one biosafety member, and two alternates.[13] (There is an absence of animal care technicians, whose viewpoint is considered by some institutions to be uniquely valuable.) In 2004, about 640 protocols were reviewed. There are two methods of review, by single designated member and by full committee. Most reviews are by a single designated reviewer; few protocols receive full committee review. Philips writes, "Animal rights groups . . . do not like the designated member review method of protocol review that is allowed by law. They would like for all protocols to be reviewed by the full committee."[14]

In the past, committee members and public observers met in the same room, but under an important new ruling they are now physically separated into two rooms.[15] Phillips stated that this change was to protect researchers' safety. Two episodes were described: In 1999, along with other institutions where primate research was conducted, the UW was a target for mail containing razor blades.[16] "Some of our researchers did receive razor blades."[17] A further threat occurred at the meeting on March 21, 2002, when, during the public comment period, tempers flared, and the life of one member was threatened by an antivivisectionist protestor who was present. As a result, "We were able to arrange to have our IACUC members meet in one room, with a separate room available for attendees. The attendees view and hear the meeting via live video. They are also still able to make comments to the IACUC at the end of the meeting, just as they did when we met in the same room. Two-way communication is available so the real difference is physical location. The first meeting in this configuration was on June 20, 2002."[18]

From that date on, public observers have not been allowed to comment during the committee proceedings or allowed to meet face to face with committee members. They are, however, allowed to make comments for up to three minutes at the end of the meeting. Public attendance has diminished to one or two observers per meeting. Representatives from the pro-animal research group The Incurably Ill for Animal Research, whom the university had previously invited to attend, now stopped coming. Phillips states that she is "very comfortable with open meetings"[19] and that there has been "no problem with the public getting information [and] . . . no tensions remain."[20]

An Animal Rights Perspective

Wayne Johnson of the Northwest Animal Rights Network went to every meeting of the IACUC from 1989 to August 2003 when he left Seattle. Thereafter other representatives from this group continued to attend through November 2005. During the time of Johnson's attendance, he was troubled by a number of research projects. For instance, in 1994–96, some baboons died from neglect. In response to a violation, the university received what he called a "slap on the wrist" from the USDA, the administrators of the Animal Welfare Act.[21] He also objected both to some psychological experiments that made rats drunk, which he found trivial, and to maternal deprivation studies of monkeys, which he found outmoded and unacceptable (see chapter 14).

At some point, Johnson applied for the nonaffiliated member slot on the committee, but he was not appointed. He said that there is "no way an animal rights person would ever be appointed."[22] With the one-room arrangement, he had come to know some committee members well, and he found the face-to-face contact important. In the one-room meeting on March 21, 2002, a person from his organization had confronted the committee, saying, "We know where you live so you'd better watch your backs."[23] The university viewed this as an imminent threat, but he said that it was intended "in a general way and not to an individual."[24] He believes that the two-room arrangement has significantly thwarted any meaningful exchange between the researchers and the public: "There is now little hope of progress."[25]

LEGAL BATTLES AND LEGAL REASONING IN PRECEDENT CASES

During the many years of the PAWS versus UW case, several other animal protection groups have taken legal action for access to information about animal experiments. Many cases are unresolved. For instance, a several-year legal battle is ongoing between In Defense of Animals and the Oregon National Primate Research Center.[26] The daily health logs of its monkeys were initially requested in 1998. To comply with this request, the center proposed charging a fee of $12,585, later raised to $151,000.[27] An appellate court concluded that both fees were excessive and were assessed incorrectly, without regard to the public's interest in the records. In September 2005, this case was remanded back to the Oregon Circuit Court for further consideration.

Legal Decisions That Allow Closed IACUC Meetings

In five U.S. states in which closed IACUC meetings are permitted by law, the precedent legal reasoning in five cases was as follows:

1. In 1988, a Virginia circuit court denied Students for Animals access to meetings of the University of Virginia's IACUC. The law applies only to meetings in which public policy is made, and the IACUC was not considered to meet this test even though its policies are for a state institution. The Richmond, Virginia, Circuit Court compared the IACUC to the university basketball or football coaching staff meetings and wrote, "To require meetings of such groups to be treated as public meetings would be to carry the idea of government in the 'sunshine' to an absurd extreme."[28]
2. In 1991, a Massachusetts State Appeals Court reversed lower court decisions and found that since IACUC meetings are held to ensure compliance with state and federal animal care regulations and not to discuss or formulate public policy, they are exempt from the state open meeting laws.[29]
3. In 1991, a four-judge panel of the New York Supreme Court, Appellate Division, unanimously decided that the IACUC of the State University of New York, Stony

Brook, is not a "public body," as defined by New York law. This committee acts only as an advisory body and is not involved in "deliberations and decisions that go into the making of public policy," and therefore does not perform a "government function."[30]

4. In 1989, an Alameda County Superior Court judge ruled that the University of California's ten campuses were not subject to the state's open meeting law because the university system was exempt from the law's requirements. However, in a separate action brought under the Public Records Act, the court ruled in 1992 that the University of California must copy and turn over to In Defense of Animals uncensored autopsy reports on lab animals that had died in its care.[31]

5. In 1991, an Oregon Circuit Court judge ruled that PETA lacked legal standing to seek judicial review of the University of Oregon's ban on public attendance at their IACUC. To obtain standing—here meaning standing to sue—the party that complains of unlawful conduct must show that its interests have been invaded.[32]

In these cases, an argument used by the defense was that the interests of universities would be harmed by public disclosure. For example, there are security risks in permitting the presence of animal rights sympathizers. If they were allowed to go on inspection tours of animal facilities (a legally required activity of IACUC members), then knowledge would be gained about the locations of rooms where animals are kept that could potentially be used for future raids. Also, disclosure of names of committee members and university research investigators could result in harassment or litigation. Publicity about committee discussions or records could stifle the review process and make its members more guarded in their comments—as appears to have happened at the University of Washington. Also, more widespread knowledge about animal experiments could result in public protest and the possible stoppage of biomedical and behavioral experimentation. Because science is a competitive endeavor, creative ideas should not be usurped by premature disclosure.

Legal Decisions That Require Open IACUC Meetings

In addition to Washington State, other states in which public disclosure laws have been interpreted to cover IACUCs include Florida, Kentucky, North Carolina, Texas, and Vermont. The fundamental rationale is that social issues are a matter of concern for the whole of society. Scientists are not immune to public scrutiny, and neither research scientists nor university officials have an overriding expertise in social values. Therefore, they should have no authority, by themselves, to determine what standards are to prevail regarding how animals are treated in scientific endeavors. State universities and other animal research facilities that accept public funding do not qualify for the independence from public scrutiny that they would have were they funded privately. In publicly funded institutions, ethical standards of scientists are subject to public scrutiny. An assessment of what is socially acceptable can be made only if information is freely available to the public and if the public is involved in decision making.

The basic case for opening IACUC meetings to the public was stated by counsel for the American Society for the Prevention of Cruelty to Animals:

> True, the information learned at meetings may be distorted by some [members of the public,] but few would argue that our press should be censored, or freedom of speech denied because some people in the media distort the truth now and then. The same reasoning

should apply here. Furthermore, in the event this does occur, there are laws regarding defamation and harassment. . . . One can argue that to deny information merely gives the interested public few options, one being to break in and actually see what is going on. To deny access . . . could encourage the unlawful behavior that many scientists and administrators at research institutions are so concerned about.[33]

The USDA's administration of the Animal Welfare Act was audited by the U.S. Office of the Inspector General[34] and a report released in September 2005. It focused on how well IACUCs were monitoring animal care activities and review of protocols. The report states, "Some IACUCs are not effectively monitoring animal care activities or reviewing protocols. From 2002 through 2004, the number of research facilities cited for violations of the AWA has steadily increased. . . . There are still problems with the search for alternative research, veterinary care, review of painful procedures, and the researchers' use of animals."

ETHICAL ISSUES

What Does the Public Have a Right to Know?

It is easy to understand why sunshine laws are popular. Without information, critics and reformers have no basis for action. They cannot seek public support regarding specific allegations of wrongdoing; they can merely complain about the secrecy of the activity. Lack of information can therefore be a death blow to the activities of watchdog organizations.

The University of Washington is publicly funded and is thus legally and politically accountable to citizens. UW officials employed several different arguments in their defense of a policy of nonaccess. They believed that they had no moral or legal obligation to give information about animal experiments to those who object to certain or all animal procedures. (No distinction appears to be made between animal welfarists, who seek reforms, and antivivisectionists, whose objective is to terminate work at the institution.)

UW officials also argued their point on the grounds of academic freedom, which consists of the absence of, or protection from, restraints or pressures that may inhibit the freedom of scholars in studying, discussing, lecturing, or publishing ideas and opinions. Such freedom "implies protection from . . . attempts to intimidate, no matter whence they come."[35] UW lawyers commented after quoting this source, "Thus, the core values of academic freedom are unfettered inquiry and dissemination of knowledge."[36] They defended what they considered the important social goods of unconstrained scientific inquiry and dissemination of knowledge.

On a strong interpretation of this view, the value of unfettered scientific inquiry takes precedence over all other values. However, a compelling contrary perspective is that at least some animal experiments are morally wrong because the experiments infringe the rights of the animal or cause unwarranted animal pain and suffering. PAWS supporters claimed that they were defending the rights and welfare of both animals and the public. Whatever the power of the moral values of academic freedom and privacy in universities, protecting the interests of animals and the public are moral values that are at least as powerful. From this perspective, the case of PAWS versus UW pits the rights and welfare of animals and the public's right to know against the rights of investigators and the value of academic freedom.

Scientists have a right to express beliefs and judgments about many matters, but if their statements or actions violate the moral rights of others (including, possibly, animals), then the latter's right might override the investigator's right to freedom of inquiry and expression. The defenses found in some contemporary writings and legal briefs of unrestrained freedom in science or in academia do not consider the full range of moral rights and responsibilities that confront free expression. Likewise, those who claim a right to information—the public's or their own—should be cognizant of the fact that competing values may, in certain circumstances, have moral weight equal to or greater than those rights.

Assessing Animal Pain and Suffering in Protocol Reviews

Investigators or oversight review committees have a responsibility to weigh and assess pain and suffering, but nationwide IACUC assessments are far from uniform. Protocol forms may or may not provide much information, and the investigator's narrative description of the project often does not describe in detail the degree of animal pain or suffering. Typically, a rough assessment of pain and suffering can be made by examining the descriptions of the experimental methods to be used. However, the full protocol is not necessarily shown to the committee or to observers. (See the introduction, pp. 30–31, 35.)

As part of the U.S. national statistics gathered annually, animal research facilities must report to the government whether an anesthetic is or is not used in experiments involving certain species of animals. This provision was added to the Animal Welfare Act in 1971 when anesthesia was not always used when needed. Decades later, changes have occurred; the use of sedation, anesthetics, and post-surgical pain relief have markedly improved. This has led some to believe that this "yes" or "no" system is outdated.[37] There is no ranking of the degree of animal harm, nor do current data capture information about distress, sensory or social deprivation of the animal, the debilitating effect of infections, or whether surgery itself is minor or major.

Some hold that the most informative system is use of a "pain scale" that ranks the degree of pain and suffering as none, minor, moderate, or severe.[38] This system is used by the University of Washington and several other American universities. The system has become national policy in several countries, including the United Kingdom, Canada, and the Netherlands.[39]

At the time of its court conflicts, the University of Washington's ACC categorized each submitted protocol according to potential discomfort or pain to the animal on a 1–4 scale of increasing severity of the procedure. Category 1 projects involve "little or no discomfort"; category 2 projects involve "some distress or discomfort"; category 3 projects involve "significant distress or discomfort"; and Category 4 projects involve "severe pain."

In 1995, after years of observing ACC meetings, PAWS publicly charged that the ACC was underestimating animal pain in the case of some protocols. Lower estimates allowed review for these projects to be conducted out of the public eye and without serious scrutiny; full committee review was circumvented by an unjustifiable designation of a lower pain category. In 1994, seven years after being granted observational status and access to ACC documents, PAWS analyzed the committee procedures and concluded that some projects involving cats and dogs had been incorrectly ranked. Because of flawed rankings to five projects, full committee review had been avoided. The university conceded that one project was ranked too low, but it held that others were accurately ranked. Issues remain, however.

Community Representation in Decision Making

Another moral problem is whether representatives of animal protection groups should be allowed a voice in decision making about animal research, possibly a vote or a right to file dissenting opinions about the acceptability of the research. Both PAWS and the Northwest Animal Rights Network tried unsuccessfully to become the assigned "community member" of the IACUC, thus providing a vote and a right to file a dissenting opinion on project approvals. But this failure does not answer moral questions about whether such representation is justified.

Within the scientific community, opinions are mixed regarding the degree to which the public, let alone animal advocates, should participate in day-to-day decision making on animal experiments. The most contentious issue in the passage of the 1985 amendments to the Animal Welfare Act was the inclusion of a nonaffiliated member. The biomedical community worried that a nonaffiliated member might disclose information detrimental to the institution. In the end, Congress decreed that a member must represent "general community interests in the proper care and treatment of animals." Congress made no stipulation about who that member should be. Since appointments are made by the institution's chief executive office or other designated official, the community itself has no say in who will represent the public's interest.

A few American IACUCs have voluntarily appointed representatives of animal protection organizations and occasionally even antivivisectionists. An unusual in-house policy was established at the Wisconsin Regional Primate Research Center, stating, "Advocates of animal rights, along with scientific peers, will be appointed by the Director to participate with full voice and vote."[40]

A different picture exists in many European countries, where national laws commonly specify that oversight committees for animal experimentation must include representatives of animal welfare organizations. For instance:

The 2005 Norwegian Animal Welfare Act requires seven specific competencies to be represented on regional review committees for animal experiments, of which one person must be a representative from an animal welfare organization.[41]

The 1991 Swiss Law on Animal Welfare (Article 18) requires that cantons (equivalent to states) institute commissions for review and approval of animal experiments. Each commission must include representatives from animal protection organizations.

A 1988 Swedish law[42] stipulates that half of the members of the "ethical" institutional review committees for animal experiments must be laypeople; within this group, representatives of animal welfare organizations must be included.

A 1987 Danish law on animal experimentation mandates a ten-person national oversight committee that must include four persons proposed by animal welfare organizations.

The 1986 German First Amendment to Animal Protection Law requires the national oversight committee to have 12 members, of whom one-third are experts from national animal welfare organizations.

In the United States, a common view in the animal research community was voiced in a 1996 article in *Physiologist*.[43] The author advises that "activists must not be given access to any research activities because . . . their goal is destruction of animal-based biomedical research." Another view is seen in a 1991 informal survey of interviews with 16 hard-to-find animal advocates who served on IACUCs. High on the list of complaints of these community members was a sense of frustration in effecting any change. Many viewed IACUCs as "rubber stamps."[44]

Conflict of Interest in the Review of Protocols

Conflict of interest is an important, albeit little discussed, moral problem about the review of research. A conflict of interest occurs when a member of an animal care committee has been in a relationship, past or present, with administrators or research investigators that would reasonably be expected to exert an influence on the member's judgment when he or she is called on to vote on a research protocol. A conflict of interest is present whenever the researcher's role obligation or personal interest in accommodating an institution, in job security, in personal goals, and the like compromises or threatens to compromise obligations to others who have a right to expect objectivity and fairness. The conflict of interest could be either financial or nonfinancial.

In the present case, having investigators and university administrators decide about either the welfare of animals or the legitimacy of the interests of animal welfare supporters seems to involve a conflict of interest. They have a financial interest in seeing the research go forward at their institution, and the research protocols they review are generally those written by their colleagues, who are often their friends or collaborators. Such relationships are not allowed in deliberations and opinions issued in courts of law, on the grounds that these relationships introduce bias and threaten discriminatory treatment. The same problem of bias and discrimination can occur in an IACUC.

However, the problem of conflict of interest is two-sided. Persons with strong animal rights or animal protection interests would also be involved in a conflict of interest if they were to review protocols. Consider an analogy. In some universities, one of the relationships that is specifically prohibited by rule under conflict of interest provisions is this: When serving on committees that involve faculty evaluation, a member of the committee may not have served as the lawyer, advocate, or trustee for the faculty member being evaluated. Analogously, a member of an animal rights or animal welfare group has a commitment to represent the interests of vulnerable animals, and therefore would serve as a kind of advocate or trustee for the animals whose welfare is at stake.

Is there a solution to the review of animal research that is relatively free of bias and conflict of interest? Perhaps the person appointed for the community slot, or even a majority of the committee, should be more independent—for example, a lawyer, a teacher of ethics, or a businessperson from the community. There is a general recognition among IACUC members at many institutions that having some sort of community representative is beneficial when they are informed and truly free of conflict of interest. They bring a fresh perspective and also bring credibility to committee deliberations. An outsider can keep the scientists alert to community concerns and remind investigators to explain in laypersons' terms what they are doing and why—possibly even making scientists more introspective about their work.

The risks present in appointing committee members from the community is that they often have no special expertise in either animal welfare or the science involved in the protocol being reviewed. One could argue that assessment of biomedical research, like treatment at the hands of a veterinarian, is a task that belongs to persons with a certain professional expertise and commitment—including a commitment to the welfare of animal subjects. From this perspective, expertise in the relevant profession will involve the ability to review both the science and the comfort of the animals, which is the immediate business at hand. If animal researchers can be both unbiased in their scientific expertise and morally sensitive in their use of the animals, then perhaps scientists should be the sole reviewers. But can they be objective and impartial in the face of a conflict of interest?

It is clear that many challenges remain about how to establish an environment in which animal researchers, animal activists, and government officials can make responsible and impartial decisions that will gain the confidence of a now wary and polarized public. These tensions may never cease.

NOTES

1. Physicians Committee for Responsible Medicine, *Your Right to Know: Understanding Animal Experiments in Your Community* (Washington, DC: PCRM, 2006). This advice preceded the University of Washington court battles and is regularly updated; see pcrm.org/resch/anexp/your_right.html.

2. For reports on this case, see A. Anderson, "U.S. University Told to Reveal Unfunded NIH Application," *Nature* 359 (September 1992): 98; and T. Adler, "APA Files Amicus Brief in Grant Application Case," *Monitor* (American Psychological Association) 24 (September 1993): 26.

3. The decision was by trial court, with no published opinion.

4. Sally Macdonald, "Animal-Rights Group Wins Order Opening UW Research Meetings," *Seattle Times,* March 20, 1987, p. B1.

5. "Suit Concluded, Dispute Drags On," *PAWS News* (February 1988): 40.

6. For information about this case, see *Progressive Animal Welfare Society v. University of Washington,* 114 Wash.2d 677,790 P.2d 604 (1990).

7. *Progressive Animal Welfare Society v. University of Washington,* 125 Wash.2d 243, 884 P.2d 592 (1994).

8. *Animal Legal Defense Fund, Inc. v. Shalala,* 104 F.3d 424 (D.C. Cir. 1997). For a discussion of this case, see Rebecca Dresser, "Scientists in the Sunshine," *Hastings Center Report* 27, no. 6 (November–December 1997): 26–27.

9. Federal Advisory Committee Act Amendments of 1997, Public Law No. 105–153, § 2(a), 111 Stat. 2689 (codified at 5 U.S.C. app. 2 § 3(2)). The statute reference is 5 U.S.C. app. 2 § 3(2) (2006).

10. National Freedom of Information Coalition, "State and Federal FOI Resources," www.nfoic.org/resources/states/.

11. Mitchell Fox, transcript of public statement made at the University of Washington Animal Care Committee meeting, May 26, 1994.

12. Ibid.

13. Nona Phillips, interview with Barbara Orlans, telephone notes, May 1, 2005, with follow-up e-mail listing IACUC membership.

14. Nona Phillips, e-mail to Barbara Orlans, June 14, 2005.

15. Nona Phillips, interviews with Barbara Orlans, telephone notes, May 1 and May 11, 2005.

16. Kathleen Holder, "Razor-Blade Threats against Researchers Put Campus on Alert," *Dateline UCDAVIS,* November 5, 1999, www.dateline.ucdavis.edu/110599/DL_letterthreats.html (accessed June 3, 2005).

17. E-mail from Nona Phillips to Barbara Orlans, May 11, 2005.

18. E-mail from Nona Phillips to Barbara Orlans, June 14, 2005.

19. Nona Phillips, interview with Barbara Orlans, telephone notes, May 1, 2005.

20. Nona Phillips, interview with Barbara Orlans, telephone notes, June 3, 2005.

21. Wayne Johnson, interview with Barbara Orlans, telephone notes, February 19, 2005.

22. Wayne Johnson, interview with Barbara Orlans, telephone notes, February 10, 2005.

23. Wayne Johnson, interview with Barbara Orlans, telephone notes, November 13, 2005.

24. Ibid.

25. Wayne Johnson, interview with Barbara Orlans, telephone notes, February 10, 2005.

26. *In Defense of Animals v. Oregon Health Sciences University*, 199 Or. App. 160, 163–167, 112 P.3d 336, 340–343 (2005).

27. Matt Rossell, outreach coordinator, In Defense of Animals, e-mail to Barbara Orlans, December 1, 2006.

28. *Students for Animals v. University of Virginia*, 12 Va. Cir. 247 (1988).

29. *Medlock v. Board of Trustees of University of Massachusetts*, 580 N.E.2d 387(Mass. 1991).

30. *Matter of American Society for the Prevention of Cruelty to Animals v. Board of Trustees, State University of New York*, 568 N.Y.S.2d 63 (1991). New York's highest court affirmed the judgment, but its reason was different. This court held that the ACC was a federal body and thus not covered by the state's public meeting law; 591 N.E.2d 1168 (N.Y.2d 1992).

31. The decisions came from trial courts with unpublished opinions.

32. *People for the Ethical Treatment of Animals v. Institutional Animal Care and Use Committee of the University of Oregon*, 312 Or. 95, 817 P.2d 1299 (1991).

33. Elinor Molbegott, counsel for the American Society for the Prevention of Cruelty to Animals, New York, transcript of a speech given in October 1989 at Rockefeller University.

34. U.S. Department of Agriculture, "Audit Report: APHIS Animal Care Program Inspection and Enforcement Activities," No. 33002–3-SF, September 2005, Executive Summary, pp. ii–iii, and Finding 4, p. 19, www.usda.gov/oig/webdocs/33022–03-SF.pdf.

35. Fritz Machlup, "On Some Misconceptions Concerning Academic Freedom," in *Academic Freedom and Tenure—A Handbook of the American Association of University Professors*, ed. Louis Joughlin (Madison: University of Wisconsin, 1967), appendix B, p. 178.

36. Tammy L. Lewis and Lisa A. Vincler, "Storming the Ivory Tower: The Competing Interests of the Public's Right to Know and Protecting the Integrity of University Research," *Journal of College and University Law* 20 (Spring 1994): 440.

37. F. Barbara Orlans. "Data on Animal Experimentation in the United States: What They Do and Do Not Show," *Perspectives in Biology and Medicine* 37, no. 2 (Winter 1994): 217–31.

38. F. Barbara Orlans, *In the Name of Science: Issues in Responsible Animal Experimentation* (New York: Oxford University Press, 1993), pp. 86–89.

39. Ibid., pp. 118–27.

40. Wisconsin Regional Primate Research Center, "Policy Statement on Principles for the Ethical Use of Animals," *American Journal of Primatology* 3 (1982): 345–47.

41. Norwegian Animal Welfare Act, Chapter 6, Section 23, as updated November 20, 2005; unofficial translation, oslovet/veths.no/act.html. E-mail from Cecilia Holman to Barbara Orlans, December 8, 2006.

42. Swedish Animal Welfare Law (1988: 534), Article 21; and Animal Welfare Ordinance (1988: 539), Article 43.

43. Michael E. Carey, "Lessons Learned from a Scientist's Personal Confrontation with Animal Zealots," *Physiologist* 39, no. 1 (1996): 9.

44. Ibid.; and Orlans, *In the Name of Science*, p. 111.

13

Can There Be Cruelty-Free
Cosmetic Testing?

In the early 1970s, as part of a study into nonsurgical treatments of squint, Alan Scott, a clinical researcher, discovered that a bacterial toxin could be used to treat abnormal muscle spasms (dystonias).[1] Such dystonias are responsible for a range of conditions other than squints, including facial spasms such as an involuntary and uncontrollable closure of the eyelid (blepharospasm). The toxin works by relaxing muscles through a local action on the nerves supplying the affected muscles. In 1987 Jean Carruthers, an ophthalmologist visiting Scott, noticed that the treatment of blepharospasm coincidentally resulted in the disappearance of the frown lines above the nose. She told her husband, a dermatologist, about this observation, and he remarked that he had been using the toxin for some time for cosmetic purposes, including the removal of these skin creases. They published a key paper in 1992, and the toxin—marketed under a variety of names such as Botox, Myobloc, and Dysport—has since found a variety of cosmetic and other uses (for 50 or so conditions, a number sure to increase), including replacing antiperspirants.[2] The FDA approved Botox for medical uses in 1989 and for cosmetic uses in 2002.

But there is a problem. The toxin has to be purified from a culture (of Clostridium botulinum), and each batch varies in strength. In order to determine the "potency" of each batch, every new batch has to be tested in mice using a lethality test from which some of the mice will die a painful death due to the paralysis of the breathing muscles, akin to asphyxiation.[3] Because of the increased cosmetic use of the toxin, the market has increased considerably since 1993, especially since the FDA approved its use for cosmetic purposes.[4] Sales of Botox may be close to $1 billion a year at present and are forecast to surge in double-digit percentages in upcoming years. It has been dubbed "the Viagra of 2002."

ANIMAL TESTING

In the past, animals were often used to test cosmetic products, but such testing is now often considered to be unjustified when the benefits are weighed against the costs to the animals involved in premarketing safety testing. When the campaign against cosmetics testing reached significant dimensions in the 1970s and 1980s, animal tests commonly caused blindness, pain, and death to rabbits, rats, and other animals. Many improvements, particularly to experimental designs, have been made to alleviate these problems. Homecare Technology Ltd. has stated, "We have produced a range of products which are 'cruelty-free,' non-toxic and environmentally safe with ingredients which are not animal tested. Organic Product Company skin care products are based on traditional herbal remedies that have been tried and tested on people not animals."[5] However, animal welfare groups, as well as some cosmetics manufacturers, remain active in pressing for a ban on testing the safety of cosmetics on animals.

One of the many protests of this testing is the June 1996 national animal rights demonstration in Washington, DC. Some 3,000 signs with the message "Against Animal Testing" were distributed to demonstrators by the Body Shop, a cosmetic retailer and a major sponsor of the demonstration. The Body Shop has tried to build a reputation in both the United Kingdom and the United States based on its condemnation of animal testing. The Body Shop's policy is that the company does not conduct animal tests and will purchase only cosmetic ingredients that suppliers have either never tested on animals for cosmetic purposes or at least not tested or retested since December 31, 1990.[6] They have established a monitoring system to enforce this policy with suppliers. This policy is noted in its marketing, and products carry the label "Against animal testing." This label is a statement of policy, not a claim that their products have never been tested on animals—a claim that is still made by various companies. Jon Entine, the Body Shop's purchasing manager, reported that 46.5% of its ingredients had been tested on animals for some purpose at some time.[7] The policy limits the Body Shop from using any newly developed ingredient (a dye or other substance) that has been tested on animals, even if this places them at a disadvantage with competitors.

Other product labels in common use are "Cruelty free" and "Never tested on animals." People for the Ethical Treatment of Animals (PETA) publishes an annual shopping guide, which includes companies such as Revlon, John Mitchell Systems, Estee Lauder, and more than 500 other companies.[8] If these companies assure PETA that they and their suppliers do not test on animals, they can then use PETA's "caring consumer" logo on their products: a rabbit in a box that says "Not tested on animals. No animal ingredients." These assurances make claims that companies using these labels are prepared to assert that the finished product contains no ingredients tested on animals by the distributor, supplier, or anyone else. Nonetheless, some consumer protection organizations and animal protection groups argue that "no animal testing" claims are misleading and deceive consumers, because almost all ingredients in use today in health and beauty aid products have been tested on animals at some time by some company, either because legislation at the time required the testing or because the ingredient is used for a purpose other than for cosmetics.[9]

In November 1995, in an effort to secure stringent product labeling standards, the National Consumers League recommended to the U.S. Federal Trade Commission (FTC) that a ban be placed on the use of product labels such as "Against animal testing," "No animal testing," or "Not tested on animals."[10] The League holds that these labels should not be allowed because they do not convey specific information that is meaningful to consumers in making choices. However, in July 1996, the FTC responded to the league by stating that they will take no action on this matter on the grounds that no consumer injury results from these product labels.[11]

THE NATURE AND JUSTIFICATION OF ANIMAL TESTING

Just about every item made by humans that we touch, smell, ingest, or to which we are exposed has been tested on animals at some time, because synthetic as well as natural chemicals will have been used in the production or preservation of these products. We now assume the safety of such products to an extraordinary degree. Most of us do not worry that the chemicals in the colored clothes that we wear might lead to skin cancer where they have been in direct contact with our bodies. Similarly, we take medicines and use deodorants, antiperspirants, shaving creams, suntan and sunblock lotions, toothpastes, or household products such as washing powders and liquids, polishes, disinfectants, and cleaners of various goods (for example, silver, brass, oven, window, floor) without fear, although many products carry warning labels. Thousands of similar examples could be listed.

Reasons for Safety Testing

Apart from safeguarding the health of the consumer, there are several reasons to implement safety testing. There is a need to protect workers in the factories producing the chemicals, a need to protect the environment from inadvertent pollution, a need to protect the user of the chemicals in agriculture, at work, in industry, or in the backyard, and a need to know what to do when a person has been accidentally exposed to a significant amount of a substance, such as children swallowing a bottle of herbicide or spilling a household chemical on themselves (that is, the need to identify organs that may be affected and the treatment of poisoning). Finally, there is a need to undertake risk assessment to figure out whether to label a chemical, either for marketing with suitable warnings on the packaging or for bulk transport when large amounts are being moved around the country on trucks or railways, to establish safe exposure levels.

What should now be tested, and how should it be tested? New chemicals, new substances, and new "improved" products are generally required by law to be tested before being marketed. The new product may use ingredients with well-known toxic or nontoxic safety profiles. Questions of risk then turn on whether there may be some unsuspected synergistic actions between the calculated "safe levels" of ingredients. New chemicals are safety tested by giving them to animals in single and multiple doses of varying size and by various routes, intended to mimic approximate human exposures. The effects on the animals are noted, such as whether the compound is an irritant (for example, to the eye or skin) and by what route (for example, oral or inhaled), and the dose at which a single dose of compound causes signs of toxicity or kills the animals (for example, Lethal Dose 50%, known as the LD50 Test).[12]

Animals Used in Safety Testing

Detailed figures on the use of animals in safety testing have been kept in the United Kingdom for decades. In 2005, 4.9% of all vertebrates used in research were used for safety testing (see table 13.1). In November 1997, the government announced that no further licenses would be issued for cosmetic finished-product testing and that existing licenses had been amended to exclude this type of work. This announcement was extended in November 1998 to ingredients intended primarily for cosmetics. As a consequence, no procedures were performed for either of these purposes in 2005. This position has not yet been adopted by all European countries, although there is a move to ban testing within the European Union.[13]

In the United States in 1980, some 14 million animals were used in the safety testing of cosmetics and household products, but available U.S. statistics lack the necessary detail, so it is impossible to obtain accurate, current information.[14]

Cosmetic Testing

The U.S. Federal Food, Drug, and Cosmetic Act defines "cosmetics" as articles intended to be applied to the human body for cleansing, beautifying, promoting attractiveness, or altering the appearance without affecting the body's structure or functions.[15] The European Directive (93/35/EEC) is more explicit and defines a "cosmetic product" as "any substance or preparation intended to be placed in contact with the various external parts of the human body (epidermis, hair system, nails, lips, and external genital organs) or with the teeth and the mucous membranes of the oral cavity with a view exclusively or mainly to cleaning them, perfuming them, changing their appearance, and/or correcting body odors and/or protecting them or keeping them in good condition."[16] Botulinum

Table 13.1. Comparison of Single Oral Dose Acute Toxicity Test Procedures

Name of Test	Numbers of Animals Used		Death as the Endpoint	Time Taken (Days)
	Minimum	Maximum		
Classical (1927)	60	80	yes	>14
OECD (1981)	30	30	yes	>14
Up-and-Down (1985)	6	10	yes	<25
ATC-BGA (1985)	6	18	yes	28
OECD (1987)	20	20	yes	>28
FDP-BTS (1987)	10	20	no	>14

Notes: The tests referred to in the left-hand column are the Classical LD50 test; the Organisation for Economic Co-operation and Development recommended standards in the years cited; the Up-and-Down test; the Acute Toxic Class—Bundesgesundheitsamt; and the Fixed Dose Procedure—British Toxicology Society.

seems not to fit in with either the U.S. or the E.U. definition, and so the term "cosmo-ceutical" has been suggested.[17]

Included in these definitions and classifications are "vanity products," although it might be argued that some of these products are beneficial and even therapeutic, such as skin creams, lotions, sunblocks or screens, suntan creams, aftershaves, perfumes, lipsticks, fingernail polishes, hardeners, and enamels, eye and facial make-up, depilatories, hair straighteners, preparations, shower gels, bubble baths, shampoos, conditioners, permanent waves, hair dyes, rinses and sprays, toothpastes, mouthwashes, deodorants, talcum powders, and soaps.

Safety testing involves a range of *in vitro* and *in vivo* assessments, and it is considered necessary only for new cosmetic substances or new combinations of ingredients that need to be more carefully evaluated.[18] The tests are designed mainly to look for skin irritation, absorption, phototoxicity (in response to UV radiation), and sensitization; eye and mucous membrane irritation; acute oral or inhalation toxicity; and any long-term effects such as carcinogenicity (cancer inducing) or teratogenicity (inducing defects in the unborn). New cosmetic *products* or formulations are examined for a "no observed effect level" (NOEL) or a "no observed adverse effect level" (NOAEL) at a dosage similar to the calculated human exposure. Cosmetic *ingredients,* on the other hand, are tested primarily for their safety to protect the industrial chemical worker. In these tests, the doses given will be increased until signs of toxicity are seen in order to obtain an idea of the level at which the substance is hazardous. Even if the test substance proves to be nontoxic in a test, it is usually necessary to subject the animals to a toxic dose of a control substance to be assured that the test is working correctly. Thus safety testing always unavoidably involves some animal pain and distress.

The Draize skin and Draize eye irritancy tests, developed in 1944, have acquired notoriety over the past 50 years because of the damaging effects on the animals tested, causing them pain, distress, and, in the early days of the test, blindness. In the skin test, the fur of the animal's trunk is clipped and the skin may then be abraded before a sleeve or semi-occlusive patch containing the test substance is applied for 24 hours. The animal and the skin are then examined at varying intervals for signs of toxicity and local injury. The skin test is used to predict sensitization of the skin and phototoxic effects (sensitization in response to light). In the past decade, these tests have been considerably modified in Europe through strategic and humane experimental designs so that the animals suffer far less than before.

The eye test used in the United States involves placing a small volume of diluted test substance in the eye of six albino rabbits and observing them for signs of irritation for up to three days.[19] If damage has occurred, animals will be followed up for 21 days to see if the damage is repaired, and if little or no repair occurs, the substance will be classified as corrosive. The eye test has been criticized because the rabbit's eye is significantly different from the human eye on several counts. For example, rabbits have a third eyelid, unlike humans; rabbits also have a slower blink reflex and a thinner cornea, and produce fewer tears than humans. Furthermore, the test has given inconsistent results between laboratories.[20] Nevertheless, the U.S. Food and Drug Administration (FDA) and the European Scientific Committee on Cosmetic Products and Non-food Products still consider the test to be useful for understanding and predicting injury to or around the human eye.[21]

Acute toxicity tests are usually carried out on white rats to determine systemic acute lethal potency. The Lethal Dose 50% test (LD50), as formulated more than 70 years ago, involved causing at least 50% of the animals to die (often a slow, painful death) from a single dose of the test substance, but this approach has now been superseded, requiring that fewer animals be used.[22] The test normally performed today accepts some *estimated* data on lethality (for example, by using data from other structurally related chemicals).[23]

Human data, if available, are used in all safety evaluations. However, it often takes several years for such evidence to accumulate from reports of routine as well as accidental exposures.

STAKEHOLDERS IN CONTROVERSIES OVER THE USE OF ANIMALS

The cosmetics industry is still expanding. In the seven major European cosmetics markets, the growth rate is around 6% per year. In the United States, Avon, Revlon, and Fabergé all have top sales in the billions of dollars. The market is currently expanding into Asia and South America.

It has become increasingly apparent that the public does not want products that have been tested on laboratory animals, so many companies have ended their testing. Some cosmetic manufacturers are so opposed to animal testing that they formed the Cosmetics Industry Coalition for Animal Welfare Ltd. (CICAW). CICAW members agree not to use any ingredient that has been tested since 1976—i.e., they adhere to a fixed cutoff date criterion, and, by so doing, they risk going out of business. In addition, a number of their key cosmetic ingredients have been superseded.[24] Other companies choose to roll the five-year cutoff date forward each year.

The general public is undoubtedly concerned about the use of animals to test cosmetic products. Polls have shown that 85–96% of the public is against animal testing of beauty, vanity, and household products.[25]

Legislation in Europe is somewhat at odds with itself as, on the one hand, it requires animal testing of ingredients for the purpose of health and safety, but, on the other, it requires that animal testing be reduced.[26] However, legislation has now been passed in Europe that is calculated to phase out animal testing without endangering human health.[27] The FDA now states that it does *not* require LD50 test data on animals to establish toxicity, and furthermore it advocates the use of various protections in the use of animal techniques.[28]

Animal rights and antivivisection organizations demand an immediate end to all animal experimentation and have campaigned for a ban on animal testing of cosmetics in particular, since cosmetics are viewed as luxury goods and cosmetic testing is viewed as a relatively easy target. Moderate animal welfare organizations, which typically promote the Three Rs concept (reduction, refinement, and replacement of animals in experiments; see chapter 1), are insistent in their claims that the use of animals for testing cosmetics is unnecessary. Some research groups established to defend the use of animals in biomedical research now accept the view that animals should not be used for testing cosmetics and certain other types of consumer products. Many products are now often tested on employees of cosmetics companies to check the safety of a new formulation whose likely toxicity could be predicted from the known changes in the new formulation from an old one. The hypothesis is that the volunteer studies would merely confirm that prediction.

ETHICAL ISSUES

Harms and Benefits in Testing

In both the United States and Europe, there is concern that we do not have adequate information on around 30,000 chemicals that are in use today. So under the HPV[29] and REACH[30] programs, there is an aim to rectify the situation and to acquire the missing information. It has been calculated that both of these studies will consume 11 million animals and will cost approximately $11.3 billion U.S.[31]

It is generally accepted that new *chemicals* should be tested, but not everyone agrees that all new *products* should be tested, especially cosmetic products. It has been suggested that the benefits to be gained from cosmetics are so trivial that the use of animals for the purpose of ensuring safety is immoral and not to be condoned, because the harms done to the animals do not compensate for the relatively small benefits to humans. Typically, animal protection organizations state that there are enough products available already and that new ones should not be developed if they involve animal experimentation.

However, if we had taken this view in 1960 and consistently practiced it, we might not have various hair conditioners, sunblock lotions, fluoride toothpastes, antiperspirants, etc., that we have today. Nor would they be available in their present range and quality. The failure to test not only runs risks of harms for humans, but also results in lost opportunities for industries and their consumers. However, this view is contestable because there is no guarantee that our knowledge base would have remained the same. It is also argued that if rules are overly stringent, whole areas of research can be brought to a standstill, with the consequent loss of the benefits of those lines of research.

Where does one draw the line regarding what will be tested as well as the harms that will be permitted in the testing? How are permitted harms to be balanced against possible benefits? In assessing such questions, we need to take account of the many types of harm and benefit that might come into consideration. For example, would pressure not to use animals to test cosmetic products preclude the safety testing of the chemical ingredients that are used to make up those same cosmetics as well as many noncosmetic products?

A related question is, "How hard should we try to use animals to mimic extreme misuses or abuses of substances by humans in order to prevent harm?" Should research be premised on the idea that someone somewhere may ignore all the warnings and take in a dose that would not normally occur if the product was used properly? Accidental ingestion and exposure by children does occasionally occur, and toxicity data *may* provide some information on what organs are affected and how to treat such persons, depending on whether the animal absorbs, metabolizes, and excretes the chemical in a similar fashion.

This problem exists with all toxicity testing in animals, because species extrapolation is an unavoidable aspect of human safety testing. However, do manufacturers go beyond what would normally be possible in dosage rates—that is, do they unjustifiably give animals dose levels that it is inconceivable that any human could reach? Evidence suggests they have done so on occasion. Leslie Fain—an animal caretaker at Gillette—witnessed rats being placed in an airtight chamber into which hair spray was then sprayed. This exposure was apparently equivalent to sealing oneself in the bathroom and spraying hair spray for one hour. The rats died of poisoning. This form of testing suggests that scientists can and should carry out more limited tests (as discussed below).[32]

Two ways forward might be to continue to try to make animal tests more humane or to replace them altogether with *in vitro* methods. The latter would be risky because our science often is not good enough to warrant this replacement. The former seems a requirement of good ethics, but how humane do the tests have to be? In other words, can we do to a rabbit only what can permissibly be done to a human?

The Alternative of Human Volunteers

Alternatives to the use of animals are often suggested as a way around moral problems in their use. The Three Rs first put forward by Russell and Burch in 1959 include *replacement alternatives* as a major moral responsibility in planning for new research.[33] (See the introduction, pp. 32–36.)

Human volunteers are now increasingly being used to test cosmetic products, just as they have long been used in biomedical research. An essential element of carrying out research on humans is not only that they should be adequately aware of the risks involved, but also that they not be manipulated or coerced into participating. Although the practice now happens, it is debatable whether an employee of a cosmetics company can take part in research testing free of manipulation by the implicit structure of rewards and punishments (salary increases, job transfers, and the like). The employee may feel that it will stand him or her in good stead for promotion or a wage increase, or keeping his or her job in times of redundancy, even though this may be explicitly disclaimed in any contract by the employer.

This shows how many moral problems concerned with the treatment of humans can arise from reflection on and requirements of alternatives to our use of animals. Though these problems are not specifically about the morality of *animal* use, associated and more general questions arise about our obligations to both humans and animals. The chief question is whether or not we are obligated to seek human volunteers to *replace* animals in cosmetic testing. If so, and if the risk is similar for both, are we obligated to use humans first or animals first? Does it matter, morally, whom we use first?

Alternatives to Using Whole Animals in Safety Tests

The U.S. Public Health Service policy on protocol review by institutional animal care and use committees states that *in vitro* biological systems to replace animals should be considered in testing. A similar approach urging scientists to "consider alternatives" has been adopted in the United Kingdom. The European Directive is more explicit and states that "an experiment shall not be performed if another scientifically satisfactory method of obtaining the result sought, not entailing the use of an animals, is reasonably and practicably available."[34]

Alternatives to the use of whole animals are currently being developed.[35] Cell culture, tissue slices, organ culture, computer modeling (*in silico*), and the use of lower organisms can all provide useful information in research and safety testing, but to date they cannot entirely replace whole animal tests, because whole animals are made up of body systems, i.e., interacting body organs, and not just cells. *In vitro* methods can reveal useful information about a chemical and its interactions with specific cell types (the scientific discipline of toxicology). For example, they can expose overt toxicity as it kills cells or alters a cellular function, and they can identify mechanisms of toxicity, sometimes more easily than can animal tests, that can be crucial for risk assessment. What *in vitro* methods cannot do is replace all the complex interactions within a whole animal. That is why such methods are often referred to as adjuncts rather than replacements.

Although animal protection organizations often suggest a greater availability of alternative tests than is actually the case, it is now clear that some alternatives can provide very useful screening techniques. For example, substances that are toxic to cells in culture may well be toxic to whole animals and need not be tested further. Studies are being carried out to seek alternatives to the Draize eye irritation test, but such alternatives are still at an early stage of development and evaluation. They include the use of isolated eyes (rabbit, chicken, bovine), complex artificial skin mixtures and skin slices, chicken egg membranes, and cell cultures. These tests still have to be fully validated for a large range of chemicals for the toxicities that we presently investigate, such as irritancy and sensitization, before being widely accepted.[36] (Some argue that the test is so inherently misleading that to use the Draize test as a standard simply replicates the errors.[37])

Humane Endpoints When Using Whole Animals in Safety Tests

Russell and Burch's Three Rs include not only the replacement alternatives outlined above, but also *refinement alternatives,* which are means by which animal suffering can be minimized, and reduction alternatives in which the fewest number of animals are used, which in turn will reduce the overall suffering of the animals. (See the introduction, pp. 32–36.) The OECD has introduced some guidance on humane endpoints so that animals can be killed before they die, i.e., when they are moribund, or death is likely, or they are in extreme pain and distress.[38] However, by the time an animal gets to this stage, it is likely to have already suffered to a considerable degree. There is also no formal procedure for updating test guidelines.[39] In the past decade, the Draize eye and skin tests have been considerably modified through strategic and humane experimental designs so that the animals suffer far less than before. In many cases suffering may be quite slight and far less severe than one might see daily in an average veterinarian's clinic. Unlike in the past, when animals were restrained in stocks for the whole of the test, the animals are now often allowed more mobility and have continual access to food and water.

However, the amount of skin exposed to the test substance can be large, and adverse effects such as irritation and inflammation can be significant during the 24-hour test period. The potential for the eye test to cause pain is considerable, and this test, like the skin test, has been modified over the past decade or so. The mucous membranes of the eye may now be anesthetized with local anesthetic before the test substance is introduced or immediately afterward, especially after the first animal has shown an adverse response. Solutions of extreme acidity or alkalinity are not tested in the eye, as they are assumed to be irritants, and substances that have already been shown to be skin irritants are not to be used in the eye (skin irritation studies precede eye tests in the tiered systems of testing now being used).[40]

Acute toxicity tests, as developed more than 50 years ago, involved large numbers of animals and required death as an integral part of the test. These tests have now been superseded. The test normally performed today accepts *estimated data* on lethality, and a major advance has been that, in some countries, regulatory authorities accept signs of toxicity rather than death as a valid endpoint.[41] The test has been further refined so that a maximum dose level is laid down, the so-called limit test, in which a maximum single dose rate of 2g/kg (in Europe) or 5g/kg (in the United States) is given. If the substance shows no toxicity at that level (interpreted as one or no animal(s) dying out of 10 given the dose after 14 days), the substance will be classified as nontoxic. If two or more animals die, then a second group will be tested at a lower dose. The complete test normally requires 10–20 rats. These tests could conceivably be further refined by reducing the number of animals and employing earlier endpoints.[42]

Michael Balls and Julia Fentem have compared the various acute toxicity tests available today, as summarized in table 13.1.[43] The data show that since 1927, significant changes have been made for various tests. In addition, the tests themselves have been refined so that they cause less pain for the animals, although it has to be questioned why three tests are accepted when they differ in their impact on animal welfare. It is a significant moral question whether authorities are obligated to choose the one that causes the least harm.

Desensitization of Animal Researchers

The vast scale on which animals are used in safety testing has, in some cases, clearly desensitized those connected with the practice. Such desensitization presents many moral problems. A duty of care extends to all animals, but discharging this obligation to the large number of animals involved in safety testing is plainly difficult.

Desensitization may occur as a consequence of being continually exposed to animal suffering, as in acute toxicity testing. An employee at Biosearch Laboratories (USA) has been quoted as saying, "Once you've been here a few days, you lose respect for all living things."[44] Oversensitization of employees toward animals may be seen by some as sentimentality, but today's rules and regulations governing the use of animals in cosmetic testing have, perhaps, yesterday's sentimentality. Management has reacted to this "sentimentality" in some laboratories by discouraging the naming of animals (an activity employees often engage in). This distancing of the researcher from the animal seems to encourage poorer care and fewer questions as to why animals are being used as they are. In other laboratories where such concerns are more openly encouraged and discussed, animals appear to be treated much better.

Ill-Gotten Gains

Because the humaneness of safety testing has increased over the past 20 years, ingredients tested during this period are likely to have caused far less animal suffering than those tested before 1986. Therefore, from the perspective of ill-gotten gains, there seems to be a moral obligation to use newer over older ingredients.

The argument of ill-gotten gains could also be applied to the importation of cosmetic products from those countries whose standards of testing are less humane. At what point should a government or a corporation decide not to import goods that have been produced by means that would be unethical or illegal in their own country? Are governments obligated to abide by such a standard in a way that corporations are not? Are individual consumers bound to the logic of ill-gotten gains in their purchases? Is "ill-gotten gains" even an important moral notion?

Mislabeling and the Ethics of Advertising

Labeling of products and advertising claims can teeter on the border of the misleading. Can integrity be retained in respect of honesty if the relevant facts are not revealed? In theory, advertising should be limited to the dissemination of information from which consumers are able to make an informed choice. If consumers are misled in the attempt to make an intelligent choice or are enticed into the choice by deception, the advertising has an enormous burden of justification. If advertisements are designed not to be rationally persuasive, but rather manipulative, we will almost surely judge them as morally inappropriate.

For many large and diversified companies, it is virtually impossible to claim that products and ingredients have not been tested on animals. What standards of disclosure, then, are appropriate in advertising their products in order that they not be deceptive? The FTC and other regulatory institutions in the United States hold that if consumers are misled by deception, the advertising cannot be justified, morally or legally. The FTC has therefore placed strict regulations on industries that produce products that are potentially harmful to humans.

Typically, both the government and consumer protection groups focus on consumer *response* to advertising and its social effects, rather than on the *intention* of the creators of that advertising. By contrast, those who defend controversial advertising often focus more on the intentions of advertising agencies and manufacturers in marketing a product, namely, the intent to sell a good product. These different emphases complicate the issues, because a product marketed with good intentions can nonetheless be advertised in a misleading way or otherwise have negative consequences. One could view the ethics of cosmetics advertisements by responsible companies as falling into this domain.

A different perspective is that of quality control. If products like cosmetics had to be certified by an independent agency as both safe and free of animal testing in order to be allowed on the market, we might care much less about the messages of advertisements or sales representatives. This view amounts to a call for higher qualitative standards in industry and regulatory branches of government as a means to resolve consumer protection issues.

Too stringent a standard of either disclosure or quality control could thwart the efforts of companies that currently are not doing animal testing, thereby frustrating the goal of preventing unnecessary animal testing. Too weak a standard runs the risks already noted, allowing fraud and causing consumers to lose any meaningful opportunity to select appropriate products.

A coalition of animal protection groups including the Humane Society of the United States, PETA, the Doris Day Animal League, and others began in 1996 to prepare an "animal testing standard" that is to be proposed to all cosmetic manufacturers to bring clarity to the terminology used on cosmetic products. The standard defines what is meant by "animal," "non-animal," and "*in vitro* testing." Individual cosmetic companies are asked to make a commitment to abide by the standard not to conduct or commission animal testing or purchase ingredients from a supplier that conducted animal testing on the company's behalf after the date of agreement. The coalition plans to publicize the names of companies so committed and to identify its products. The standard permits all companies to adopt this policy and to benefit in its marketing from this commitment. In this way, the coalition hopes to exert pressure to end animal testing on cosmetics in the future.

CONCLUSION

Professor Michael Balls, former director of the European Center for the Validation of Alternatives in Methods, suggests that the goal in cosmetic testing should be the manufacture and marketing of new, better, and safer cosmetic products containing new, better, and safer ingredients. This ideal, he thinks, can be achieved using sound cosmetic science and reliable safety assessment, and without using toxicity test procedures on laboratory animals. Balls asserts that action must be taken now to ensure that considerable progress toward this goal is made before a ban on cosmetic testing is effected. In reality, a "ban" will not likely soon be accepted, but, to minimize the criticism from animal protection organizations that will inevitably follow from postponement of a ban, the cosmetics industry and the European Community (EC) are increasingly going to have to provide evidence that they are continuing to support the development, evaluation, and validation of alternative methods of testing. That alternative tests are playing a major role during in-house development and testing of new products will, however, not be morally sufficient in the eyes of animal protection organizations—not in the EC, the United States, or other developed countries. There is certain to be renewed pressure for entirely replacing animal tests for cosmetics with validated alternatives.

NOTES

1. Krys Bottrill, "Growing Old Disgracefully: The Cosmetic Use of Botulinum Toxin," *Alternatives to Laboratory Animals* 31 (2003): 381–91. This article significantly influenced the writing of this case, especially regarding botulinum toxin.

2. J. D. A. Carruthers and J. A. Carruthers, "Treatment of Glabellar Frown Lines with C. Botulinum-A Exotoxin," *Journal of Dermatological Surgery and Oncology* 18 (1992): 17–21.

3. D. W. Straughan, "Progress in Applying the Three Rs to the Potency Testing of Botulinum Toxin Type A," *Alternatives to Laboratory Animals* 34 (2006): 305–13.

4. See *Orange Country News* source "ocregister" of November 10, 2005, www.ocregister.com/ocregister/money/yourcounty/article_760904.php (accessed March 11, 2007).

5. U.K. Royal Society for the Prevention of Cruelty to Animals, "Think Before You Shop . . . Cruelty-Free Product Guide," *Information Sheet* (1995): 22–26.

6. "The Body Shop Animal Protection Statement 95," The Body Shop International PLC, 1996, p. 21.

7. Quoted in Jon Entine, "Shattered Image," *Business Ethics* 8, no. 5 (September/October 1994): 23–28.

8. People for the Ethical Treatment of Animals (PETA), www.stopanimaltests.com/consumerProducts.asp. No posting date given (accessed March 11, 2007).

9. M. Balls, "Comments on Labeling Related to the Animal Testing of Cosmetic Ingredients and Products Manufactured and/or Marketed within the European Economic Community," *Alternatives to Laboratory Animals* 19 (1991): 302–7.

10. Karin L. Bolte of the National Consumers League, letter to the Honorable Robert Pitofsky, Chairman, U.S. Federal Trade Commission, Washington, DC, p. 9.

11. Jodie Bernstein, Director, U.S. Federal Trade Commission, letter to Linda F. Golodner, President, National Consumers' League, July 9, 1996.

12. The formal or "old" LD50 test subjected animals to increasing doses until a significant number of them died so that it was possible to compute a lethal dose of 50% by extrapolation. Normally more than 50% of animals died.

13. See American Veterinary Medical Association, www.avma.org/onlnews/javma/mar03/030301a.asp (posted March 1, 2003, accessed August 25, 2007). See also Enterprise and Industry for an up-to-date summary of the Cosmetics Directive, ec.europa.eu/enterprise/cosmetics/html/cosm_simpl_dir_en.htm (posted May 11, 2007, accessed August 25, 2007).

14. A. N. Rowan, *Of Mice, Models, and Men: A Critical Evaluation of Animal Research* (Albany: State University of New York Press, 1984). Since 1984, Rowan has reestimated the number to be nearer 4 million, but it is impossible to be precise because of poor and inadequate data in the United States.

15. U.S. Department of Health and Human Services, Public Health Service, Food and Drug Administration, "Cosmetics Handbook," 1992, www.cfsan.fda.gov/~dms/cos-hdbk.html (accessed March 12, 2007).

16. Council Directive 93/35/EEC, amending for the sixth time Directive 76/768/EEC, Article 1(1), eur-lex.europa.eu/LexUriServ/site/en/consleg/1976/L/01976L0768-20060809-en.pdf (accessed August 25, 2007).

17. See World Wide Words, created April 18, 1998, www.worldwidewords.org/turnsofphrase/tp-cos1.htm (posted April 18, 1998; accessed March 11, 2007).

18. *In vitro*, literally meaning *in glass*, is used to describe those tests that can be carried out without the use of living animals, although for some tests an animal may have to be killed to provide tissue. *In vivo* tests, on the other hand, require whole, living animals to be used.

19. The OECD test, with which the United States has agreed to comply under the Mutual Acceptance of Data, requires only three rabbits to be used. However, the U.S. Environmental Protection Agency appears to require (or at least request) that six animals are routinely used.

20. Humane Society of the United States, "The Draize Eye-Irritancy Test," *Fact Sheet*, 1993. See also DeWayne H. Walker, "Effects of the Shift to Alternatives on Industrial Practices," *Animal Welfare Information Center Newsletter* 7, no. 1 (Spring 1996), www.nal.usda.gov/awic/newsletters/v7n1/7n1walke.htm (accessed August 25, 2007).

21. The SCC (Scientific Committee on Cosmetology) was established by the European Commission to assist in examining the complex scientific and technical problems surrounding cosmetics composition, manufacture, packaging, and labeling. It has since been renamed the European Scientific Committee on Cosmetic Products and Non-food Products.

22. J. W. Trevan, "The Error of Determination of Toxicity," *Proceedings of the Royal Society of London, Series B* 101 (1927): 483–514.

23. Robert D. Combes, Ian Gaunt, and Michael Balls, "A Scientific and Animal Welfare Assessment of the OECD Health Effects Test Guidelines for the Safety Testing of Chemicals under the European Union REACH System," *Alternatives to Laboratory Animals* 34, suppl. 1 (2006): 77–122.

24. Joe Piccioni, "Welcome Address at the International Conference on Animal Welfare in the Cosmetics and Toiletries Industry," International Conference on Animal Welfare in the Cosmetics and Toiletries Industry (Cosmetics Industry Coalition for Animal Welfare Ltd., 1995), p. 1.

25. Virginia Mathews, "Putting Cruelty to the Test," *Marketing Week*, May 14, 1993, p. 21. The British Union for Anti-Vivisection (BUAV) reports that 85% (whereas the RSPCA finds that 96%) of persons surveyed were against animal testing of beauty and household products. The *UK Daily Mirror* (October 29, 1992) cited a MORI poll (Market & Opinion Research International, Ltd.) giving a figure of 87% not wanting cosmetics tested on animals.

26. D. W. Straughan, "The EU Target for a 50% Reduction in the Use of Experimental Animals by the Year 2000: What Does It Mean?" *Alternatives to Laboratory Animals* 23, no. 2 (1995): 262.

27. European Council Directive 93/35/EEC, amending for the sixth time Directive 76/768/EEC on the approximation of laws of the member states relating to cosmetic products, states that animal testing of ingredients or combinations of ingredients should be banned starting on January 1, 1998, but only if alternative methods of testing have been scientifically validated. This did not happen, and the end date was postponed. See www.colipa.com/site/index.cfm?SID=15588&OBJ=15757#cell_11523 (accessed March 11, 2007).

28. "Animal Use in Testing FDA-Regulated Products," FDA Position Paper, October 1992; see also "Current Policies on the Classical LD50," *Scientists' Center for Animal Welfare (SCAW) Newsletter* 11, no. 3 (Fall 1989): 12.

29. U.S. Environmental Protection Agency, "High Production Volume (HPV) Challenge Program," no posting date given, www.epa.gov/chemrtk/ (accessed August 25, 2007).

30. M. Balls and R. Combes, "The REACH System: Scientific and Animal Welfare Implications of EU Legislation on Chemical Testing," *Alternatives to Laboratory Animals* 34,

suppl. 1 (2006): 158; C. Grindon and R. Combes, "Introduction to the EU REACH legislation," *Alternatives to Laboratory Animals* 34 (2006): 5–10.

31. Christina Grindon, "The New EU REACH Regulation Has Finally Been Adopted," *Alternatives to Laboratory Animals* (2007) 35: 239–42.

32. "Beauty without Cruelty Cosmetic Guide," *Leaflet BWC* (Newlands, S. Africa), November 1990; and New Zealand Anti-Vivisection Society, nzavs.org.nz/mobilise/17/2.html.

33. W. M. S. Russell and R. L. Burch, *The Principles of Humane Experimental Technique* (London: Methuen and Company, 1959).

34. Council Directive 86/609/EEC on the approximation of laws, regulations, and administrative provisions of the member states regarding the protection of animals used for other scientific purposes, Article 7.2, *Official Journal of the European Communities* 29, L.358 (December 18, 1986): 1–29.

35. L. H. Bruner, "Alternatives to the Use of Animals in Household Products and Cosmetic Testing," *Journal of the American Veterinary Medical Association* 200 (1992): 669–73.

36. See European Council Directive 93/35/EEC, ec.europa.eu/enterprise/cosmetics/doc/200315/200315_en.pdf (accessed March 12, 2007).

37. M. Balls and R. Combes, "The Need for a Formal Invalidation Process for Animal and Non-animal Tests," *Alternatives to Laboratory Animals* 33 (2005): 299–308.

38. OECD Environmental Health and Safety Publications Series on Testing and Assessment, No. 19, Guidance Document on the Recognition, Assessment, and Use of Clinical Signs as Humane Endpoints for Experimental Animals Used in Safety Evaluation Environment Directorate, 2000, www.olis.oecd.org/olis/2000doc.nsf/LinkTo/env-jm-mono(2000)7 (accessed March 11, 2007).

39. R. D. Combes, I. Gaunt, and M. Balls, "A Scientific and Animal Welfare Assessment of the OECD Health Effects Test Guidelines for the Safety Testing of Chemicals under the European Union REACH System," *Alternatives to Laboratory Animals* 32 (2004): 163–208.

40. R. J. Fielder, I. F. Gaunt, C. Rhodes, F. M. Sullivan, and D. W. Swanston, "A Hierarchical Approach to the Assessment of Dermal and Ocular Irritancy: A Report by the British Toxicology Society Working Party on Irritancy," *Human Toxicology* 6 (1987): 269–78.

41. M. J. van den Heuvel, D. G. Clark, R. J. Fielder, P. P. Koundakjian, G. J. A. Oliver, D. Pelling, N. J. Tomlinson, and A. P. Walker, "The International Validation of a Fixed Dose Procedure as an Alternative to the Classical LD50 Test," *Food Chemical Toxicology* 28 (1990): 469–82; OECD Revised Guideline 401 (OECD 1987) for acute oral toxicity testing; R. D. Bruce, "An Up-and-Down Procedure for Acute Toxicity Testing," *Fundamental and Applied Toxicology* 6 (1985): 151–57.

42. K. Cussler, D. B. Morton, and C. F. M. Hendriksen, "Humane Endpoints in Vaccine Research and Quality Control," in *Humane Endpoints in Animal Experiments for Biomedical Research,* Proceedings of the International Conference, Zeist, Netherlands, November 22–25, 1998, ed. C. F. M. Hendriksen and D. B. Morton (London: Royal Society of Medicine Press, 1999), pp. 95–101.

43. M. Balls and J. H. Fentem, "The On-Going Process to Replace the LD50 Test," *Humane Innovations and Alternatives* 7 (1993): 544–47.

44. People for the Ethical Treatment of Animals, "Undercover Investigator," *The PETA Guide to Compassionate Living* (Norfolk, VA: PETA, 2007), p. 9, quoting an employee in 1988.

PART VIII

BEHAVIORAL RESEARCH

14

Monkeys without Mothers

Following approximately a six-month gestational period, a pregnant female rhesus monkey (*Macaca mulatta*) begins to show evidence of the imminent birth of her infant. If she lives in a "natural" environment such as a forest in Southeast Asia, she starts to change her usual activity patterns and may move away from the typical social pathways of her group to more secluded and quieter parts of the environment. Her group likely comprises many other adult females, males, and immature animals of varying ages and temperaments. As the time of birth nears, she shows evidence of labor by hunching, squatting, leaning on vertical surfaces, and touching her vagina frequently.

As the labor progresses, the placental sac ruptures and the head of the infant eventually emerges from the birth canal. The mother then reaches between her legs with both hands, carefully grasps the head of the baby with her fingertips, makes a gentle bending movement to the right or left and then firmly pulls the infant free. She immediately places the newborn on her chest.[1] The rhesus monkey infant is born equipped with strong grasping, rooting, and sucking reflexes that help to secure the infant to the mother and help it to locate the nipples and to suckle.

Once the infant is in place, the mother fastidiously cleans the infant, removing all traces of the blood, soil, and amniotic fluid that remain. Once the coat of the infant is dry, active grooming begins. At this time she closes her body around the infant in a warm and protective posture with her pale flesh, hands, and brown grey fur constantly in contact with the infant. The infant reciprocates by grasping the mother's flesh and fur with its hands and feet.

Under field conditions, the infant stays in this close physical bond with the mother for weeks before the loosening grasp of the mother and the emerging curiosity of the infant combine to allow it to make brief excursions, first to other parts of the mother's body and then to other parts of the physical and social environment barely inches away. By three to five months of age the infant may cautiously start to move brief distances away from the actual grasp of the mother. Here it begins to encounter other animals, including other infants.[2]

Though the infant does not go far during these excursions, the attention of the mother remains riveted on the infant. Similarly, the infant completely depends on the presence of the mother as a base of security from which these tentative expressions of independence can be safely launched. Infants are actively protected by their mothers from overly rambunctious play partners and from more aggressive and less tolerant group members; there is an absolute certainty of direct intervention should it be required. The mother responds with haste and patience to the demands of her infant. Her ministrations, more often than not, bring ease and relief to a frightened or hungry infant. Breaks in this responsiveness result in intense emotional distress and behavioral disruption on the part of the infant. Should the mother disappear or die during this early period of development, the infant, if not adopted by another female, would certainly die.

As its first year progresses, the infant spends more and more time away from the direct physical control of the mother. It becomes involved in the work of playing and bonding with other infants and group members. Yet the connection between the mother and infant remains obvious and enduring. Rest, protection, nutrition, play, and sleep are sought in the comfort of the mother's proximity and embrace. The explicitness of this attachment relationship continues at least until the birth of the next infant, which requires a more active process of weaning. Even then, and perhaps for the rest of the life of the mother, her offspring, both male and female, maintain a lifelong recognition of and deference for her, and she for them.[3]

It is clear that in the field environment, the separation from or loss of its mother is a natural and unfortunate tragedy for the rhesus monkey infant. Its consequences are played out with Darwinian directness. Because of the stark and predictable consequences of such a separation, biological mechanisms have evolved to prevent this loss or separation. Therefore, raising monkeys without mothers is virtually certain to produce profound confusion, disorientation, distress, and behavioral changes in the infants.

Yet the practice of purposely raising monkeys without access to mothers and peers has had a long history in research on the experimental psychology of development. Monkeys have been raised without or separated from mothers for various scientific reasons: to test theories of attachment, to create models of a variety of human behavioral disorders, and to test the effect of certain medications proposed to treat those human disorders, to name just a few.

HARLOW AND HIS MONKEYS

Perhaps most notable among those researchers who have used this rearing procedure as a central part of their work was the late Harry F. Harlow (1905–81) of the University of Wisconsin. While other researchers have separated infant monkeys from their mothers for research purposes, Harlow has perhaps received the greatest amount of attention from the animal protection community, at least in part because of the acclaim he received from many of his scientific peers.[4] Harlow's motives for using this procedure have been characterized by elements of the animal protection community as expressions of sadism or at least extreme indifference, and his research has been declared redundant and irrelevant.[5] Others have staunchly defended his character and his work, pointing out its major and enduring significance.[6] It is fair to say that both the man and the work have been at the vortex of ethical debate since at least the mid-1970s.

Any discussion of the science and the ethics of Harlow's work must begin by acknowledging that he was a most productive and professionally acclaimed psychologist. He published over 300 articles and books and graduated 36 PhD students over an active research career that spanned nearly 50 years. Along the way he received virtually every significant prize for scientific achievement available. For example, he received the Gold Medal from the American Psychological Association in 1973, membership in the American Philosophical Society, and was the first psychologist to be elected a member of the National Academy of Sciences. He received the National Medal of Science from President Lyndon Johnson in 1967 and the Kittay Award from the psychiatric community in 1975.

The historical context in which Harlow's work proceeded is also important. He was an early soldier in the profession of experimental psychology's campaign to be acknowledged as a natural science. This acknowledgement was judged to require the adoption and application of a strictly scientific methodology, then widely interpreted to mean the explicit use of experiment and controlled observation.[7] Inference from uncontrolled observation was not sufficient.

Harlow's work was extensively chronicled in scientific journals, the popular press, and TV documentaries. He traveled and spoke constantly to large and small audiences at scientific meetings, interest groups, and thousands of introductory psychology students who attended the University of Wisconsin. He rarely turned down any serious group who made a request for him to discuss his ideas. He was proud of his work and actively exposed the form, structure, and proposed implications of his research to the scientific community and lay public.

Soon after he joined the faculty of the University of Wisconsin, he initiated a research program concerned with learning abilities of nonhuman primates. In this program he adapted for animal use some of the evaluation techniques of the human intelligence testing movement. As the results of this research program proved successful, he found it necessary to establish his own facilities where he could specify more precisely the conditions of housing and testing.

THE MIND OF THE RHESUS MONKEY

Harlow's work on the process and manner by which monkeys learn to solve discrimination problems began to attract interested attention in the 1940s. The attention came as he began to defend an unpopular theoretical position. He proposed that monkeys solve discrimination problems by developing various hypotheses about the solution and then by testing them; the process of learning occurs as incorrect hypotheses are steadily eliminated in favor of the correct approach.

In some of these experiments, monkeys were tested in an apparatus in which they were presented with two three-dimensional objects that differed from one another in a variety of ways (e.g. color, shape, and size). One of the objects was randomly selected as "correct." The objects were presented to the monkey on a sliding tray, which was moved to within the monkey's reach when the trial was to begin. The monkeys were trained to make their choice by pushing the object to one side. If the monkey chose the correct object, a small piece of food would be revealed beneath it in a small, shallow well. The food was then quickly eaten or stored in the monkey's large-capacity cheek pouches to be consumed at another time. The position of the correct object would be changed at random from one side of the tray to the other. Each separate problem would be presented for a fixed number of trials, usually six.

The monkeys were tested on literally hundreds of these problems over the course of several months. As the monkeys' experience proceeded, it was observed that their performance improved to the point where they eventually made errors on only the first trial of a new problem. In Harlow's words, the monkeys had "learned how to learn" by applying a "win-stay, lose-shift" strategy: If on the first trial of a new problem the monkey "won," that is, was rewarded for its choice, it should "stay" with that object in whatever position the object appeared on the tray during the following trials. If, on the other hand, the monkey "lost" on the first trial, it learned to shift to the other object on all succeeding trials.[8]

Harlow's hypothesis was controversial for a number of reasons. First, it flew in the face of the rather mechanistic explanations of animal learning then favored by the dominant behaviorist school. This mechanistic perspective tried to explain the changes seen during learning as the result of the connection or disconnection of small response units to specific stimuli through the action of contiguity, reward, non-reward, and punishment, not as the development of cognitive strategies. In addition, the whole process of learning was thought to be motivated by the need to reduce internal biological drives like hunger and thirst.[9]

Clearly Harlow's notions painted a very different picture of primate learning and the "mind" of the monkey. He described monkeys as having complex cognitive abilities that involved the existence of intentions, curiosity, and solution plans. This was not a description of the insensate automata implied by the behaviorist explanations. As for the drive reduction theory of motivation, Harlow revealed that he fed the animals in his experiments their normal day's ration of food *before* he tested them on his discrimination problems. He described the monkeys as participating in these problems with their cheek pouches full of food, swallowing bits of that food after having made either correct or incorrect responses.[10] This picture was devastating to purely behavioristic interpretations, which depended on differential drive reduction to account for behavior change and correct responding.

Harlow encountered criticisms of his interpretations on methodological grounds as well. One of the foundational criticisms was that because the monkeys in Harlow's experiments had been captured and imported as adults from the forests and cities of southern Asia, one could not be certain that the responses observed during the laboratory experiments were not acquired previously in the complex natural environments from which these animals had been snatched.

Harlow reasoned that in order to respond to the criticism he had to establish experimentally the ontogeny (course of development in the individual) of learning abilities in rhesus monkeys. He would then be able to determine empirically the point in time when various learning abilities emerge. Together with A. J. Blomquist, Harlow developed a protocol[11] in which infant rhesus monkeys could be separated from their mothers at or soon after birth and raised in a nursery where their life experiences could be tightly controlled for as long as required by the experimental design.[12] At this point, ethical problems began to be discernible in Harlow's work.

The Motherless Monkey as Experimental Control

The first step required a procedure in which the gestational stage of pregnant females could be known. With this information the experimenters would know when to be present to separate the infant from the mother as soon after birth as possible. Once the infants were separated they would be housed alone in small wire mesh cages where they could be fed and cared for according to strict schedules. During the first months after birth, the singly housed infants were placed in a setting modeled after a human nursery. The cages with Plexiglas and wire mesh walls were arranged so that the monkeys could see and hear other infants but could not contact one another physically. A staff of technicians prepared formula and bottle fed the infants around the clock.

During the initial feedings the small infants were wrapped snugly in a gauze cheese-cloth that restrained the monkey firmly without injury while it was hand-held and trained to drink from a bottle. This human-infant contact was maintained only for the minimum amount of time required to complete the feedings. Once the feedings were completed, the infant was placed back into its individual wire cage with a clean cloth provided as insulation against the barren metal cage floor. The monkeys tended to wrap themselves in this cloth while they were alone in their cages, a fact that would change the course and purpose of raising monkeys without mothers at a later time.

Once the infants had gained strength and mobility, the formula was presented to the monkeys on a small inclined rack. The rack mimicked the feeding position of mother-reared infants. It provided the infants with an apparatus that would support their weight and climbing abilities and that further reduced the amount of necessary contact with human handlers. Once the monkeys were old enough, they were weaned to a cup and then to solid food. They were moved to larger individual cages and into standard holding rooms. There the animals stayed for months or years until they were assigned to a learning experiment. They were removed from their "home" cages for weekly weighing, cage cleaning, occasional health checks, and regular TB testing. The monkeys could see and hear other monkeys but could not physically contact them.

At this point in history, rearing monkeys without access to mothers and without physical access to peers was considered by Harlow to be a procedure whose main purpose was to standardize the pre-experimental ages and histories of the monkeys to be used in his experiments on learning. These procedures were viewed as a legitimate and sound way for an experimentalist to control the effects of variables that could potentially confound the interpretation of an experiment. From an experimental perspective, the procedures proved useful. Harlow and his associates detailed the learning capacities of rhesus monkeys beginning within the first week after birth until sexual maturity. The results supported his earlier descriptions of monkey learning.[13]

Harlow did not intend to "do" anything to the monkeys in this work in order to change them. Nor did he want to produce a defect or injury in them, since this would only serve to complicate further the results of the experiments that the procedure was intended to clarify. Less clear, however, is whether or not Harlow believed that raising monkeys in the prescribed manner would produce distress and discomfort, and whether this risk mattered to him. The only hint of an answer to this question is that in his writing he takes pride in the fact that the mortality rates of his nursery-reared animals were lower than in the wild as well as in infants reared by their own mothers in the laboratory environment. He almost seems to be boasting that he and his staff were better monkey mothers than were monkey mothers.[14]

RAISING MONKEYS WITHOUT MOTHERS AS AN INVESTIGATIVE PROCEDURE

The initial reason Harlow raised monkeys without mothers was to standardize life histories and ages of animals in experiments in order to eliminate potential problems in his research. However, a significant shift occurred in this intention: Harlow began to use the motherless rearing protocol as a way to learn something about the psychological make-up of the animals. Harlow now wanted to discover the factors that contribute to the attachment bond that so obviously exists between a mother and her infant. Clearly human and nonhuman offspring alike maintain proximity to the mother and seek out her protection at times of stress and danger. But what mechanisms account for the connection? Pursuit of this question became a turning point in Harlow's research career and moved him from the ranks of the respected psychological researchers to the rarefied atmosphere of the famous and, to some, the infamous.

In the 1950s, explanations of the basis of development of the early attachment bond between human mothers or caretakers and their infants consisted of four positions:

1. The theory of secondary drive. According to this perspective, the infant becomes attached to the mother because the mother's actions meet the infant's pressing physiological needs.
2. The theory of primary object sucking. Here the infants are considered to possess an inborn need to relate to the breast and to suck it.
3. The theory of primary object clinging. Under this explanation, the infant is believed to possess a built-in need to touch and to cling.
4. The theory of primary return-to-womb craving. Here the infant is seen as resenting its expulsion from the womb and seeking to return there. Therefore, the infant stays in close proximity to the mother.

The first two explanations stress the importance of the early feeding situation. The act of feeding the dependent infant, thereby reducing its hunger drive, establishes through reinforcement the behaviors of approach, contact, and maintenance of proximity by the infant. These attachment behaviors are then considered to be "derived" from the more basic and essential action of drive reduction. Elements of these explanations were favored by proponents of both the behavioristic perspective and certain psychoanalytic traditions, two groups who tended to agree on almost nothing. On the other hand, members of the psychoanalytic tradition called the British Middle Group believed in the third alternative and the innate importance of contact and clinging in the development of attachment. Prominent among these theorists was psychoanalyst John Bowlby.[15] The fourth position also had prominent adherents.

To test these differing conceptualizations in the format of a traditional experiment would require an approach that could determine the effect of feeding independently from these other factors. One obvious complicating factor was that a living mother or caretaker could not easily be created that could feed an infant without also holding it. The act of holding an infant to the breast or cradling the infant during bottle feeding automatically exposed the infant to a host of other factors. Prominent among these were body heat, skin, surface texture, heart sounds, and vocalizations. Thus, an experiment that was to test the feeding explanation of early attachment would require that feeding occur in the absence of all or most of those other factors. If such a situation could be created, one then could assess whether attachment developed or not. But how could such an experimental arrangement be created?

THE DEVELOPMENT OF THE MOTHER SURROGATE

According to Harlow's own description of the development of the experimental approach, the solution to the problem came to him in a vision: in late 1957 Harlow was returning to Madison, Wisconsin, from a business trip to Detroit, Michigan. He was still in need of a topic for his presidential address to the American Psychological Association, which he would deliver the next year. He wanted something strong, dramatic, and critical of drive reduction theorists who remained very influential in psychology. It was late, and he had consumed a fair amount of complimentary airline champagne. As he turned to look out the window above Lake Michigan, he visualized in the empty seat next to him a fully formed mechanical mother surrogate: "As I turned to look out the window, I saw the cloth surrogate sitting in the seat beside me with all her bold and barren charms."[16] The mother in the vision had a cylindrical body that leaned back at approximately a 45-degree angle. In the upper third of her chest was an aperture where a feeding bottle could be inserted. It was also clear that the cylindrical body could accommodate coverings of various textures from soft and warm to cold and rough.

The visualized model seemed to contain all the attributes necessary to test the nutritional theory of early attachment in monkeys. Contact comfort could be presented with or without feeding, and rough-textured "mothers" could be made to be the source of nutrition. Harlow already had an idea that the monkeys would attach to soft-textured mothers. As mentioned earlier, the basic nursery-rearing protocol had included presenting a soft cheesecloth gauze pad to the newborn infants that were held in individual wire mesh cages. The monkeys invariably wrapped themselves up in those cloths and showed clear signs of disturbance when the cloths were removed; the monkeys grabbed onto them tightly, resisting the technicians' attempts to take them away. Once removed, the infant monkeys screeched and jerked convulsively in protest. When a clean cloth was returned, the disturbance calmed immediately as they recontacted the cloth.[17]

These observations were powerful, but they were not definitive, and they did not meet the requirements of a "true" experiment, which requires specificity and controlled comparisons. Casual observations in an uncontrolled setting like a nursery would not do, especially for a presidential address to the American Psychological Association, an association deeply involved in the continuing struggle for recognition as a "hard" science.

The Initial Mother-Surrogate Experiments

After his vision, Harlow soon commenced conducting a series of mother surrogate experiments designed to test the central controversies. The present discussion will focus on the report published in the journal *Science* in 1959.[18] *Science*, the oldest American scientific publication, has been devoted to the dissemination of new, provocative findings; it has been said that publication in this journal can make a research career. Therefore, competition for publication in this periodical is fierce. For a psychologist like Harry Harlow to have a paper accepted for publication in *Science* would indicate the potential significance of the experiments and would show that psychology is in reality a scientific enterprise in the same way that biology, physiology, and chemistry are legitimate scientific enterprises.

Harlow's paper in *Science* reports the results of 14 distinguishable experimental tests. The experiments were divided into the core demonstration of the effect of nutrition on the preference for an inanimate surrogate, fear-challenge tests designed to determine the initial existence of an attachment, and whether the attachments maintained their strength over time. The article reports that the cloth mother was constructed from a cylinder of wood covered with a sheath of terry cloth, whereas a wire surrogate mother was constructed of a hardware-cloth cylinder. The cylinders were mounted on an aluminum base situated at a 45-degree angle. Each surrogate had a distinctively different wooden head.

Dual Surrogates

In the initial experiment, eight newborn rhesus monkeys were separated from their mothers and were placed individually in standard laboratory cages. Attached to each cage were two booths containing a cloth surrogate and a wire surrogate. For half of the monkeys, their total nutrition was obtained from bottles available on the cloth surrogate, while the nutritional allotment for the remaining monkeys was available from the wire mother. A gauze-covered heating pad was also available to all the monkeys on the floor of their cages, positioned away from the surrogates during the first 14 days of the experiment. The mean number of hours each monkey spent in contact with the two different surrogates was recorded for a minimum of 165 days.

Results showed that by day 25, all the monkeys chose to spend nearly 18 hours a day in direct physical contact with the cloth surrogate regardless of the surrogate from which the monkey received its feedings. Contact with the wire mother was minimal throughout the experiment, stabilizing at about one and one-half hours per day with no difference between the monkeys fed on the wire surrogates or those fed on the cloth surrogates. On the surface, it appeared that the nutritional theory of attachment had been defeated by this rather simple demonstration. However, Harlow recognized that the observed differential contact time between the cloth and the wire mothers might simply reflect the fact that the cloth mothers were a more comfortable "nest" and not that an actual psychological bond had been established. In other words, attachment and comfort explanations both fit the data.

Fear-Challenge Tests

In order to eliminate this ambiguity, Harlow arranged a series of challenges in which the monkeys were exposed to stimuli and situations known to produce fear in infant monkeys—the kind of fear that would, under normal rearing situations, drive an infant to seek protection and contact from an attachment object like a "real" mother, but not from another object. What would these surrogate-reared monkeys do when faced with these circumstances?

Fear-challenge tests involved introducing fear-provoking objects (e.g., a mechanical toy bear) into the home cage of the infant monkeys living with the cloth and the wire surrogates and observing their response. The introductions occurred three times during the first 22 days of age and then every 20 days afterward. Two types of data were recorded: first, the type of the surrogate to which the monkey retreated when first exposed to the intruder; and second, the quality of the response made once the chosen surrogate was contacted. Results showed that when the infant monkeys were exposed to a fear stimulus they strongly tended to retreat to the cloth surrogate, regardless of the feeding arrangements they had experienced. In addition, once the monkeys were in contact with the cloth surrogates their fear responses rapidly reduced, to the point that some of them ventured back toward the stimulus and explored it.

Single Surrogates

Other experiments involved animals that were raised with the experience of only one surrogate. One group of four monkeys was raised with and bottle fed from a single wire surrogate. A second group of four monkeys lived with a cloth mother who did not provide nutrition. By raising monkeys with only a feeding wire surrogate, Harlow was attempting to determine whether a bond could be nutritionally created with a wire surrogate if the infant was provided no opportunities to experience a cloth surrogate providing contact comfort.

Results showed that, consistent with the previous experiments, monkeys raised with nonfeeding cloth surrogates spent nearly 18 hours per day in contact with the surrogate. Monkeys raised with only feeding wire surrogates increased their time in contact with the surrogate from 6 to 12 hours per day over the course of 165 days. These findings suggested that under certain circumstances an attachment bond could be derived from a feeding relationship. The nutritional theory once again had to be reconsidered.

Did this nutritionally based relationship confer the kind of protections or reassurances that had been observed for the cloth surrogate monkeys? Home cage challenge tests showed that though the wire surrogate infants retreated from the fear objects in the direction of their surrogates, the monkeys did not embrace them. Nor did they show a reduction in fear that had been seen for the cloth surrogate groups. Instead, these animals clutched themselves, body-rocked, called out, and screamed until the fear object was removed. These findings were interpreted as further evidence against the nutritional theory of attachment. In other tests, it was found that monkeys reared in the dual or single cloth surrogate conditions worked to gain visual access to their cloth surrogates and to a live monkey to an equivalent degree. Single-wire-reared monkeys with no cloth surrogate experience strongly preferred to view the live monkey.

Open Field Challenge and Attachment Retention Tests

Drawing on previously published tests of human children on the effects of attachment, Harlow compared the behavior of single-surrogate-reared monkeys with monkeys raised without surrogate experience in a novel open field environment. The open field was a small room filled with unusual objects and toys. The monkey's surrogate was present in the environment on half of the open field exposures. It was found that monkeys raised with single cloth mothers used their surrogate mothers as bases of operation from which they explored the novel environment. Monkeys raised with single wire surrogates were found to be highly emotional and distressed even when their surrogate was present in the field. Due to their highly typical rocking and huddling, Harlow likened their behavior to that of autistic "institutionalized human children."

Harlow also continued to assess the nature and strength of the attachment bond by checking the responsiveness of the various groups to their mother surrogates once they had been permanently separated from them. He found that the monkeys raised with access to the cloth surrogates continued to work to gain visual access to her form for at least the next 15 months. Monkeys raised with wire surrogates alone showed no such maintenance. Similarly, retention tests conducted in the open field showed that monkeys reared with cloth surrogates continued to contact the surrogate when tested over the three-month period following separation and showed reduced emotionality in the novel environment. Wire-reared infants, on the other hand, showed no such preference, and did not have ameliorated levels of emotional distress.

In a variant of the open field challenge, Harlow placed the monkey's surrogate in a Plexiglas box that blocked direct contact. Harlow reports that following several "violent crashes," cloth-surrogate-reared monkeys adjusted to the condition and continued to show levels of reduced emotionality. These results supported the idea that the infants benefited from the presence of the surrogate even though direct contact was prevented. Little of that kind of benefit was observed for the wire-reared monkeys. In other challenge tests, Harlow found that the monkeys would travel a more "dangerous" route to get to the cloth surrogates.

In summary, there are four core findings from these experiments:

1. Infant monkeys preferred to maintain contact with surrogates with a soft body texture regardless of the feeding arrangements.
2. When exposed to fear-provoking situations, monkeys both sought physical proximity to the cloth surrogates and also appeared to calm in their presence.
3. Infant monkeys raised with cloth surrogates would learn to operate a lever in order to get even a brief visual glimpse of their surrogate.
4. After separation from the surrogates, monkeys raised with cloth surrogates showed retention of these indices of attachment for at least the next year.

An additional finding was that the monkeys raised with wire surrogates and exposed to the fear situations showed a host of bizarre and clearly abnormal behaviors like body-rocking and self-clasping. Harlow again likened these behaviors to those seen in severely disturbed and institutionalized autistic children. This finding was to be experimentally exploited to a great extent later as the animal-model approach to the study of abnormal behavior gained support and attention. It was also later discovered that all the surrogate-reared females showed deficient social and maternal behavior when they became pregnant some years later.

ETHICAL ISSUES

These behavioral observations of monkeys reared with surrogate mothers profoundly influenced the acceptance of psychology as an experimental discipline. The moral problems surrounding the research are no less important, as has been widely recognized. The descriptions and pictures of monkeys clinging tightly to cloth-covered cylinders or writhing in distress in the absence of any form of comfort made, and continues to make, an indelible impression on readers, students, and scholars of the discipline.

Research Benefits

Although these experiments were conducted nearly 50 years ago, virtually all modern-day introductory psychology texts prominently discuss their relevance in sections concerned with explanations of human development. Teachers commonly find that the facts of these experiments consistently elicit a strong response. The reality and meaning of maternal attachment is laid bare and is made unmistakable by the data and the pictures. The pedagogical force of the experimental demonstrations and their ability to communicate important developmental concepts has been repeatedly demonstrated. Many believe that this work profoundly influenced the way modern psychology is conceived as a scientific discipline and its relevance to important issues such as child-rearing practices.

As discussed earlier, the central focus of the surrogate work was on the debates concerning theories of attachment. Seriously flawed notions about the development of human attachment were refuted by this experimental work. We learned that good mental health itself is essentially dependent upon the parent and child establishing and learning to maintain proper attachment relationships. Contact comfort and expression of parental love for the infant were shown to be fundamental ingredients for an adequate rearing environment. In one observer's view, the discovery of this conclusion "may be compared to that of the role of vitamins in physical health."[19] Interpreting the attachment process as a side effect to feeding had helped to maintain blindness to this fundamental principle, with potentially disastrous consequences for the promotion of proper child-rearing practices and the treatment of mentally ill children.[20] It is important to keep in mind that beliefs about appropriate child rearing practices in the early part of the twentieth century were dominated by notions about the importance of strict discipline and scheduling, not the nurturance of parental infant-child attachment. For example, the prominent psychologist John B. Watson claimed in 1928 that warm nurturing interactions were actually a danger. He wrote: "When you are tempted to pet your child remember that mother love is a dangerous instrument. An instrument which may inflict a never healing wound, a wound which may make infancy unhappy, adolescence a nightmare, an instrument which may wreck your adult son or daughter's vocational future and their chances for marital happiness." He suggested that parents shake hands with their children rather than hug or kiss them.[21] Harlow's work is seen by many as providing a crucial data-based counterforce to this tradition. Harlow put it this way: "Remember, for every mistreated monkey there exist a million mistreated children; if my work will point this out and save only one million human children, I really can't get concerned about ten monkeys."[22]

Harlow's experiments have also revealed a great deal about the cognitive and emotional life of monkeys. The pictures of infant monkeys cuddling and rubbing their bodies on the soft surrogate mothers or crying out in fear and distress during the challenge tests, coupled with the findings from the learning experiments, filled the behaviorist's empty animal with feeling and thought. The meaning of Darwin's concept of mental continuity in the species in nature (see the introduction, pp. 11–14) was illustrated in clear relief. Others have argued that advanced appreciation of human-like characteristics and rearing requirements of monkeys provided by these experiments eventually helped to improve the welfare of laboratory animals as the findings informed the evolution of animal husbandry techniques.[23]

Costs and Harms to the Animals

These benefits must be placed in context with the substantial costs and harms to the animals that resulted from a variety of sources. There were, for example, background costs associated with establishing a breeding colony, which required the purchase and importation of monkeys trapped in the forests of Southeast Asia. There was the stress and pain of trapping, separation from group members, injury, disease and death of animals in transport, and the stress of adaptation to a laboratory environment upon arrival. Standard laboratory existence consisted of individual housing in stark metal cages with little or no opportunity to interact socially; adaptation for an animal that had spent its entire life in a social context was quite difficult. Once the females gave birth there was the stress of the separation experienced by both the mother and the infant.[24]

During the first experiments designed to test the preferences for the wire and cloth surrogates, while being provided the fundamental elements of warmth, postural support, and nutrition required for survival, the infants were deprived of the common maternal care responses such as holding, cleaning, and grooming. They were required to live alone in individual cages, a condition completely alien to the evolutionary preparation of the species.

In terms of the challenge experiments, the direct examination of the effects of stress and fear was to a great extent the purpose of the experiments. Attachment, by definition, is a process that is revealed by behavior generated by stressful situations. Therefore the initial and retention challenge tests are described as purposely producing reactions in the infant monkeys such as crouching, rocking, convulsive jerking, self-clutching, and freezing, or, as Harlow himself put it, "abject terror."[25] One could ask whether the entire array of tests was necessary to make the point that attachment had been established and maintained with the cloth mothers. The later experiments seem to depict a hunt for an ever more dramatic demonstration of an already demonstrated attachment finding.

As several psychologists have maintained, it is not clear whether Harlow discovered anything new, or at least anything that could not have been discovered without the use of the monkeys involved. Even Bowlby, one of Harlow's staunchest supporters, seems to suggest that the work had primarily a rhetorical effect on debates that were already under way.[26] For example, the philosopher Theodor Adorno, a fugitive from Nazi Germany, wrote a book in 1950 titled *The Authoritarian Personality* in which he argued that rearing children in strict, coldly disciplined homes helped to create the ground from which bigoted and authoritarian adults emerge. Further, others have pointed out that the importance of permissive, warm rearing environments were already being widely promoted in venues such as the pamphlets by the Department of Labor's Children's Bureau and Benjamin Spock's book *Baby and Child Care*, both of which were published before 1950. Spock's book sold more than 28 million copies over the course of its history.[27] Is a new "emphasis" in a field a discovery worthy of the suffering of the animals in these and related experiments? Must we adhere to the entrenched belief that a scientific theory requires a controlled experiment for acceptance?

We might also ask whether we would approve this work if it were proposed today and came before an institutional animal care and use committee. What modifications would be needed? Is a dramatic demonstration and powerful teaching tool worth the discomfort and suffering of an intelligent and emotionally complex animal?

The Problem of Retrospective Moral Judgment

When reviewing Harlow and his work, we should recall the assumptions of the period in which the work was done. The Animal Welfare Act did not exist until 1966 and did not directly influence experimental designs until 1985. It is today widely believed, as the chairman of the Chemical Manufacturers Association once put it, that "you cannot judge people or a company based on today's standards or knowledge for actions taken 40 to 60 years ago."[28] This thesis suggests that people who use animals cannot be held responsible for catching, transport, and research practices that were deemed professionally appropriate a half century ago. But is this thesis right? Can we not judge Harlow and the institution where he worked at all?

It may help here to introduce a distinction between judging the *rightness or wrongness* of an action and judging the *blameworthiness or praiseworthiness* of the agents who perform those actions. In many circumstances, it is reasonable to say that an action was wrong but that the agent had no basis for knowing that it was wrong and therefore is not blameworthy. Blame is often mitigated by lack of factual information, cultural beliefs, a person's good character, and perhaps by institutional expectations. But were these mitigating conditions in place in the case of Harry Harlow? On the more fundamental level, is there any basis even for judging that he did anything wrong?

NOTES

1. O. L. Tinklepaugh and K. G. Hartman, "Behavioral Aspects of Parturition in the Monkey (*Macaca rhesus*)," *Comparative Psychology* 11 (1932): 63–98.

2. R. A. Hinde, T. E. Rowell, and Y. Sencer-Booth, "Behavior of Socially Living Rhesus Monkeys in Their First Six Months," *Proceedings of the Zoological Society of London* 143 (1964): 609–49.

3. R. A. Hinde and Y. Spencer-Booth, "The Behavior of Socially Living Rhesus Monkeys in Their First Two and a Half Years," *Animal Behavior* 15 (1967): 169–96.

4. L. A. Rosenblum, "Harry F. Harlow: Remembrance of a Pioneer in Developmental Psychobiology," *Developmental Psychobiology* 20 (1987): 15–23.

5. See M. Stephens, *Maternal Deprivation Experiments in Psychology: A Critique of Animal Models* (Jenkintown, PA: American Antivivisection Society, 1986).

6. See W. S. Gilmer and W. T. McKinney, "Early Experience and Depressive Disorders: Human and Nonhuman Primate Studies," *Journal of Affective Disorders* 75 (2003): 97–113; and D. Blum, *Love at Goon Park: Harry Harlow and the Science of Affection* (Cambridge, MA: Perseus, 2002).

7. See E. G. Boring, "The Validation of Scientific Belief," *Proceedings of the American Philosophical Society* 96 (1952): 535–39.

8. H. F. Harlow, "The Formation of Learning Sets," *Psychological Review* 56 (1949): 51–65.

9. See K. W. Spence, "Cognitive versus Stimulus-Response Theories of Learning," *Psychological Review* 57 (1950): 159–72.

10. H. F. Harlow, "Mice, Monkeys, Men, and Motives," *Psychological Review* 60 (1953): 23–32.

11. Based on the previous work of Gertrude van Wagenen; see E. J. Farris, *The Care and Breeding of Laboratory Animals* (New York: Wiley, 1950).

12. A. J. Blomquist and H. F. Harlow, "The Infant Rhesus Monkey Program at the University of Wisconsin Primate Laboratory," *Proceedings of the Animal Care Panel* (April 1961): 57–64.

13. See H. F. Harlow, "The Development of Learning in the Rhesus Monkey," *American Scientist* 47 (1959): 459–79.

14. See H. F. Harlow, "Of Love in Infants," *Natural History* 69 (1960): 18.

15. J. Bowlby, "The Nature of the Child's Tie to Its Mother," *International Journal of Psychoanalysis* 39 (1958): 350–73.

16. H. F. Harlow, M. K. Harlow, and S. J. Suomi, "From Thought to Therapy: Lessons from a Primate Laboratory," *American Scientist* 59 (1971): 539.

17. Observations recorded by the nineteenth-century evolutionary theorist Alfred R. Wallace on the strong attachment of an orphaned baby orangutan to a "mother" made of a roll of buffalo skin had previously captured this intuition. See D. Blum, *The Monkey Wars* (New York: Oxford University Press, 1994), p. 89.

18. H. F. Harlow, "Affectional Responses in the Infant Monkey," *Science* 130 (1959): 421–32. We have chosen this paper for three reasons: First, because the paper is a quite complete description of the initial surrogate experiments written for a wide scientific audience and not just for psychologists; second, because it introduces the use of observational methods and illustrative photography, which were to become keynotes of Harlow's work during this period; and third, because of the very nature and stature of the journal in which the report appears.

19. J. Bowlby, *Child Care and the Growth of Love* (Harmondsworth, England: Penguin Books, 1953), p. 69.

20. See J. Bowlby, *Maternal Care and Mental Health* (Geneva: World Health Organization, 1951); R. Spitz, "Hospitalism: An Enquiry into the Genesis of Psychiatric Conditions of Early Childhood," *Psychoanalytic Study of the Child* 1 (1945): 53–74.

21. J. B. Watson, *Psychological Care of Infant and Child* (New York: W. W. Norton, 1928), p. 87.

22. D. Blum, *Love at Goon Park*, p. 292.

23. See G. C. Ruppenthal and D. J. Reese, *The Nursery Care of Nonhuman Primates* (New York: Plenum Press, 1979).

24. It is important to note that the establishment of primate laboratories also creates health risks to humans brought about by disease transmission, bite wounds, etc. For example, since 1932 at least 40 laboratory and animal care technicians have contracted a meningoencephalitis caused by B-virus infections contracted from laboratory-housed rhesus monkeys, with a mortality rate of 70%. The most recent case was reported in 1997 at the Yerkes Regional Primate Research Center. See A. E. Palmer, "*Herpesvirus Simae*: Historical Perspective," *Journal of Medical Primatology* 16 (1987): 99–130; and Centers for Disease Control and Prevention, "Fatal *Cercopithecine herpesvirus 1* (B Virus) Infection Following a Mucocutaneous Exposure and Interim Recommendations for Worker Protection," *Morbidity and Mortality Weekly Report* 47 (1998): 1073–76.

25. H. F. Harlow, "Affectional Responses in the Infant Monkey," p. 423.

26. J. Bowlby, *A Secure Base* (New York: Basic Books, 1988), p. 26.

27. N. P. Weiss, "Mother, the Invention of Necessity: Dr. Benjamin Spock's *Baby and Child Care*," *American Quarterly* 29, no. 5 (1977): 519–46.

28. "Ex-Owner of Toxic Site Wins Ruling on Damages," *New York Times,* March 18, 1994, p. 5B.

15

The Experimental Study of Animal Aggression

Can aggression be studied in an ethical manner? Aggression is a behavior found almost universally in the animal kingdom. It is defined as a hostile act that poses a threat to another creature. It is exhibited in many ways, including threatening body movements, vocalization, fighting, wounding and inflicting pain, sexual attack, and killing. Commonly, animals act aggressively to exclude others from their territory, to capture food, or to control populations. Displays of aggression are influenced by age (newborns and infants below a certain age do not show aggression), by the physical environment, by previous social experience, and by the aggression level in a particular community. One manifestation of aggression is infanticide—the killing of infants by adults. It occurs in several species of animal. Human infanticide is practiced in several cultures to control population, to favor the birth of a particular sex (usually male), and in waging war.

THE HISTORICAL BACKGROUND OF THE
SCIENTIFIC STUDY OF AGGRESSIVE BEHAVIOR

In the eighteenth and nineteenth centuries, biologists reported anecdotal observations of infanticide in both male and female wild animals. But it was not until the mid-twentieth century that scientific experiments about aggressive encounters including fighting, infanticide, and predation were reported in the scientific literature. The study

231

of animal behavior was then a newly established discipline. Much interest was aroused when researchers identified a hierarchy of dominant and submissive animals. Several avenues were investigated to address Darwin's concept of sexual competition in selecting a mate. In animals, infanticidal behavior has been described as a type of social pathology induced by overcrowding and by intense competition for scarce resources. Some investigators suggested that infanticide may be a genetically influenced aspect of an animal's "normal" behavioral repertory—an adaptive strategy in circumstances of food shortage, for example. Under those conditions, maternal culling of the litter could be so considered.

Many biological variables remain uncontrolled in field studies, making it difficult to state unequivocally that the observed infanticide was attributable to a particular underlying mechanism. So some animal behavior researchers turned to laboratory-based studies in which conditions could be more readily controlled. Rodents became a commonly used species because they breed readily in the laboratory, and individuals or entire litters of neonates can be introduced to male or female test subjects. In the mid-twentieth century, the focus was on understanding more about the subject animal, but, as time passed, many began to consider the possible applications of this research to aggressive behavior exhibited by humans.

Laboratory-based studies of infanticide in themselves were controversial because they were manipulated by humans. But additional worries focused on the possible cruelty of the experimental procedures being tried. For instance, strong electric shocks were given to paired rats, guinea pigs, and hamsters to test if aggression was induced by an insult to the nervous system.[1] Male mice were castrated at birth and females were given large doses of injected testosterone to investigate pup-killing behaviors in male and female mice.[2] An estimated 795 newborn mice were used as victims in a series of experiments on infanticide, testing social status and sexual experience of adult aggressors.[3] These experiments and others were reported in several different scientific journals.

INFANTICIDE RESEARCH IN A LABORATORY

Robert W. Elwood, a zoologist, worked for many years on aggression in gerbils and published his findings in *Animal Behaviour*. This is the journal of two sister organizations, the Association for the Study of Animal Behaviour (ASAB) in the United Kingdom and the Animal Behavior Society (ABS) in the United States. In 1977, Elwood reported his observation that male Mongolian gerbils killed pups they had not fathered.[4] It was unclear how this killing could be beneficial. He suggested that perhaps it was because the pups provided food.

Later, he worked in laboratories at Queen's University of Belfast, in Northern Ireland. He assembled information from many sources, including his own experiments, to show that adult males of at least 11 different mammalian species killed infants genetically unrelated to them.[5] These species included baboons, lions, macaque monkeys, squirrels, hamsters, and mice.

In 1980, Elwood conducted experiments showing that male gerbils housed with their pregnant mates would not harm pups. There was a clear inhibition against pup cannibalism by males housed in these circumstances. However, in previous work he had found that male gerbils housed alone or those housed with nonpregnant females would indeed kill stranger pups when tested. Housing conditions were an important factor in this aggression.

Just why the males killed pups was not understood. A suggested evolutionary explanation was that a male increases his reproductive success at the expense of competitors by killing a competitor's offspring and then mating with the mother and becoming the father of his own litter.[6] Perhaps this inhibition is mediated at least in part by genotype and is thus heritable. But if an adult male is to successfully perpetuate his genotype, it is imperative that any infanticidal tendencies be inhibited prior to the birth of his own offspring.

In 1980, Elwood also found that while sexually naive (never copulated) gerbils tended to cannibalize pups, similarly housed experienced males (those that had reared at least one litter) did not harm test pups. He suggested that maybe the inhibition of infanticide is dependent upon the physical presence of the pregnant female and infanticide is reestablished if the female is removed. Maybe a pheromone in the urine or sebaceous glands of the pregnant female was involved in inducing the infanticidal behavior of males; the effectiveness of the pheromone is temporary unless renewed. In keeping with this, some researchers suggested that the male might learn certain features of the female, such as the odor of her urine, that discourage him from killing in her presence.[7]

Whether copulation was or was not involved in influencing infanticidal behavior was unresolved. One researcher had suggested that the experience of copulation alone was sufficient to suppress infanticide among male mice.[8] Elwood in 1987 had considered copulation as a possible mediating mechanism, but he rejected that hypothesis because there appears to be a gradual inhibition during the mate's pregnancy that becomes effective only in the final six days of her pregnancy. Nonetheless, other researchers had found decreased infanticide by males immediately after copulation.

Does copulation itself inhibit infanticide, or is cohabitation an essential factor? There was no consensus answer. Elwood decided to investigate these issues with a colleague, Malcolm C. Ostermeyer. Their study was designed to distinguish between two hypotheses: copulation in male mice inhibits infanticide, or it is cohabitation with the pregnant female that is necessary. According to the answer, difference mechanisms would be involved. They reported their work in *Animal Behaviour*.[9]

Experimental Procedures and Results

Since sexual history could influence the results, these investigators chose sexually naive (never copulated) CS1 strain mice approximately three months old. The animals had been individually housed for 18 days. Not all mice demonstrate infanticidal behavior, so a pre-experimental (baseline) Test 1 identified "killers" and "nonkillers." The test for infanticide was to place a stranger pup in with the adult male for up to 36 hours and record whether the pup was or was not killed. There was no possibility of escape for the newborns. About 60% of the males killed the stranger pup, "usually with a swift bite to the head or thorax." These were named "killers." The others who did not kill were named "nonkillers." Then three matched experimental groups were formed, each containing eight killers and six nonkillers. This formulation represented the proportion of 60% killers to 40% nonkillers established in Test 1. Additional tests for infanticidal behavior (as before) were made at different time intervals: Test 2 was on the day of mating, and Test 3 was 18 days after mating.

Three different housing situations were compared, as follows:

1. The males in Group 1 were each paired with virgin females and tested again (Test 2) with a pup immediately after a vaginal plug was found. (Such a plug indicated that copulation had taken place; the females were checked each morning.) The females were removed from the cage during this test. Whether the pup was killed was reported. The two animals continued to cohabitat and 18 days later, when the female was near to giving birth, the male was tested again (Test 3) with another pup and "yes" or "no" for infanticide was reported.
2. Males were treated as for Group 1, but the females were removed permanently after the vaginal plug was found.
3. Males in Group 3 were kept isolated and just received baseline Test 1 and Test 2 18 days later.

For this study, 42 adult mice had been used (3 groups each containing 14 animals). Groups 1 and 2 had three opportunities to kill pups, and Group 3 had two opportunities. So 112 newborn pups were offered as victims. The authors stated that "on ethical grounds, numbers of animals used were kept to a minimum consistent with statistical validity."[10]

The results showed that there was no significant difference in infanticide between those that had recently copulated (Test 2, Groups 1 and 2) and those that had not (Test 2, Group 3). There was, however, a decline to zero infanticide if the female remained with the male (Test 2 versus Test 3). Thus copulation alone has no effect on the perpetration of infanticide. Only the males that continued to live with the females showed an inhibition. These results were in agreement with Elwood's previous work on gerbils.[11] The precise stimuli from the female responsible for producing this behavior was not investigated in the study.

Decision of a Journal's Ethical Committee

When the manuscript of the article was being considered for publication, the journal's "Ethical Committee" deliberated about how to proceed. Publication was approved subject to the condition that it be accompanied by an editorial note stating, "The Ethical Committee of the ASAB considered this paper and was satisfied that the killing of the pups was instantaneous and that no suffering was involved."

It was only a footnote, but such an editorial note marked the first pronouncement of prepublication ethical scrutiny. Readers would see that studies published in *Animal Behaviour* were being formally reviewed for ethical concerns in the use of animals and that specified standards were being enforced. This note became an event of historical importance in ethical review of any scientific journal, and its publication opened the door to additional debate on what a researcher should or should not do in conducting studies of infanticide, aggression, and predator-prey relationships, as well as what should or should not be published.

Mounting Ethical Concern

Questions about aspects of experimental procedures on animal aggression had been raised for some time. Growing concern about methods used to study animal behavior had resulted in the formulation of first-ever guidelines for such research in 1981.[12]

This policy was prepared by the two sister professional associations in the United Kingdom and the United States. It was this policy that was being enforced in Elwood and Ostermeyer's 1984 paper. Over the following years, some manuscripts involving aggression have been rejected by *Animal Behaviour* for reasons pertaining to ethics.

A number of other professional associations have established guidelines on animal welfare, but their enforcement has not been a matter for public reflection because there is no indication that they are being enforced. Among professional associations, these animal behaviorists are unusual in having established timely guidelines and significant methods of enforcement.

Animal behaviorist Felicity A. Huntingford was an important force in promoting ethical studies of animal behavior and was a strong contributor of ideas on how to refine experimental procedures to reduce harm to the animals. She analyzed the articles on aggression (and the related issue of predator-prey relationships) published in *Animal Behaviour* in the years 1979, 1980, and 1981.[13] Her article was published in the same 1984 issue as the Elwood and Ostermeyer paper. There were a total of 46 papers concerning aggression, of which 28 used artificially staged encounters of captive animals. Among her major concerns were avoiding trivial research, extracting maximum information from each encounter, and minimizing suffering. She felt that, wherever possible, the question under consideration should be answered by observations in the wild.

Ethical debate regarding aggression research is ongoing today, and many new ideas have emerged since the early 1980s. Elwood himself has contributed to this discussion, and *Animal Behaviour* has published a number of other such articles.[14] Other significant papers were reprinted in a 1992 booklet titled *Ethics in Research on Animal Behaviour*.[15]

Since 1981, when the first animal behavior guidelines were issued, several revisions have occurred, most recently in 2006.[16] These updates have incorporated new methodologies that reduce interference or harm to the animal subjects. Each revision has extended the range of topics, kept pace with shifts in the fields of interest, and demonstrated sensitivity to ethical considerations.

DO NONHUMAN STUDIES SHED LIGHT ON HUMAN AGGRESSION?

The Elwood-Ostermeyer project had no intent of shedding direct light on *human* aggression, but modern developments in biological research have discovered that there is some potential for explanation in humans. Some aggression investigations on animals appear to reveal a better understanding of human aggression, especially if one is willing to assume that the continuum of life forms is strong. Nevertheless, extrapolating the relevance of nonhuman animal studies to an understanding of human behavior is a matter of substantial moral and scientific controversy.

According to one view, animal studies have limitations in contributing to our understanding of human violence. Human aggression involves complicated social and environmental factors that are not and cannot be duplicated by animal studies. Aggression is mediated by cultures that are not duplicated in captive, nonhuman animals. The unpredictable and sometimes explosive manner in which the trait of human aggression is displayed provides little basis for trying to replicate these situations in nonhuman, captive animals.

Some psychologists have questioned the clinical value of laboratory research on animals. Among them is J. A. Kelly, who examined the 1984 volume of *Behavior Therapy*, a journal specializing in behavioral intervention and therefore likely to report human studies that draw on prior animal studies.[17] He found that of the 1,132 citations, only 2% referred to animal studies. Similarly, the results of a large-scale 1996 survey of psychologists conducted by S. Plous showed that mental health workers rarely or never use findings from psychological research on animals.[18] Nearly 95% of these psychologists indicated that they would not be seriously hampered by an absence of animal research.

Research efforts to induce or aggravate aggression are often controversial and are frequently criticized. For instance, it has been repeatedly demonstrated that stress induces aggression in both animal and human studies. Research on mice has shown that isolation, sleep deprivation, or immobilization can induce marked increases in aggression. Critics argue that these studies merely confirm observations that are readily available from humans and add little, if anything, to our knowledge.

Over time, the substance and credibility of these criticisms have fluctuated, as has federal funding. The funding fluctuations have mirrored the level of scientific understanding of the links between rodent and human aggression. According to a 1994 report, the National Institutes of Health (NIH) funding for animal aggression studies reached a peak in 1975 when the Division of Neuroscience and Behavioral Science of NIH funded 27 studies at a total cost of $900,000.[19] The report stated that this level has since "steadily declined due to waning interest, because exact causal relationships were difficult to prove."

Nonetheless, some tempting links to understanding human aggression have emerged from animal studies. Factors known to influence nonhuman animal aggression include hormones such as testosterone, various drugs including alcohol, modulation of neuroanatomic sites and neurotransmitter systems (including serotonin and norepinephrine), and genetic conditions.

More recently, links between nonhuman and human aggression have slowly become more secure and, as a result, federal funding has increased. The greatest surge has come from the tremendous advances in our understanding of genetics. It has long been known that animals can be selectively bred for aggressive strains, but it was not until the 1990s that new methods of genetic manipulation became widely used. Genetic structure has now been identified and aggressive tendencies modified. Since the mid-1990s, more than 15 genes have been identified in male mice with effects on offense-type aggression.[20] These genes have homologues in humans, with similar effects on molecular and cellular biology.

In 2003, a mouse gene called Pet-1 was discovered to be essential for normal levels of anxiety and aggression. When this gene is removed or "knocked out" in a mouse, aggression and anxiety are greatly elevated compared with control mice.[21] This research opened a new door to the study of mood disorders in humans. Some investigators believe they have identified "good mouse models to study the development of antisocial behavior in mice that may be relevant to humans."[22] A 2005 study provides the first example of a human gene correcting aggressive mouse behavior, and the authors at the University of British Columbia suggest that the "mechanisms underlying the 'fierce' mouse may be similar to the mechanisms found in humans."[23]

Still under study are applications of these nonhuman animal studies to the nature and regulation of aggression in humans. Development of useful therapeutic interventions that relieve human antisocial behaviors may be possible, but this is not likely to be known for many years.

ETHICAL ISSUES

The Justification of Experiments with Animals

Does the knowledge that comes from basic animal behavioral research provide a sufficient justification for killing 112 newborn animals, as happened in the Elwood and Ostermeyer case, even when there is no known application of the knowledge that will provide benefits to either animals or to humans? This work made a contribution to knowledge about the paternal behavior of male mice and infanticide and its inhibition. An underlying assumption was that knowledge about infanticide in mice could be relevant to the social structure of other groups. If this thesis is correct, would such a contribution then be sufficient to justify the research?

It has never been entirely clear in the evaluation of this kind of research which criteria should be used for judging the significance of experimental results. A provision of *Animal Behaviour*'s then-current guidelines states: "If animals are confined, constrained, harmed or stressed in any way, the investigator must consider whether the knowledge that may be gained justifies the procedures. Some knowledge is trivial, and experiments must not be done simply because it is possible to do them." So, presumably, when the journal permitted publication of this study, the ethical committee's opinion was that these infanticide studies were not trivial and therefore that the knowledge gained justified the harms to the animals.

From a moral point of view, was this judgment correct? It is always possible that some specific knowledge of animal behavior could be put to use to help protect a species or its environment—such as human understanding about migratory instincts or preferred routes. We often do not see the utility in scientific experiments until some time well after their completion. The key question when knowledge gained contributes to an understanding of the animal world is this: If there is no clear application of or rationale for use of the information, should we declare it trivial or should we say that we rarely understand exactly how future scientists will use information and must therefore not judge science on the basis of immediate benefit?

This is a more important question than it may at first appear to be, because it reaches beyond animal aggression studies. A vast amount of both behavioral and biomedical research involving animals is *basic* research with no clear line(s) of application. While much of this research causes only trivial harms or uneasiness in animals, much of it is as deeply invasive and harmful as the killing involved in some animal aggression research.

Scientific Merit and the Choice of Laboratory Studies or Field Studies

The experimental subjects in the Elwood and Ostermeyer research were "male CS1 mice," indicating that these were captive-bred mice of a particular strain. The 1981 guidelines for the ASAB/ABS state that whether or not the subject animal has spent "a lifetime in captivity" can be of "profound importance."

Are studies of natural behavior (such as natural instincts) using caged animals scientifically valid and representative of normal behavior? Or do the captive raising and caging itself so influence behavior that the caging is the crucial causal condition, thus suggesting that there is no scientific value? And if the studies are scientifically uninteresting, are they then unethical?

Animals that are singly caged throughout their lives behave in many deviant ways. From this it follows that the results of such experiments may be questionable and stand in need of independent verification. Is an encounter between two animals in the environment of a cage really a faithful duplication of naturally occurring conditions? Psychologist Lewis Petrinovich has stated: "The essential artificiality of the laboratory and the usual lack of any essential relationship of the laboratory setting to an organism's adaptive capacities do violence to the integrity of behavioral [studies]. . . . If the situations are not representative . . . then no analytical method is of much value."[24] It is a matter of careful scientific inquiry and judgment whether prearranged infanticide or any similarly induced behavior is representative of normal behavior. The controversial character of science done in this way has often been noted in evaluations of scientific studies.

In addressing the ethics of aggression studies, observational field studies of naturally occurring events of aggression have been consistently recommended, as opposed to laboratory studies, under ASAB/ASB guidelines. But field studies also have limitations. Unlike laboratory studies, they cannot be standardized, which is often a crippling methodological problem. Furthermore, manipulation of the environment is often not possible, nor is it desirable, because any human interference may alter an animal's natural behavior and thus be subject to the objections just mentioned. Laboratory studies make it possible to regulate the experimental situation by controlling potentially relevant variables and to replicate the experiment. Thus the underlying mechanisms can be understood more precisely.

Elwood and Ostermeyer chose to do the infanticide study in the laboratory because they could manipulate the animals and standardize the tests in ways that would be impossible in the field. Yet their ultimate objective was to understand normally occurring infanticidal behavior that would be relevant to the species, and potentially even beyond the species, so that the results are generalizable to other mice and their wild counterparts. If this assumption is not supported by independent scientific evidence, the research may be scientifically unsound and therefore unethical.

One of the basic principles of research involving both human subjects and animal subjects—accepted universally in both science and ethics—is that research lacking scientific merit also lacks moral justification. So the question is whether much of the work on animal aggression and in many other areas is of this description.

Adequacy of Committee Review

It has been argued that if the purpose of an experiment is trivial, then no infliction of harm or distress in animals whatsoever is justified.[25] These early 1981 guidelines encouraged review by those who were "in a different discipline" as being especially likely to be helpful since they "will not share all the investigator's assumptions," including any biases that an individual investigator or a discipline as a whole may have. Those outside the animal behavior discipline are more likely than those within it to raise questions. The Elwood and Ostermeyer paper was reviewed by the United Kingdom's ethical committee, which reviews European-based work. (In the United States, the ABS reviews other geographical areas.) This committee believed there was value in answering the hypotheses posed in the study. But was the review adequate?

Questions about the ethical review of animal research by researchers in the field were demonstrated in a survey of all licensed biomedical animal researchers conducted by Frans R. Stafleu[26] at Utrecht University in the Netherlands. Each licensee was asked about the justification of several well-designed protocols, some of which involved significant animal pain. The results showed that respondents *always* assumed that the experiment was justified. Even procedures involving considerable harm to monkeys were not challenged. According to this report, respondents, all of whom were biomedical researchers, agreed with the acceptability of the research goal as an "incontestable fact." Whether this would be true of animal behaviorist researchers has yet to be studied.

Nevertheless, it would be too quick to dismiss review by peers as so contaminated by conflict of interest as to be worthless. The fairness of the review appears to depend heavily on the persons involved, the resources and training given to the committee, and the environment in which it operates. For example, the 1984 ethical committee seems to have been of high quality. So there are serious moral questions about the appointment and composition of the committees responsible for the ethical review of research.

A recent development since the 1980s is to appoint representatives of animal protection groups to committees involved in setting policy or reviewing animal research. Of interest is the composition of the ASAB ethical committee as of early 2007. On this 14-member committee, not only are other disciplines represented, but one member represents an animal welfare organization, the Universities Federation for Animal Welfare.[27] The sister organization in the United States does not as yet include such representation on its Animal Care Committee, but it is reportedly working on this issue.[28]

Most research investigators believe that a research institution cannot allow outsiders to determine the acceptability of its research, but others see the situation as a classic case of the fox guarding the chicken coop. Perhaps there exists some morally acceptable compromise.

Alternative Strategies Using the "Three Rs" Framework

Of all the scientific disciplines, the animal behaviorists are arguably the keenest proponents of conducting research in an ethical manner. The ASAB and ABS have exhibited clear sensitivity to ethical issues. The cornerstone of this sensitivity is the commitment to seek alternatives in animal research.

Their first guidelines in 1981 demonstrated immediate recognition of the concepts of the Three Rs. These guidelines state that "Alternatives to animal experiments should be considered," referencing the 1978 book by D. H. Smyth, *Alternatives to Animal Experiments*.[29] Smyth's book was inspired by, and did much to draw attention to, the famous earlier book of William Russell and Rex Burch, which began this framework of seeking alternative research methods to minimize animal harms (see chapter 1, pp. 32–34).[30]

This framework is structured around the following categories: replacement (the choice of species and non-animal alternatives); reduction (the number of individual animal subjects); and refinement (the efforts to design and conduct the studies to minimize suffering to animals). This framework will now be used to analyze some possible alternative strategies to the assessment of research involving animals.

Replacement

In behavioral research, replacement with a non-animal procedure is, understandably, the least feasible approach because live animal subjects are generally essential in behavioral research. However, non-animal alternatives such as video records from previous work or computer simulations can sometimes be used, and replacements may sometimes be used for teaching purposes. Another alternative that some find morally preferable—though this is controversial—is to use a less-sentient organism. According to Huntingford in her 1984 paper, aggression experiments should be conducted with invertebrates rather than vertebrates, and among vertebrates, with fish rather than birds or mammals.[31] These preferences are thought to pose fewer ethical problems because the simpler the nervous system an animal has, the less it is likely to experience suffering.

Reduction

For reduction, the 1981 guidelines require that investigators keep the number of animals to the minimum to accomplish the experimental goals. Elwood and Ostermeyer claimed that "on ethical grounds the numbers of animals used were kept to the minimum consistent with statistical validity."[32] Was the reference exclusively to the 42 adults, or did it include the 112 pups that were either killed by infanticide or presumably died for other reasons?

Researchers are frequently not careful about stating the methods of how they conform to the ethical obligation to reduce the numbers of animals to the minimum necessary. The advice of a biostatistician is required. According to geneticist Michael F. W. Festing, it is still relatively rare for investigators to state specifically that they have considered reducing the number of animals used.[33] There is a need for "improved experimental design and statistical analysis" of animal experiments if they are to be considered "ethically acceptable."[34]

Refinement

The most important reforms of the Three Rs so far developed have come from the refinement of laboratory methods to keep pain and suffering to a minimum, commensurate with valid experimental design (see chapter 1, pp. 32–36). In 1981, refinements were not well developed; this concept was a relatively new idea. But as the animal behavior guidelines have evolved over the years, these ideas have become basic and central to policies on humane animal experimentation.

In the 1984 paper, Elwood and Ostermeyer did address the issue of pain but gave an incomplete account of the potential sources of animal pain or suffering. Only one potential source was addressed: the manner of death at the moment when an adult kills a pup. The researchers reported that death "usually" came about from a swift bite to the newborn pups' head or chest. Elwood defended the use of day-old pups on the grounds that death came swiftly and that older pups have greater perception of discomfort and pain. Without elaboration, the ethical committee judged that the deaths were "instantaneous and that no suffering was involved." Not mentioned, however, were the harms potentially coming from the pups who were not killed but were left in the males' cages for 36 hours. Were they alive when the researchers removed them? If so, by what method were the pups humanely killed? Questions might also be raised about whether the mothers suffered from the loss of their newborn pups. Answers to these questions would not automatically render the research unjustified, but they would presumably make impartial reviewers more informed and less certain to find the research justified.

Improved ethical concern by researchers is also taking place, as shown by the fact that some authors include their own "ethical notes." As an example, one article's authors' note pointed out that "effective refuge" was provided for house mice who were being used as potential victims of intruder aggression.[35] The 2006 guidelines for ASAB/ASB include an unusual provision: the fact that a species being studied is classified as "vermin" in the country concerned "does not free the researcher from normal obligations to the experimental animals."[36] The different moral status of vermin mice from laboratory mice in varying situations is elegantly addressed by Harold A. Herzog.[37]

Another refinement in the 2006 guidelines is the selection of strain: With current understanding of refinements, the ASAB/ABS advises that the researcher should use the strain that is believed to be "the least likely to experience" pain or distress.[38] Instructions to authors submitting papers to ASAB/ABS in early 2007 are extensive and are intended to encourage reflection "from an ethical point of view" of procedures they have used.[39] For example, if the study involved potentially harmful manipulations, such as infanticide, then "full details of the procedure" are needed in the manuscript. If a procedure or experimental manipulation could potentially cause distress or pain or have any other adverse effect, then experimenters must "justify its use and explain any measures taken to minimize such effects. Did the experimenter have plans to intervene if adverse effects were severe, and if so, were intervention measures ever implemented?" Requiring information on intervention is exemplary.

In some circumstances, protecting prey from injury is as simple as removing the prey before the onslaught of attack. In situations in which there is a long latency before an attack, there may be time for the researcher to recognize an imminent attack (by the animal's posture and behavior) and rescue the victim. In 1991, Elwood stated that with gerbils, he considered intervention to be essential because otherwise adults would cannibalize a pup even before it had been killed.[40] In these cases, Elwood removed the pups in his experiments and "immediately" and humanely killed them. In this setting and using this methodology, rescue is impossible: To return the pup to its original litter after human handling and interference would likely result in the rejection of the pup by its mother.

In much of the scientific literature, there has been a tendency to magnify certain potential benefits of research while downplaying the animal harm resulting from experimental procedures.[41] This tendency has the effect of making the research seem justified, even though a more measured approach might find that the data on animal harm recorded by scientists are not as thorough as they should be. The inclusion of more information about the condition of experimental animals, the severity and duration of their pain or distress, and how adverse states are to be alleviated should produce better forms of review than those that often occur.

When live animals are used, an obvious refinement is to prevent injury to either the victim or the predator. In 1989, Glenn Perrigo and his associates commented on the "escalating public and scientific concern" about studies of infanticide where live pups are used to measure behavior.[42] These authors developed a wire mesh tube in which the pups are effectively protected from serious injury. Afterward, all pups are returned safe and uninjured to their mothers. In some studies, placing an intervening transparent partition between an aggressor and a victim has been used with apparent success.

Thus there appear to be alternative ways in which behavioral studies of nonhuman animal aggression can be conducted that are more morally sensitive than methods have been in the past. However, these alternatives are not obvious and require careful reflection in light of each scientific protocol.

The Problem of Retrospective Moral Judgment

It is widely believed that it is morally inappropriate to judge people or institutions based on *today's* moral standards for actions taken many years ago. The belief is that people cannot be judged or held responsible for research practices that were common and never seriously challenged until recently. In looking back on the Elwood and Ostermeyer and related experiments and attempting to evaluate their moral acceptability, we need to take into consideration the assumptions of the period in which the work was done, especially the kinds of ethical standards that were relevant to the evaluation of experiments involving animals, such as basic principles, government policies, and rules of professional ethics. In 1984, the newly devised 1981 ASAB/ASB guidelines were still untested, institutional committee review was not common (it was not mandated in research involving animals until 1985), and professional journals rarely, if ever, subjected manuscripts to ethical review for animal welfare concerns prior to publication. The ethics of animal behavior research was still an emerging field.

Today's professional standards and climate are very different. There is more professional society involvement and an increased awareness throughout the relevant professions of the three-R alternatives. If relevant standards and duties were largely or even entirely undeveloped at the time, this fact becomes exculpatory for persons accused of wrongdoing. Such circumstances would be very different from a situation in which there existed well-developed and officially endorsed policies for research involving animals.

In making retrospective moral judgments about mid-twentieth-century work, it helps to distinguish between evaluating the moral quality (in particular, the *wrongness*) of actions, practices, policies, and institutions in contrast to evaluating the blameworthiness (culpability) of agents. Sometimes officials and investigators are blameworthy for not having had policies and practices in place to protect animal subjects in research, but sometimes there are mitigating conditions that shield them from blame, even though we recognize moral deficiencies. For example, the scientific culture of the time may have fostered certain forms of moral ignorance or moral blindness, or a research institution's division of labor and designation of responsibility may have been diffuse. These mitigating conditions might exculpate the persons involved even though wrongdoing occurred. This problem has never been seriously studied or even mentioned in research involving animals, though it has been a significant concern in research involving human subjects. Research on both animal and human aggression continues. In the 1990s, scientific interest in aggression was stimulated by efforts to place laboratory animals in communal houses in contrast to keeping them alone in small cages that offered no opportunities for social contact with other animals. Group housing has been attempted with varying degrees of success in an effort to comply with a 1985 amendment to the Animal Welfare Act that requires that the "psychological well-being" of primates be addressed, a norm that has now been extended to other laboratory species. However, coping with aggression has been a considerable problem in these efforts to provide group housing.[43]

Today biomedical researchers continue to use nonhuman primates as models for human antisocial behavioral states. Examples include investigations of increased aggression resulting from substance abuse of cocaine or alcohol, which study the biobehavioral effects of drugs used clinically to treat violent aggression in humans. Since researchers continue to study aggression and violence in both animals and humans, the challenge remains to design experiments that are ethically sound.

NOTES

1. R. E. Ulrich and N. H. Azrin, "Reflexive Fighting in Response to Aversive Stimulation," *Journal of the Experimental Analysis of Behavior* 5 (October 1962): 511–20.

2. Owen Samuels, Gregory Jason, Martha Mann, and Bruce Svare, "Pup-Killing Behavior in Mice: Suppression by Early Androgen Exposure," *Physiology and Behavior* 26 (1981): 473–77.

3. U. William Huck, Robin L. Soltis, and Carol B. Coopersmith, "Infanticide in Male Laboratory Mice: Effects of Social Status, Prior Sexual Experience, and Basis for Discrimination between Related and Unrelated Young," *Animal Behaviour* 30 (1982): 1158–65.

4. Robert W. Elwood, "Changes in the Responses of Male and Female Gerbils (*Meriones unguiculatus*) towards Test Pups during the Pregnancy of the Female," *Animal Behaviour* 25 (1977): 46–51.

5. Robert W. Elwood, "The Development, Inhibition, and Disinhibition of Pup-Cannibalism in the Mongolian Gerbil," *Animal Behaviour* 28 (1980): 1188–94.

6. Frederick S. vom Saal, "The Regulation of Infanticide and Parental Behavior: Implications for Reproductive Success in Male Mice," *Science* 215 (March 5, 1982): 1270–72.

7. Huck, Soltis, and Coopersmith, "Infanticide in Male Laboratory Mice," 1161–62.

8. J. B. Labov, "Factors Influencing Infanticidal Behavior in Wild Male House Mice (*Mus musculus*)," *Behavioral Ecology and Sociobiology* 6 (1980): 297–303.

9. Robert W. Elwood and Malcolm C. Ostermeyer, "Does Copulation Inhibit Infanticide in Male Rodents?" *Animal Behaviour* 32 (1984): 293–94.

10. Ibid., p. 293.

11. Ibid.

12. "Guidelines for the Use of Animals in Research," *Animal Behaviour* 29 (1981): 1–2.

13. Felicity A. Huntingford, "Some Ethical Issues Raised by Studies of Predation and Aggression," *Animal Behaviour* 32 (1984): 39–46. An appendix was added in 1992.

14. Robert W. Elwood, "Ethical Implications of Studies on Infanticide and Maternal Aggression," *Animal Behaviour* 42 (1991): 841–49; Robert W. Elwood and Stefano Parmigiani, "Ethical Recommendations for Workers on Aggression and Predation in Animals," *Aggressive Behavior* 18 (1992): 139–42; Paul Frederic Brain, "Comments on Laboratory-Based 'Aggression' Tests," *Animal Behaviour* 32 (1984): 1256–57; Glenn Perrigo, W. Cully Bryant, Lee Belvin, and Frederick S. vom Saal, "The Use of Live Pups in a Humane, Injury-Free Test for Infanticidal Behaviour in Male Mice," *Animal Behaviour* 38 (1989): 897–98.

15. Marian Stamp Dawkins and Morris Gosling, eds., *Ethics in Research on Animal Behaviour* (Amsterdam: Elsevier, for Association for the Study of Animal Behaviour and the Animal Behavior Society, 1992).

16. A succession of joint guidelines for the Association for the Study of Animal Behaviour and the Animal Behavior Society has been published, as follows: *Animal Behaviour* 29 (1981): 1–2; *Animal Behaviour* 34 (1986): 314–17; *Animal Behaviour* 47 (1994): 245–50; *Animal Behaviour* 65 (2003): 249–55; and *Animal Behaviour* 71 (2006): 245–53. Also current as of early 2007 are "A Guide to Ethical Information Required for Animal Behaviour Papers," www.elsevier.com/framework_products/promis_misc/ethyanbe.doc (accessed March 20, 2007), and "Guidelines for the Treatment of Animals in Behavioural Research and Teaching," www.elsevier.com/framework_products/promis_misc/ASAB2006.pdf (accessed March 20, 2007).

17. J. A. Kelly, "Psychological Research and the Rights of Animals: Disagreement with Miller," *American Psychologist* 41 (1986): 839–41.

18. S. Plous, "Attitudes toward the Use of Animals in Psychological Research and Education: Results from a National Survey of Psychologists," *American Psychologist* 51 (November 1996): 1167–80.

19. "Report of the Panel on NIH Research on Anti-social, Aggressive, and Violence-Related Behaviors and Their Consequences" (Bethesda, MD: National Institutes of Health, April 1994).

20. Caroline Blanchard, "IS-2 Genes and Aggression: From Mice to Humans," paper presented at the Fourteenth World Meeting of the International Society for Research on Aggression, July 9–14, 2000

21. T. J. Hendricks, D. V. Fyodorov, L. J. Wegman, N. B. Lelutiu, E. A. Pehek, B. Yamamoto, J. Silver, E. J. Weeber, J. D. Sweatt, and E. S. Deneris, "Pet-1 ETS Gene Plays a Critical Role in 5-HT Neuron Development and Is Required for Normal Anxiety-like Aggressive Behavior," *Neuron* 37 (January 2003): 233–47.

22. "Toward an Animal Model for Antisocial Behavior: Parallels between Mice and Humans," *Behavior Genetics* 33 (2003): 563–74, www.springerlink.com/content/xq4304143v733162/

23. Brett S. Abrahams, Melvin C. H. Kwok, Eric Trinh, Saeed Budaghzadeh, Sazzad M. Hossain, and Elizabeth M. Simpson, "Pathological Aggression in 'Fierce' Mice Corrected by Human Nuclear Receptor 2E1," *Journal of Neuroscience* 25 (2005): 6263–70. doi:10.1523/JNEUROSCI.4757-04.2005.

24. Lewis Petrinovich, "Probabilistic Functionalism: A Conception of Research Method," *American Psychologist* 34 (1979): 383, 388.

25. See, for example, Patrick Bateson, "When to Experiment on Animals," *New Scientist*, February 20, 1986, pp. 30–32.

26. Frans R. Stafleu, "The Ethical Acceptability of Animal Experiments as Judged by Researchers," PhD thesis, University of Utrecht, Netherlands, 1994, p. 83.

27. E-mail from Angela Turner, Managing Editor, *Animal Behaviour,* to Barbara Orlans, February 27, 2007.

28. E-mail from Todd M. Freeberg, Chair, Animal Care Committee, Animal Behavior Society, to Barbara Orlans, March 1, 2007.

29. D. H. Smyth, *Alternatives to Animal Experiments* (London: Scolar Press, Research Defence Society, 1978).

30. William M. S. Russell and Rex L. Burch, *The Principles of Humane Experimentation Technique* (London: Methuen and Company, 1959; repr. Dover Publications and Potters Bar, Universities Federation for Animal Welfare, 1992), altweb.jhsph.edu/publications/humane_exp/het-toc.htm.

31. Huntingford, "Some Ethical Issues Raised," p. 41.

32. Elwood and Ostermeyer, "Does Copulation Inhibit Infanticide," p. 293.

33. Michael F. W. Festing, "Reduction of Animal Use: Experimental Design and Quality of Experiments," *Laboratory Animals* 28 (1994): 212–21.

34. Michael F. W. Festing and Douglas G. Altman, "Guidelines for the Design and Statistical Analysis of Experiments Using Laboratory Animals," *ILAR Journal* 43 (2002): 244–58, www.frame.org.uk/atlafn/statsguidelines.pdf.

35. Samantha J. Gray, Susanne Plesner Jensen, and Jane L. Hurst, "Effects of Resource Distribution on Activity and Territory Defence in House Mice, *Mus domesticus*," *Animal Behaviour* 63 (2002): 531–39.

36. "Guidelines for the Treatment of Animals in Behavioural Research and Teaching," *Animal Behaviour* 71 (2006): 245–53, www.elsevier.com/framework_products/promis_misc/ASAB2006.pdf.

37. Harold A. Herzog, Jr., "The Moral Status of Mice," *American Psychologist* 43 (1988): 473–74; repr. *ILAR Journal* 31, no. 1 (1989).

38. "Guidelines for the Treatment of Animals in Behavioural Research and Teaching," p. 246.

39. For current author instructions, see "A Guide to Ethical Information Required for Animal Behaviour Papers," www.elsevier.com/framework_products/promis_misc/ethyanbe.doc (accessed February 23, 2007).

40. Elwood, "Ethical Implications of Studies on Infanticide," p. 843.

41. David B. Morton, "A Fair Press for Animals," *New Scientist* 1816 (1992): 28–30; Lynda Birke and Jane Smith, "Animals in Experimental Reports: The Rhetoric of Science," *Society and Animals* 3 (1995): 23–42.

42. Perrigo et al., "The Use of Live Pups in a Humane, Injury-Free Test," p. 897.

43. Group housing of laboratory animals enhances environmental enrichment, but it can also lead to unwanted aggression and, as a result, negative effects on the well-being of the animals and on the validity of experimental results. In a review, the following authors make practical recommendations for providing environmental enrichment for housing male mice which include, among other things, optimizing group size to three animals per cage. P. L. P. Van Loo, L. F. M. Van Zutphen, and V. Baumans, "Male Management: Coping with Aggression Problems in Male Laboratory Mice," *Laboratory Animals* 37 (2003): 300–313.

PART IX

WILDLIFE RESEARCH

16

The Death of a Vagrant Bird

On a hot August day in 1991, several amateur bird watchers were encamped in southern New Mexico at a place called Rattlesnake Springs, just inside Carlsbad Caverns National Park. This small oasis, located in the midst of the parched Chihuahuan desert, attracts a large number of bird species and had become a popular observational area. For some time the attention of many members of a bird-watching group had been drawn to the sight and song of a lone, small olive and yellow bird about six inches long that seemed oddly out of place. Descriptions and taped recordings of its song strongly suggested that the bird was a Yellow-green Vireo.

As far as anyone knew, the established range of this species was from Central America to Mexico. In an arresting use of language, individual birds sighted out of their established geographical context are referred to as "vagrants." One common use of the noun "vagrant" is meant to designate someone who travels "idly with no means of support, such as a drunkard,"[1] but the usage here is a direct derivation from the Latin root *vagari*, meaning "to wander." Many circumstances lead vagrant birds to be out of place, and they are associated with different degrees of scientific importance. For example, the bird may have overshot its migration target, been blown off course by a chance encounter with a storm, hitched an unintended ride on a boat or plane, or be in an active search for a new habitat.

While there had been scattered rare sightings of vagrant Yellow-green Vireos in southern Texas and southern Arizona in the 1970s, there was no record of the bird having ever been sighted as far north as Carlsbad, New Mexico. The status of the Yellow-green Vireo in South America is somewhat uncertain because it has a strong resemblance to the closely related Red-eyed Vireo, and their populations are sometimes confused. Accurate identification takes a careful look, because both species have yellow flanks, an olive crown, and head striping.[2]

The sightings in the Southwest had raised interesting questions of whether the species was in the initial stages of a northern expansion and, if so, why? Might it be because of a loss of habitat? In the bird's home range, it inhabited canopy, forest borders, and lighter woodlands, terrain all under ecological challenge. According to reports, this single vagrant bird remained in the vicinity of Rattlesnake Springs until September 1991, when it precipitously disappeared. It was concluded that the bird had either died or had migrated back to Central America for the winter.

On July 1 of the following year, another bird resembling a Yellow-green Vireo was once again sighted in the same vicinity. Several observers who had made the 1991 sighting believed that this bird was the identical bird observed the previous year. The sighting was reported on the Rare Bird Alert hotline, a service managed and used by the amateur bird-watching community, or "birders" as they are also known. Shortly after the posting on the hotline, bird watchers began to arrive from around the United States in hopes of observing the bird.

KILLING AND COLLECTING

On July 8, 1992, John Trochet, a graduate student in ornithology from the University of California at Berkeley who was collecting goldfinches for his dissertation research, traveled to Rattlesnake Springs. Once there he engaged in conversation with several birders who informed him of the presence of the vireo. He eventually sighted the bird and recorded its distinctive song with his portable tape recorder. At some point soon after the sighting, Trochet made a decision to "collect" this bird.

The term "collect" refers to the practice of killing a bird with a shotgun or capturing it in a trap or net and then killing it. The bird is then converted into a specimen for deposit and study in an ornithology museum. The tradition in museum ornithology involves the creation of a repository of information by preserving large numbers of specimens of existing groups of birds. The collections are composed of three types of specimens: mounts, skins, and "alcoholics." Mounts are specimens on pedestals in lifelike poses. Skins are specimens in which the skeleton (other than the legs and wing bones) and internal organs are removed, leaving intact the skin and feathers, head, and beak. The term "alcoholics" refers to the internal soft parts, which are preserved in solution. These collections are then used to study differences and similarities between species and between populations within a species.

Trochet's Problem

John Trochet possessed a legal permit to collect any non-endangered bird species in the state of New Mexico for scientific purposes, but by federal law collecting is not permitted in national parks. National parks have the legal status of being sanctuaries for the wildlife contained within their borders, but only as long as they remain within those borders. If Trochet aimed to legally collect the vagrant vireo, he would have to wait until it flew out of the park. This could be a long wait with little chance of success.

Whereas there is a clear prohibition about interfering with animals on park land, there is no specific wording in the regulations that in fact prevents someone from luring an animal out of the park. Apparently aware of this distinction and not willing to adopt a more passive and chancy waiting strategy, Trochet used the tape recording he had made of the bird's own song and began to play it aloud at the springs. This technique is frequently used by ornithologists to stimulate a bird that they can hear but not see clearly to reveal itself. The bird hears the recording and reacts as if the sounds were coming from another bird and seeks it out in a territorial display. According to Trochet's own account, the procedure worked: The vagrant vireo flew out of the canopy and began to search for the source of the song. Trochet continued to play the song to the vireo as he walked off the protected property of the National Park and toward a private ranch where he had set up a trap of mist nets.[3] On private land the bird was no longer legally protected, and Trochet's collecting permit was in force.

After following the replay of its taped song out of the park and flying one quarter of a mile to the ranch site, the vireo was quickly captured in Trochet's nets. Trochet removed the bird from the net and noted that it was indeed a male Yellow-green Vireo in excellent nesting condition. After the examination, Trochet grasped the body of the vagrant in the palm of his hand, closed his fingers around it, and squeezed tightly. The hand pressure prevented the bird from breathing and it soon died of suffocation. The procedure is called "thoracic compression" and is commonly used to kill birds in the field. Once the bird was dead, Trochet prepared it as a specimen and sent it back to the University of California ornithology museum.

The Reaction

The reaction of the various interested parties to the collection of this vireo was swift and robust. The ensuing debate between professional ornithologists, birders, and the public at large highlighted the relationship between the legal and the ethical, as well as the costs and benefits of the perceived need of some scientists to chronicle an unexpected occurrence contrasted with the wishes and enjoyment of the public. Trochet and other "professionals" asserted the authority and obligation of science to swiftly and accurately describe, record, and explain nature as it exists and changes, even if it means stretching the overall intent of a formal regulation. Birders were outraged that the scientist either failed to consider or undervalued their interests in seeing this unique individual bird alive. Other members of the public who commented on the death of the bird seemed to be upset that the bird was killed, regardless of Trochet's permit or the legality of the action. They seemed to take the position that the value of the vireo's life was independent of the uses the scientists attached to the specimen or the birders attached to the observation of a living Yellow-green Vireo. Others expressed surprise that there was furor about the death of a single bird.

Despite the many disagreements between the parties, there was agreement about certain aspects of the vireo incident. All parties eventually agreed that luring a bird off the protected confines of a national park was ethically inappropriate, even though not illegal. Park regulations only speak to animals being killed or disturbed on actual park land, and therefore no legal action was possible. Nonetheless, the action was seen as violating the spirit of the law and as morally dubious.

Before we consider the more significant ethical conflicts presented by this case, we need to review briefly the various conceptual and value frameworks of the participants.

THE PURPOSE AND VALUE OF ORNITHOLOGICAL MUSEUM COLLECTIONS

In an often-quoted article, Kevin Winker of the Bell Museum of Natural History at the University of Minnesota reviewed the traditional historical and modern justification for bird collecting.[4] In the most general sense, collecting is the primary way the avian record of biodiversity is preserved. It records and maintains exemplars of what has been seen, where it has been seen, when it has been seen, and under what conditions, and it serves as a resource for research and education. Examination of the skins and tissues using the comparative method helps to reveal the variations and similarities that are an expression of the process of evolution.

The discovery of the theory of evolution itself was in part dependent upon the process of classifying and comparing the morphological relationships of birds collected by Charles Darwin in the Galapagos Islands. Although painted illustrations and photographs also have served this function, they have always been considered inferior to an actual specimen that can be handled, visualized, measured, and remeasured. Scientists point out that collecting must continue because nature is dynamic and our knowledge of it requires constant updating. Ranges expand and contract, populations become isolated from one another, and morphological variations arise or are newly recognized. During the 10-year period between 1980 and 1990, for example, over 600 new species of birds were identified and verified using the process of observation, collection, and comparison.[5]

North American museums house upward of 3 million bird specimens that have been collected over the past century, but the development of newer genetic analyses has rendered many of the older specimens obsolete.[6] Also, some techniques of preservation interfere with these new biochemical procedures. Nonetheless, comparison of morphological and genetic information helps sort through the problem that species membership is often obscured by morphological similarity. Accordingly, scientists still have a need for collections that foster meaningful comparisons.

Specimens provide information beyond that required to detail the variation within the bird world and to study evolution in the process of speciation. These data may also offer information important to conservation efforts. The argument is that precise knowledge of bird diversity is required in order to develop strategies to protect species. In a related use, museum collections helped to establish the disastrous impact of DDT on avian reproduction as well as the emergence patterns of important zoonotic diseases like hanta virus and Lyme disease.[7] Therefore, as long as collection does not threaten the well-being of a *population*, the judicious collection of *individual* birds is in the interest of the overall population. The information potentially provides important insights into our understanding of the processes of evolution, speciation, and biogeographical distribution. In addition, the information may inform conservation and protection plans.

Nonetheless, the practice of museum ornithology and collecting in general has long been waning.[8] In 1980, Robert Ricklefs pointed out that specimens were being acquired at a very low level even though many important taxonomic questions remained unanswered.[9] He suggested that the museum tradition in ornithology was dying and being replaced by the study of ecology, ethology, and physiology—something of a paradigm shift in scientific investigation. Yet students of ornithology today still recognize the importance of the collection tradition and the fact that data relevant to new forms of study are present in collections. The collections are not merely anachronistic dust collectors.

But how much valid scientific information can be acquired by collecting and examining the specimen of the particular vagrant vireo discussed above? The scientist in this case took the expected position of inquiring about whether the individual seen and heard was in reality a Yellow-green Vireo. Science is about accuracy, and because it is well known that the Yellow-green Vireo is difficult to distinguish from the Red-eyed Vireo, photographs and taped song data were not sufficient for species identification. If it were found to be a Yellow-green Vireo other questions would arise, such as, "Which of the subpopulations has it come from?" Answers to such questions often require a closer look than that provided by a photograph or audiotape. The final determination of species or subpopulation membership may require biochemical analysis, which involves a significant amount of tissue and, accordingly, the "sacrifice" of the bird.

Specific identification of the vireo is important for reasons other than mere taxonomic considerations. Collection permits the acquisition of additional data such as age, sex, fat condition, diet (from stomach contents), general health, pesticide level, parasite load, and existence of injuries and disease. Was the vagrant among an initial wave of pioneering individuals expanding the species range? If so, why the expansion? Are there problems associated with habitat loss in the home range? Is there an overabundance of individuals that cannot find suitable mates or nest sites? The implications of these alternatives might inform further investigation and might contribute to conservation and protection activities important to the professional and the public alike.

THE PURPOSE AND VALUE OF BIRDING

The phenomenon of birding has emerged from many corners of interest. Fascination with bird life and behavior is widely shared and tends to express respect for the values of conservation and protection. At one end of the continuum, birders are represented by those who simply place feeders on their window sills to attract members of the local bird community, and they take pleasure in the observations. A classic exemplar of this perspective is presented in the book *Wings at My Window,* by Ada Clapham Govan.[10] In her book she recounts how as a housebound invalid she became fascinated with birds when a chickadee visited her window feeder. She eventually became so involved and gained so much pleasure from this pastime that it helped relieve her chronic incapacitating arthritis. Her book continues to motivate many to adopt the hobby.

There are also those who plant special trees and shrubbery around their homes in order to attract a larger or more specialized array of species. Still another level of interest is found in "listers." They are motivated to observe and identify as many species of birds as possible. Lists of sightings are scrupulously kept, personally compared with those of other birders, and turned into local and national organizations as census devices. In this manner birding contributes to a fundamental purpose of museum ornithology, the description of what species have been seen and where they were seen. However, some professional biologists have questioned the validity of list-derived data, on the grounds that many birders are not sufficiently experienced in the application of the accepted methods of species identification.[11]

It would be inaccurate to say that, as a group, birders oppose all specimen collecting. Most acknowledge that a certain amount of collecting is necessary. The illustrated field guides on which they depend for accurate identification are themselves constructed by examining trays upon trays of specimen skins in museum collections. However, their interest is decidedly on the observation and identification of living birds. Frank Chapman, a major shaping force in birding and a long-term editor of the magazine *Bird-Lore,* instituted the traditional creation of "Christmas Lists" in 1900 as a way of distracting people away from shooting birds and toward counting and observing them.

Like scientists, birders are interested in the rare and unique, and the appearance of a vagrant bird is certainly that. The presence of vagrants has the effect of stimulating social and educational interactions among interested people. The situation not only offers the opportunity to observe a member of a species not normally accessible, but it also represents a challenge to the birder's identification skills. A single individual must be located, observed, and identified; a needle must be found in the avian haystack. The length of and pride in one's lifetime list is increased by a potentially once-in-a-lifetime observation. Other more tangible benefits are also recognized. While in search of the prize, birders get moderate levels of exercise and spend money. They buy film, digital cameras, audiotape, meals, gas, airline tickets, and motel rooms. What has become known as "ecotourism" is good for the economy and can be extremely important even inside the boundaries of national parks. In short, many lives are enriched by the presence and continued life of a vagrant bird. Once it is a tagged specimen skin in a drawer filled with other dead vireos, all this activity ceases.

ETHICAL ISSUES

By the end of the day on July 8, 1992, a scientist was in possession of a specimen, birders were without a fascinating object of observation, and a single Yellow-green Vireo was dead. The conflicts are by now clear. How shall these conflicts be viewed? Was a moral rule or a law broken? Was a covenant with the sanctuary status of the national parks broken? Was the understanding of an important issue in a realm of science advanced? Were the interests of birders unnecessarily frustrated? Were the interests of the various parties properly considered and, if necessary, balanced? Was a moral wrong done to a vulnerable individual? Was the bird killed humanely?

The Birder-Scientist Conflict

It has been generally acknowledged that Trochet broke an "unwritten" rule by using information acquired from birders actively observing the vagrant to make a scientific collection. No less important are some issues raised by an open letter dated September 28, 1992, written by Professor Ned K. Johnson, curator of ornithology at the University of California at Berkeley. He was Trochet's dissertation advisor. He wrote, "My personal rule is that the collecting of vagrant individual birds that birders have been observing and enjoying is unwise. Despite the fact that it is often scientifically desirable, and perfectly legal under many permits, too much ill-will is generated by such an act." Obviously, Trochet disregarded this unwritten rule in the incident under discussion.[12]

The choice of the terms "unwise" and "ill-will" in Johnson's letter is revealing. These terms imply that the matter is one of public relations and unnecessary bad feelings, rather than one of the moral justification of the action. The unwritten rule to which Johnson refers has to do, in his interpretation, with prevention of ill will and not the weighing and balancing of the interests of scientists and nonscientists or the individual bird. One implication of the statement would seem to be that as long as birders are currently unaware of the existence of a vagrant, and collection by a scientist would therefore not cause a reaction of ill will, their concerns and interests need not be considered.

It could, however, be argued that the collection of a vagrant sets in motion consequences that affect the lives of birders and others whether they have seen or know about the collection. Some consequences are more tangible than others. For example, some vagrants are no longer available to be discovered and enjoyed, and the legitimate interests of birders in seeing living nature have been thereby terminated. It may be that the claims of scientists should take precedence in such a situation. However, final determination of a priority of interests can be justified only if it takes into account the claims of all affected parties, not merely those aware of a specific situation. This is all before any consideration of the value of the life of the bird, from the bird's perspective.

Following the vireo incident, the New Mexico Department of Game and Fish scheduled a meeting at which ornithologists and birders could openly discuss their concerns. It was expected that the meeting would result in the development of a set of policies that would be adopted by the department and serve as guidelines for professional and public conduct. On February 19, 1993, a set of regulations made the following points explicit and was officially adopted:[13]

1. The taking of wildlife for scientific and educational purposes is a highly important activity but must not be harmful to wildlife populations and must not abridge the legitimate "rights" of others who use wildlife.
2. The sacrifice of vagrant birds solely for the purpose of documentation of occurrences is "discouraged."
3. No vagrant birds appearing on the Rare Bird Alert hotline shall be collected. An individual who violates this provision will be assessed one violation point. The accumulation of three points will result in a suspension or revocation of his or her collection permit.[14]
4. All collected specimens are to be considered state property and are to be deposited in an approved institutional museum where they can be inspected by members of the public as well as scientists.
5. Professionals with collecting permits must make their status and purposes known to those with whom they come in contact in the field.

While affirming the importance of scientific and educational collecting, the regulations clearly state that there are others who "use" wildlife; their interests must also be considered. In the case of vagrant birds, the interests of birders are allowed, under these regulations, to take priority over the interests of scientific collectors. While protecting the activities of the amateur naturalist, the provision seems to question whether scientists as a group can be trusted to take the interests of others into account as they conduct their work.

Alternatives to Killing

Birders in this case argued that the vagrant was more important to them and their activities than it was to the scientists, and therefore their interests deserved priority. From this point of view, the scientific benefits of collection must be shown to outweigh these and other related benefits. Whether or not this point of view is correct, we can ask whether the increased certainty of identification that underlies the collecting of the vireo is worth the losses to the birders and others. From the birder perspective, the answer is decidedly "no." But is this judgment impartial and morally appropriate?

It was widely believed by the New Mexico birder community that a reasonably certain identification could have been made without killing the vireo. Field notes, photographs, and audiotapes of the song most likely could have served as an adequate foundation for species identification. If confusion existed about identification, the bird could have been captured, examined, photographed, and then released. If additional biochemical analyses were needed, they could have been done on a retained feather or a small blood sample drawn from a wing vein, procedures quite common in ornithological field research.

As an alternative to killing the bird, the vireo might have been banded or "ringed." In this procedure, the identifying information of a particular bird is registered to an identification number that is embossed on a small aluminum band placed harmlessly on the leg of the bird. In the United States, once the bird is banded, the identifying information is filed with the Fish and Wildlife Service in Washington, DC. The plan is that if the bird is found again, its location and condition are reported to the service and relayed to the individual who first banded the bird.

Although only about 5% of banded birds are returned and reported, this procedure potentially provides important information regarding migratory movements, longevity, and geographical distribution. If banding had occurred in this case, future sightings might have shed light on whether this bird was the same individual that had been returning for two years to Rattlesnake Springs. If it were, the case for accidental vagrancy would have been weakened in favor of the scientifically significant range expansion hypothesis. A serious consideration of these alternatives would have required planning and a consideration of the interests of other people pursuing the vireo. But how much do their interests count? And do these considerations outweigh the interests of scientists in collecting and amassing information? When interests conflict in this way, is there any way to determine whose interests count the most?

The Significance of a Life

The interests we have just been discussing are *human* interests where different human interests have come into conflict. What about the bird's interests, including the bird's life? Are these really "interests"? If so, can these interests legitimately compete with and even override human interests?

Common Assumptions about the Significance of a Bird's Life

Many common arguments in science and beyond downplay the significance of the death of a bird, even when it is killed without a clear, warranting purpose—e.g., when a bird is killed merely because it is an object that can be hunted. These arguments sometimes derive from views about the importance of the death of an individual when that event is compared with the size of the overall population and the number of deaths from other causes. From this perspective, since the estimated North American bird population is between 5 and 20 billion, the death of any given vagrant bird may not seem a significant event.[15]

Other human-caused bird mortalities account for an enormous number of deaths, dwarfing the losses brought about by scientific collecting. These deaths include an estimated annual loss of 148 million birds due to collisions with windows and motor vehicles and 18 million fish-eating birds killed under federal permit in order to protect fish hatcheries.[16] The practice of sport hunting is another source of purposeful bird deaths. For example, it has been estimated that in 1970 and 1971, 5 million Mallard ducks were killed by hunters,[17] and the annual hunt of Mourning Doves kills somewhere between 11 and 42 million birds.[18]

It is also well known that migrating birds like the vireo are often killed in large numbers as they encounter natural disasters such as storms. For example, David and Melissa Wiedenfeld[19] calculated that a single tropical storm that roared across Grand Isle, Louisiana, in April 1993 killed an estimated 40,000 birds, affecting 45 species of neotropical migrants just as they were about to reach the end of their spring trans-gulf flight.

A variant of this argument is that the death or deaths of members of a population or species have significance only if the deaths adversely affect the integrity or existence of a population or species. Therefore, the death of a single individual from a large population is insignificant. By this reasoning, the death of a vagrant is of no real significance. Since the likelihood of the vagrant returning to its native population is low, in a reproductive sense the animal is already dead. Killing the individual only hastens this established reality.[20]

Arguments from the Intrinsic Value of a Life

From another perspective, however, the life of a bird has intrinsic value. The heart of the concept of the *intrinsic value* of a life is the claim that the value of an animal is not limited to an analysis of its usefulness to humans. The value of something that is a means to an end is an *extrinsic value*. For example, a bird may have economic value in that its feathers can be sold and made into a form of adornment, and its flesh can be sold for food. In less material forms of instrumental value, a bird may bring pleasure to one who observes it or hears its song, or it may provide data for a scientific investigation. The intrinsic value of a bird, by contrast, is found in its own experiences of flying, resisting death, eating, nesting, reproducing, relating to other birds, and the like. Clearly a bird has its own ends (goals, objectives) and cannot be reduced in value merely to a status as a means to the ends of humans.

As we saw in the introduction to this volume (see pp. 24–25), the concept of inherent value has been related by some philosophers directly to questions of the rights and the moral standing of animals. From the utilitarian perspective, philosophers such as Jeremy Bentham, Tom Regan, Raymond Frey, and Peter Singer view animals as having experiences that are good in themselves—for example, through whatever pleasures and feelings of association they experience. They therefore have a significant stake in how their lives are played out. From this perspective, the bird's moral status requires us to give moral weight to the bird's life and experiences. Regan (see pp. 24–25) argues that any animal that is the "subject of a life" has intrinsic or inherent value.

Still others base their justification for the value of animals in the nature of the biological world itself. According to this conception, moral sentiments of considering the value and well-being of other beings have evolved from natural selection and the reproductive advantage of social integration. Social living requires some degree of constraint of self-interest. Among social mammals, these required constraints have taken the form of other-oriented sentiments such as respect, love, sympathy, and regard. As we have come to understand that all living beings are biologically interdependent, the circle of other-directed concern that we recognize in creatures has broadened. This line of thinking pushes us to ask whether the idea of the intrinsic value of a living creature as an end in itself may in the final analysis be a philosophical abstraction from primitive sentiments—some of which, such as love, are seemingly moral. These sentiments seem to be found in many creatures.[21]

Both scientists and birders have often incorporated this concept of intrinsic value into how they conduct themselves and speak of animals. To them, the fact that the collection of a vagrant Yellow-green Vireo might help to demarcate in time and space a population expansion to the southwestern United States or might bring pleasure to group of birders or money to motel owners is not to the point. The bird is an end in itself and not a "thing" that gains in value by giving pleasure to birders or by satisfying the questions of an ornithologist. Its interests as a living being must also be considered with equal weight along with the interests of others involved. From this perspective, crushing the life out of the bird to make it a museum piece is an immoral act even if scientific value results from the "collection."

The Means to Death

A consideration of both the value of the bird and alternatives to killing it suggests the need for an assessment of the means of death. Although published news reports of the vireo incident claimed that the bird died "in a few seconds," implying that the manner of death was insignificant, this claim has been disputed.

A panel of the American Veterinary Medical Association (AVMA) has evaluated the appropriateness of euthanasia techniques on a set of dimensions that defines the concept of a "good" or relatively pain-free death as well as the acceptability of a practice. The scales include: (1) ability of the procedure to induce loss of consciousness and death without causing pain, distress, anxiety, or apprehension; (2) time required to induce unconsciousness; (3) reliability; (4) irreversibility; (5) compatibility with subsequent evaluation, examination, or use of tissue; (6) safety of personnel; (7) compatibility with requirement and purpose; (8) emotional effect on observers and operators; (9) compatibility with species, age, and health status; (10) drug availability and human abuse potential; (11) ability to maintain required equipment in proper working order; and (12) safety for predators/scavengers should the carcass be consumed.[22]

The 2000 AVMA panel report "conditionally" accepts thoracic compression as a euthanasia technique for small birds when other techniques are unavailable and the operator is well trained. The procedure that they specifically describe requires that the operator grasp and compress the bird's thorax with the thumb and forefinger of one hand from under and behind the wings while the forefinger of the other hand compresses the sternum. In theory, if done properly, loss of consciousness occurs in several seconds, and death shortly thereafter. If the procedure were done by an inexperienced person the bird may be able to struggle, thereby delaying the loss of consciousness and death. Further, if the pressure is not properly coordinated and maintained for a sufficiently long time, reversibility can easily occur, requiring that the procedure be reinitiated. Finally, there is a strong chance of a negative emotional impact on observers and operators. Published descriptions of the vireo's death leave questions about whether the specifics of this conditionally approved procedure were the same ones followed by Trochet.

The AVMA panel also acknowledges that the requirements of field research may not always be compatible with the pain-free death of experimental subjects. Field researchers use the words "collecting," "killing," or "harvesting" and not "euthanasia" in part to mark this distinction. However, published guidelines for the use of wild birds in research state that thoracic compression is appropriate only to complete the killing of birds already wounded by gunshot.[23] The options recommended for killing birds collected by net or trap include the use of various anesthetic agents or physical means such as cervical dislocation or decapitation, all of which either reduce anxiety and fear or rapidly induce unconsciousness.

In February 1993, Trochet closed the matter with a letter of apology to the New Mexico Department of Game and Fish in which he said: "Though it probably further reflects badly on me, I must say that I did not realize in advance that the collection of the Yellow-green Vireo would create such a fire-storm of protest. As in all previous instances when I elected to collect a bird, I made the decision wholly on the basis of the scientific merits. Making such a narrowly focused assessment is not a mistake I will make again."[24]

Despite the passage of time after this case was closed, a mention of the incident still today induces deeply felt reactions among scientific collectors, birders, and proponents of the intrinsic value of animals. Despite new regulations, anger and mistrust prevail. No new Yellow-green Vireos have been sighted at Rattlesnake Springs, or at least none has been publicly reported. The skin of the vagrant vireo lies flat in a small specimen tray in the Museum of Southwestern Biology at the University of New Mexico in Albuquerque. Records kept on the use of specimens at the museum show that no one has examined the skin since 1992 for research purposes. However, it has been used twice in educational contexts while discussing the specifics of this particular incident. A literature search does not uncover any published scientific research based on the sighting. In a contact with Trochet in 2006, he indicated that he had nothing to add to his previously published statements.

In what some might regard as a surprising outcome, Trochet today regularly participates in bird counts and leads birder groups on field excursions in the central valley of northern California. He was part of the team that in 2004 made a sighting of the Ivory-billed Woodpecker, a species long thought to be extinct. He also writes site guides pertaining to the habitats and sightings of a large number of species.[25]

NOTES

1. *Merriam-Webster's Collegiate Dictionary,* 10th ed.

2. R. S. Ridgely and G. Tudor, *The Birds of South America* (Austin: University of Texas Press, 1989), p. 150.

3. Mist nets are constructed of thin nylon fibers that are virtually invisible to flying birds. Once the birds strike the net, they become entangled in the webbing and are unable to escape.

4. K. S. Winker, B. A. Fall, J. T. Klicka, D. F. Parmelee, and H. B. Tordoff, "The Importance of Avian Collecting and Need for Continued Collecting," *Loon* 63 (1991): 238–46.

5. See C. Sibley and B. Monore, *Distribution and Taxonomy of Birds of the World* (New Haven: Yale University Press, 1990).

6. R. Ricklefs, "Old Specimens and New Directions: The Museum Tradition in Contemporary Ornithology," *Auk* 97 (1980): 206–7.

7. K. S. Winker, "Natural History Museums in a Postbiodiversity Era," *BioScience* 54, no. 5 (2004): 455–59.

8. J. Spalding, *The Poetic Museum: Reviving Historic Collections* (London: Prestel, 2001).

9. R. Ricklefs, "Old Specimens and New Directions," pp. 206–7.

10. Ada Clapham Govan, *Wings at My Window* (New York: Macmillan, 1953).

11. J. Remsen, "Use and Misuse of Bird Lists in Community Ecology and Conservation," *Auk* 111, no. 1 (1994): 225–27.

12. R. Burnson, "Man Who Killed Bird Apologizes," *Las Cruces Sun News,* September 29,1992, p. A4.

13. "New Mexico Department of Game and Fish Conditions and Provisions for the Taking of Wildlife for Scientific and Educational Purposes," State Records Office, Santa Fe, New Mexico, 1993, www.wildlife.state.nm.us/conservation/documents/wildlifeforscientificeducation.pdf (accessed February 11, 2007).

14. While there is no documentation to support the contention, it was widely believed in the birder community that they could personally authorize the collection of a vagrant appearing on the hotline.

15. American Ornithologists' Union, "Report of the *ad hoc* Committee on Scientific and Educational Use of Wild Birds," *Auk* 92 (1975): 1A–27A (3, Supplement).

16. J. Remsen, "Emotionalism is the Epitaph for Enlightenment," *Birding* (April 1993): 129–32.

17. R. C. Banks, "Human Related Mortality of Birds in the United States," U.S. Fish and Wildlife Service, Special Scientific Report, Wildlife, 1979, p. 215.

18. Winker et al., "The Importance of Avian Collecting," pp. 238–46.

19. D. Wiedenfeld and M. Wiedenfeld, "Large Kill of Neotropical Migrants by Tornado and Storm in Louisiana, April 1993," *Journal of Field Ornithology* 66, no. 1 (1994): 70–80.

20. Remsen, "Emotionalism Is the Epitaph for Enlightenment."

21. See J. C. Baird, "Intrinsic Value, Quantum Theory, and Environmental Ethics," *Environmental Ethics* 7 (1985): 257–75.

22. See "Report of the AVMA Panel on Euthanasia," *Journal of the American Veterinary Medical Association* 218, no. 5 (2001): 669–96. The AVMA cautions that this report has been widely misinterpreted; see www.avma.org/issues/animal_welfare/euthanasia.pdf (accessed February 11, 2007).

23. American Ornithologists' Union, "Report of the Committee on Use of Wild Birds in Research," *Auk* 105, suppl. 1 (1988): 1A–41A.

24. "Game and Fish OKs Rule on Bird Collecting," *Albuquerque Journal,* February 20, 1993, p. A4.

25. See John Trochet, "Site Guide Reprinted from the Central Valley Bird Club Bulletin, Cosumnes River Preserve," www.cvbirds.org/SiteGuides/CRP.pdf (accessed February 11, 2007).

PART X

EDUCATIONAL USES OF ANIMALS

17

Should Frog Dissection Continue?

Clear and reliable national data on the number of frogs killed for dissection in middle schools and high schools are lacking, but some data do exist. There are roughly 30 million students in grades 7–12 in the United States. About 80% of teachers who responded in a 2004 survey reported that they use dissection to teach biology.[1] There is therefore no doubt that over a million frogs are killed each year for this purpose.

College and high school students as well as biology teachers are divided over issues surrounding dissection. Some believe that dissection is an important part of education and should be retained, but others have their doubts. A key event in the history of recent discussions of dissection was the objection of a student in California named Jenifer Graham, who refused to dissect a frog in her high school biology class. This case opened many questions about what is and what is not morally defensible in dissecting frogs and other animals for educational purposes.

A REFUSAL TO DISSECT: JENIFER GRAHAM'S PROTEST

Graham, a 15-year-old student in Victorville, California, refused to dissect a frog. She said that her refusal was based on her respect for life and that her ethical position had nothing to do with teenage squeamishness. Graham instead offered to substitute college-level research on amphibian behavior, but this offer was refused. The school downgraded Graham's grade from an A to a D, later upgraded to a C. A notation was added on her official transcript for college admission stating, "This student refused to participate in the dissection portion of this class."

Graham challenged the grade in a state court and ultimately in the California Supreme Court. Lawyers appointed by the Humane Society of the United States tried to negotiate a settlement. The school argued that there is no substitute for the actual dissection experience; it is "necessary for college."[2] Lawyers for the school board argued that the educational objectives of learning the internal anatomy of a frog cannot be achieved with models or films. No agreement was reached.

The case attracted worldwide media attention. In the U.S. District Court in Los Angeles, Graham's lawyers argued that her ethical beliefs are equivalent to a religion and that the school district had violated her right to freedom of religion under the first amendment of the U.S. Constitution. The *Los Angeles Times* pronounced these arguments weak because no specific religious teaching speaks out against dissection, nor were Graham's objections truly *religious* in character.[3] Her moral position was that she wanted no part in the harming and killing of an animal for the sake of her education. Though she was only 15, she seemed to have thought through a general moral position on the use of animals to the point that she also had become a vegetarian, did not wear leather, and did not use personal care products tested on animals.

In June 1988, the District Court ruled that the state education system does not require dissection in preparation for admission to its colleges and universities, thus undermining one of the high school's arguments for refusing to allow credit for alternative areas of study. Later, the California Supreme Court dismissed the case in Graham's favor and also offered a compromise: Graham's knowledge of frog anatomy and dissection should be tested by using a frog that had died of natural causes. This ruling, as Juliana Texley sharply put it, "led biologists to conjure images of frantic teachers hovering in swamps waiting for the untimely demise of amphibians."[4] Graham graduated from high school and the matter became moot.

As these events were occurring, humane organizations were supporting a bill before the California state legislature permitting conscientious objection by students who objected to dissection. Graham testified on behalf of the bill and played a role in the bill's passage. The governor signed the Student's Rights Bill into law: Beginning in January 1989, science teachers were required to accommodate non-animal alternatives if the student objected to a curriculum requirement to dissect. This was the second U. S. law of its kind to be passed. More problems were to come.

National media attention was soon enhanced by Graham's participation in a controversial television advertisement. In October 1987, Apple Computer had developed "Operation Frog," one of the first computer programs marketed as an alternative to actual dissection. The commercial, narrated by Graham, lasted 30 seconds. The full text was:

Last year in my biology class, I refused to dissect a frog. I didn't want to hurt a living thing. I said I would be happy to do it on an Apple computer. That way, I can learn and the frog lives. But that got me into a lot of trouble, and I got a lower grade. So this year, I'm using my Apple II to study something entirely new—constitutional law.[5]

This last was said with a twinkle in her eye, and it was an obvious reference to her then-ongoing court battle.

This advertisement was criticized by several pro-animal-research organizations. For instance, the California Biomedical Research Association circulated an "action alert" stating that the ad was "in very poor taste and offensive" to science educators; it urged that protests should be sent to Apple President John Sculley.[6] A spokesperson for the Association of American Universities said that the advertisement "was a cute market-able commercial for anti-vivisection."[7]

A DISPUTE ABOUT EDUCATION IN SCIENCE

Graham's case had intensified a long-simmering dispute. From one point of view, objec-tions to dissection are a most serious threat to science, because doubts about dissection suggest doubts about animal experimentation more generally. To support dissection is to support experimental science and to reject antivivisectionism. The American Medical Association, a keen defender of animal research, announced that it would step up its efforts to keep dissection in the classroom—a story on the front page of *USA Today* on April 2, 1991. The Graham case had escalated into a national controversy cast as animal experimentation versus antivivisection.

Although dissection is still widely used today, it is generally accepted that alterna-tives such as computer simulations, various forms of multimedia, models, and other non-animal alternatives are increasingly being used, often displacing dissection. Interest groups (mainly humane associations), educational institutions (such as the Center for Alternatives at the University of California), and software manufacturers have a multi-tude of alternatives and advice to offer.[8] Many of these alternatives include information about animal behavior and ecology along with the details of anatomy. Some also include interactive examination modules that can be modified by teachers.

In 2007, some of these interest groups reported increases in the use of their programs providing alternatives to dissection. Animalearn[9] and the Physicians Committee for Responsible Medicine[10] showed significant increases over previous years. Since 2006, the Physicians Committee for Responsible Medicine has offered, free of charge, its ver-sion of a dissection program called Digital Frog.[11]

In 2007, there were nine state laws in the United States and assorted resolutions to allow students to refuse to participate in dissection.[12] Typically, schools from the earli-est grades through twelfth grade are required to notify parents or students beforehand of the option to decline dissection. Instructors must allow alternative assignments. The National Science Teachers Association (hereafter Science Teachers) has been opposed to these laws on the grounds that they "eliminate an educator's decision-making role" and deny students the opportunity to learn through an actual animal dissection.[13] Despite this concern, adoption of conscientious objection policies nationwide has continued to increase.

THE LEGACY OF THE STUDENT PROTESTS

Inspired by Graham's actions, other students refused to participate in classroom projects that caused harm or death to sentient animals. Ironically, the students most emboldened by her lead were in college or in veterinary or medical school, not students in high school. Undergraduate students refused to dissect frogs or give repeated electric shocks to rats; veterinary students refused to conduct nontherapeutic surgery on dogs and cats and demanded only beneficial surgery as part of their training; and some medical students objected to classes requiring multiple major practice surgeries on the same animal (as many as 10 surgeries spaced out over several weeks). Like Graham, they proposed that they be allowed to pursue an alternative that did not harm animals; when not permitted to do this, a number of these students went to court.

Within a few years of the decision in the Graham case, decisions came down from courts that almost uniformly favored a student's right to alternative forms of study. Teachers at the collegiate level and above quickly learned not to refuse such requests by their students.

A decline in harmful and fatal animal use as well as general acceptance of Three R alternatives (refinement, reduction, and replacement of animal procedures) has been notable in U.S. veterinary and medical schools. Training veterinary students has shifted from highly consumptive use of animals to more humane ways that benefit the animals.[14] In medical schools, a 2001 survey showed a dramatic decline in the use of live animals in pharmacology, physiology, and surgery courses, thereby establishing a continuous decline since 1985.[15]

In contrast, high schools show a much slower pace. In many schools, students did not feel emboldened to speak up with their objections. In addition, both of the two major teachers' professional associations (the Science Teachers, as previously mentioned, and the National Association of Biology Teachers—hereafter Biology Teachers) have promoted and strongly preferred actual animal dissection.

Lynette A. Hart, director of the University of California's Center for Animal Alternatives, has been instrumental in gaining acceptance of alternatives in veterinary schools. She comments that the "limited use of alternatives in secondary education contrasts with the concerted adoption of alternatives in veterinary curricula."[16] As we have seen, this is due in part to the different goals that high school teachers have for their students. Some believe that it is essential that students experience the actual "act" of dissection such as cutting skin, reflecting back muscles, moving organs, and the like. If this is the educational focus, there is likely no adequate alternative available. However, if the goal is more general—that is, the learning of anatomy (e.g., structure names, functions, and appearance)—this information can be learned in a variety of ways. Unfortunately, these differences in goals are usually not clearly articulated. This fragmentation, separating university instructors from those in high schools, continues today and seems likely to continue for some time.

Mixed Messages Sent to Biology Teachers

For the two years following Jenifer Graham's court case, in 1989 and 1990, the Biology Teachers boards of directors announced official policies that encouraged acceptance of alternatives for dissection and animal experiments. The directors maintained that dissection was given too much laboratory time and that a general reexamination of high school lab curricula was needed. They proposed to use animals in teaching that would provide opportunities to "introduce ethical concerns and an ecological appreciation of animals."[17] The boards provided literature, workshops, and other means to implement increased use of alternatives.

Despite clarifications aimed at explaining that actual dissection was not disallowed and that "we do not see our guidelines as precluding the use of animals in biomedical research,"[18] there was considerable misunderstanding within the ranks of the Biology Teachers. Court cases had not yet run their course, and teachers named in legal suits were understandably angry. Soon the Biology Teachers withdrew their monograph on dissection alternatives and stopped their workshops. The pro-alternatives policy was then overturned by the group's new board of directors. A subsequent policy in 1993 stated that "NABT acknowledges that no alternatives can substitute for the actual experience of dissection and urges teachers to be aware of the limitations of alternatives."[19] This policy has persisted and remains the official policy as this book goes to press.

In the meantime, discussion of alternatives to dissection has languished in some corners of teacher education. Teachers' conferences and professional literature avoid these thorny topics as far as possible. It is as if dissection, like abortion, has become so controversial a topic that no one is willing to address it in polite conversation.[20]

A Crack in the Ice?

Nonetheless, there have been developments. The Massachusetts State Department of Education recently cooperated with Theodora Capaldo, the president of the New England Anti-Vivisection Society, to conduct a survey of teachers' practices and attitudes regarding dissection.[21] Such a cooperative relationship with an antivivisection association has historically been unusual. It suggests some reduction, however minimal, in the polarization of viewpoints and a step in the direction of cooperation. As a result of this survey, the Department of Education passed a resolution permitting student conscientious objection. The resolution allows dissection to be openly discussed and ethical issues addressed to the satisfaction of teachers.

ETHICAL ISSUES

Many general issues about harming and killing animals are discussed in chapter 1 of this book. The issues raised below are specific to the use of animals in education.

Harms to Animals: Death, Pain and Distress, and Use of Nonnatural Environments

Causing pain or distress and taking an animal's life are serious matters, even when the purpose is the advancement of science education. They require moral justification. In general, justification rests on balancing the importance of the enterprise's goal, the anticipated benefits, and the likelihood of achieving these benefits. For those who believe that dissection is not a necessary condition of anatomical knowledge, there is a deep worry that the purpose behind the entire enterprise is morally problematic. If causation of harm or killing occurs for no compelling reason, the conduct seems pointless and unethical. Is there a compelling reason?

To illustrate the seriousness of the decision to implement the dissection process, consider the impact on the animals themselves. In preparing for a dissection exercise, frogs arrive in the classroom either alive or dead. If the frogs are caught in the wild, there are ethical concerns about how they were captured and transported and possibly about conservation and disturbing the ecosystem where they were caught. When wild-caught frogs are collected, they are placed with many other frogs in bags where they may experience dehydration, contract disease, or suffocate before arriving at a biological supply house. Since the economic value of the animal often remains unchanged whether the animal is alive, sick, or dead, there are no financial incentives to motivate improved treatment.

Many frogs are the product of an industry inside supply houses that breed frogs for human purposes. While this industry reduces problems of using wild populations, it also precludes the possibility that the animals will live in a way that is natural for the species. In addition, there are few rules to ensure that frogs will be humanely (rapidly and painlessly) killed, either in the field, in supply houses, or in the classroom.

Negative Impacts on Students

Psychologist Kenneth J. Shapiro reports that some students find dissection personally and emotionally disturbing.[22] Students often recoil not only at killing but also at the prospect of handling a dead body. Some students and parents view even the cutting up of a body as a kind of desecration, defilement, or sacrilege. Strong negative feelings can remain into adulthood and can be damaging. These feelings can also adversely affect a student's attitude toward the further study of biology. These kinds of reactions may be further enhanced if the dissection is poorly done, yields little educational benefit, or takes place in a disrespectful atmosphere.

The potential for desensitization is a related matter in the education of young, often emotionally immature students. Some adults recall initially approaching frog dissection with strongly negative feelings. However, they found that they could get themselves to participate if they averted their attention away from their compassionate feelings and proceeded. However, the wisdom of suppressing compassion while facilitating the infliction of pain or death on sentient animals has been questioned. Douglas Allchin, who has taught both high school and college biology, is disturbed about dissection because it is, by its very nature, destructive; "each organism is removed and discarded in turn."[23] He believes that there is nothing more important than that a student learn respect for life, and he is personally opposed to dissection.

Some recent research has linked harm directed toward animals with disrespect for, and often violence directed at, other humans.[24] This rationale is specifically invoked in a 2005 New York State Assembly bill to prohibit dissection of cats and dogs in secondary schools.[25] Those who have such worries about a spillover from disrespect for animals to disrespect for humans appear to be in agreement with a famous argument once advanced by philosopher Immanuel Kant (whose views are explicated in chapter 1). Kant says that "if a man shoots his dog because the animal is no longer capable of service . . . his act is inhuman and damages in himself that humanity which it is his duty to show towards mankind."[26]

Not everyone agrees, however. Many teachers find dissection a rewarding experience and not one that damages their students. They find their students excited and attentive. As mentioned above, the Biology Teachers' policy current in 2007 states that there is "no substitute" for actual dissection. Similarly, the Science Teachers promote dissection in their official policy current in 2007.[27] According to some, the emotional impact of dissecting can be a valuable experience that stimulates learning through hands-on experience.

One high school teacher reports that "I can still remember my first dissection of a mammal. It was a mouse. What ensued was a tremendous explosion of consciousness and understanding. All the things I had been learning were suddenly real. It was a profound experience. But it was something more. By confirming all the things I had been taught, it helped me understand that the world was a rational place, and that knowledge and understanding can come from serious study of real specimens and real data. I see this same kind of learning in my own students."[28]

Academic Freedom for Biology Teachers

Different teachers are effective in different ways, and individual teachers' academic freedom should, as a general rule, be respected because it ultimately benefits the student. Each teacher has a position, based on personal experience, about what has proved effective in the classroom. One unusual high school teacher conducts an elective biology course that consists solely of dissecting various animals, first a fetal pig, then a chicken, a cat, an animal heart, and finally a sheep brain.[29] Suppose that such a teacher is very able at his or her craft, and suppose the students love the course. Would a teacher be inappropriately thwarted by not being able to include dissection or even to extol the virtues of dissection when he or she is convinced of its value? Should teachers be forced by a court's mandate to change the way they run their classrooms?

Biology teachers in public schools have a professional responsibility to observe national science education standards. These standards are intended to ensure that the key concepts of modern biology are transmitted to students. One 2007 standard for life science teaching requires that students in grades 9–12 develop an understanding of the cell, the molecular basis of heredity, biological evolution, interdependence of organisms, the organization of living systems, and the behavior of organisms.[30] Does dissection fit into the achievement of any of these goals? Should it be required? If a teacher were not allowed to use dissection as a method of teaching these topics, would this constraint constitute a serious breach of academic freedom?

To cast light on this discussion in the United States, it is worth noting that dissection has been banned in several countries including the Netherlands, Switzerland, Poland, and Israel.[31] National policies in England, India, and Italy support dissection choice. The laws in Germany, England, Sweden, and Denmark prohibit animal experimentation by pre-college students. The German law is notably precise: "Only persons with the requisite expertise may conduct experiments on animals. Only persons who have completed university studies in veterinary medicine, medicine, or natural sciences may conduct experiments on vertebrate animals."[32] Are such policies overly restrictive and a serious impediment to science education? Can such views be made coherent with the idea of academic freedom?

Conscientious Objection

What are the options if a student—or, for that matter, a teacher—objects to dissection? Punishing a student has proved a risky response, and schools generally try to avoid this strategy. One option is to require a student to observe a dissection done by others. Here a student presumably learns without having to take actions that he or she views as offensive. However, this solution has proved not to work for those students who conscientiously object to all forms of participation in or observation of dissection. They object to dissection itself.

Yet another option is to make a course elective, with teachers forewarning students about its content. This option has the value of preserving freedom of choice for teacher and student alike. However, it will not be satisfactory to students who object to dissection occurring in their school. Are these students rebels without an adequate cause, or is there much to be said in their favor? Are they in the mold of great conscientious objectors, or are they more like troublemakers?

One suggested policy is that a teacher should first question a student who refuses to dissect an animal.[33] These authors propose that if a student or parent objects, a private meeting should be scheduled to discuss the matter. If an agreement cannot be reached, then the matter should be referred to an administrator who is knowledgeable regarding legal, ethical, and educational issues

This procedure requires a young student (perhaps with the support of his or her parents) to defend a developed moral position and explain the moral or religious foundations on which his or her beliefs are based. One problem with this policy is that students are generally not well trained in how to represent and defend the moral and religious foundations of their thinking. Young persons can be intimidated by questions posed by school authorities, and the entire process can be an ordeal. Moreover, there is an ethical issue here about burden of proof. Should only those who object to dissection be called upon to explore their motives and reasons? Is it unfair to require conscientious objectors to justify their position but not to ask the same of students who willingly dissect?

We know that Jenifer Graham's defense of her views by appeal to her "religious" views created problems, but it has never been resolved exactly which sorts of appeals would count for or against the acceptability of her stated convictions. In the end, her case never resolved the question, "Where should authorities and teachers draw the line in allowing students to appeals to their personal sense of conscientious objection?"

NOTES

1. Lesley A. King, Cheryl L. Ross, Martin L. Stephens, and Andrew N. Rowan, "Biology Teachers' Attitudes to Dissection and Alternatives," *ATLA* 32, suppl. 1 (2004): 475–84.

2. Juliana Texley, "Doing without Dissection," *American School Board Journal* 179, no. 1 (January 1992): 24–26.

3. Editorial, *Los Angeles Times*, August 7, 1988, pt. V.

4. Texley, "Doing without Dissection," p. 25.

5. Constance Holden, "Apples, Frogs, and Animal Rights," *Science* 238 (December 4, 1987): 1345, www.sciencemag.org (accessed January 25, 2007).

6. Ibid.

7. Ibid.

8. The Physicians Committee for Responsible Medicine at www.dissectionalternatives.org provides information about alternatives that are available commercially, online, and through humane association loan programs (accessed August 21, 2007). An additional source for dissection alternatives for pre-college science education is the University of California's Center for Animal Alternatives at www.vetmed.ucdavis.edu/Animal_Alternatives/ (accessed August 22, 2007).

9. E-mails from Laura Duccheschi, Animalearn, to Barbara Orlans, December 20, 2006, and February 6, 2007.

10. E-mail from Laura Yin, Physicians Committee for Responsible Medicine, to Barbara Orlans, January 10, 2007.

11. Digital Frog 2, Physicians Committee for Responsible Medicine, support.pcrm.org/site/PageServer?pagename=dissalt_digital_frog2 (accessed August 22, 2007).

12. The nine U.S. states with laws, along with the dates established, are Florida 1985; California 1988; Pennsylvania 1992; New York 1994; Rhode Island 1997; Illinois 2000; Virginia 2004; Oregon 2005; and New Jersey 2006. The additional five states with Department of Education or state resolutions requiring school districts to provide dissection alternatives are Maine 1989; Louisiana 1992; Maryland 1997; Massachusetts 2005; and New Mexico 2005. A summary of these policies is available at www.hsus.org/animals_in_research/animals_in_education/dissection_laws.html (accessed August 22, 2007).

13. National Science Teachers Association, "Responsible Use of Live Animals and Dissection in the Science Classroom," adopted by the NSTA board of directors, June 2005, www.nsta.org/positionstatement&psid=44 (accessed August 22, 2007).

14. In a succession of surveys ongoing from the 1980s, the Association of Veterinarians for Animal Rights has documented a shift toward more humane methods of animal use in veterinary schools. Detailed results are published as available in their newsletters and some information is available at www.avar.org/tech_school_animalused6.asp (accessed August 22, 2007). See also Lynette A. Hart, Mary W. Wood, and Hsin-Yi Weng, "Mainstreaming Alternatives in Veterinary Medical Education: Resource Development and Curricular Reform," *Journal of Veterinary Medical Education* 32, no. 4 (2005): 473–80.

15. For a survey showing that 68% of U.S. medical schools do not use live animals in their courses, see Lawrence A. Hansen and Gerry R. Boss, "Use of Live Animals in the Curricula of U.S. Medical Schools: Survey Results from 2001," *Academic Medicine* 77, no. 11 (November 2002): 1147–49.

16. Lynette A. Hart, Mary W. Wood, and Hsin-Yi Weng, "Three Barriers Obstructing Mainstreaming Alternatives in K–12 Education," *Altex* 23, special Issue (2006): 13–16.

17. National Association of Biology Teachers, "The Responsible Use of Animals in Biology Education, Including Alternatives to Dissection: A NABT Policy Statement," approved by the NABT board of directors, October 25, 1989, in *American Biology Teachers* 52 (1990): 72.

18. National Association of Biology Teachers, "NABT's Policy on the Responsible Use of Animals in Biology Classrooms: A Clarification," approved by the NABT board of directors, November 11, 1990, in *American Biology Teacher* 53 (January 1991): 71.

19. National Association of Biology Teachers, "The Use of Animals in Biology Education," adopted by the NABT board of directors, May 2003, www.nabt.org/sites/S1/index.php?p=60 (accessed January 22, 2007).

20. Hart, Wood, and Weng, "Three Barriers Obstructing Mainstreaming Alternatives," p. 13.

21. Current Curriculum Frameworks, Massachusetts Science and Technology/Engineering, Dissection Survey Results (Malden: Massachusetts Department of Education, 2006), pp. 133–39, www.doe.mass.edu/frameworks/current.html (accessed December 18, 2006).

22. Kenneth J. Shapiro, "The Psychology of Dissection," *Science Teacher* (October 1992): 43.

23. Douglas Allchin, " 'Hands Off' Dissection," *American Biology Teacher* 67, no. 6 (August 2005): 369–74.

24. Randy Lockwood and Frank Ascione, *Cruelty to Animals and Interpersonal Violence: Readings in Research and Application* (West Lafayette, IN: Purdue University Press, 1998). See also "The Link between Cruelty to Animals and Violence toward People," www.animalink.ab.ca/HumaneEducation/indexviolencelink.htm (accessed February 6, 2007).

25. New York State Assembly Bill A00922, "An Act to Amend the Education Law, in Relation to Dissection of Dogs and Cats" (June 21, 2005).

26. Immanuel Kant, "Duties in Regard to Animals," in *Animal Rights and Human Obligations*, 2nd ed., ed. Tom Regan and Peter Singer (Englewood Cliffs, NJ: Prentice Hall, 1989), pp. 23–24.

27. National Science Teachers Association, "NSTA Position Statement: Responsible Use of Live Animals and Dissection in the Science Classroom," adopted by the NSTA board of directors on June 2005 and again in early 2007; see www.nsta.org/about/positions/animals.aspx (accessed August 23, 2007).

28. Susan Offner, "The Importance of Dissection in Biology Teaching," *American Biology Teacher* 55, no. 3 (March 1993): 147–49.

29. Valerie Strauss, "When Cutting Up in Class Is Okay," *Washington Post*, March 5, 2007, pp. B1–2.

30. National Science Education Standards, Life Science, Content Standard C, books.nap.edu/readingroom/books/nses/ (accessed February 21, 2007).

31. New England Anti-Vivisection Society, www.neavs/org/esec/legislation (accessed August 21, 2007).

32. German Law on Animal Protection, Federal Minister of Food, Agriculture and Forestry, Bundesgesetzblatt, pt. 1, Bonn, August 22, 1986. English translation by the Services of the Commission of European Communities, p. 36.

33. Margaret D. Snyder, Nadine K. Hinton, J. Fredrick Cornhill, and Ronald L. St. Pierre, "Dissecting Student Objections," *Science Teacher* (October 1992): 40–43.

Index

Three Rs and animal, 32–34
transparency of, 188–90, 194–97
See also Animal Welfare Act; Codes of
   ethics; Institutional Animal Care and Use
   Committees; Research; Review and
   oversight of experimental procedures;
   Three Rs
Extinction, 109, 116, 163–69. *See also*
   Bonobos; Conservation; Death; Ecology;
   Species

Fabergé, 206
Factory farms,
   cheaper products from, 48, 53, 56–57, 79–80
   chicken farms, 74ff
   harms caused by, 35, 47, 54–56, 58, 64, 67,
      78–84
   hog farms, 47ff
   processes at, 50–52, 64–66, 75–78
   veal farms, 61ff
   See also Chickens; Meat; Pigs; Veal calves
      and farming
Fain, Leslie, 207
Farinato, Richard, 113
Fear,
   in birds, 80–82, 92, 259
   in calves, 67
   in elephants, 113
   the emotion of, 18, 80–82, 172, 224–28
   expressions of, 9, 12, 18, 37, 54, 67, 80–82,
      122, 150–51, 224–28
   Fear-Challenge Test, 224–28
   in monkeys, 219ff
   in pigs, 54
   thresholds of, 29–30, 157
   See also Distress; Emotions; Monkeys
Federal Food, Drug, and Cosmetic Act, 204
Federal policies (U.S.),
   on animal sacrifice, 152–54, 157
   on availability of information, 190–96
   governing the cosmetics industry, 202–11
   on inspection of laboratories, 34, 123,
      177–81, 186
   on minimizing animals' pain, 34, 36–37,
      57, 157
   See also Animal Welfare Act; Cosmetics;
      Federal Trade Commission; Public
      Health Service
Federal Trade Commission, 203, 212
Feld Entertainment, 120
Fentem, Julia, 210
Fertilizer, 49–50
Festing, Michael F. W., 240
Fighting
   bonobos and, 165
   cockfighting, 91–105

morality of, 23, 91, 98–105, 144, 157
See also Aggression; Chickens; Cockfights;
   Predators
Fish and fishing, 3, 14, 74, 137, 152, 154,
   165, 168, 240, 257
Fish and Wildlife Service, 256, 260
Food and Drug Administration (FDA), 201–2,
   205–6, 213
Food Safety and Inspection Service, 52, 59
Fox, Mitchell, 189, 191
Foxes, 82
Francione, Gary, 180
Freedom,
   academic, 194–96, 269–70
   animals' losses of, 20, 37, 67, 114, 123–25,
      182
   of information, 190–96
   of religion, 154–55, 264
   See also Autonomy
Freedom of Information Act, 190–91
Free-range chicken, pigs, and veal, 49, 53,
   66, 84. *See also* Chickens; Pigs; Veal
   calves and farming
Frey, R. G., vi, 21–23, 25, 257
Friedman, Milton, 55
Frogs, 263–68
Fur, 3, 139, 142, 154, 205, 217. *See also*
   Hunting; Leather; Trapping animals

Galleros, 93, 103
Gambling, 102–3. *See also* Cockfights
Gamecocks, 93, 96. *See also* Chickens;
   Cockfights; Roosters
Gameness, 96, 101
Garcia, Jerry, 103
General Agreement on Tariffs and Trade
   (GATT), 84
Genetics
   and breeding, 79, 94, 97, 104, 116–17
   and farming, 53, 62, 66
   genetic conditions, 77, 140, 236
   genetic diversity in, 167, 169
   genetic manipulation, 142, 236
   genetic similarity between species,
      164, 184
   See also Breeders; Species
Gennarelli, Thomas A., 178–85
German First Amendment to Animal
   Protection Law, 197
Gestation crates, 51–53, 64. *See also* Crates;
   Pigs
God, 9–10, 12, 15, 24, 91, 150, 154. *See also*
   Religion; Ritual; Theology
Gorillas, 40, 82. *See also* Apes
Gourmet writers and chefs (ethics of), 66,
   69–70

CPSIA information can be obtained at www.ICGtesting.com
Printed in the USA
BVOW031745011212

306945BV00002B/5/P

9 780195 340198